# Case-Based Eye Diseases and Disorders

# Case-Based Eye Diseases and Disorders

Editor: Brayden Burton

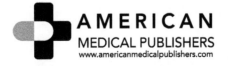

AMERICAN
MEDICAL PUBLISHERS
www.americanmedicalpublishers.com

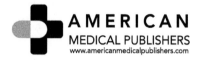

**Cataloging-in-Publication Data**

Case-based eye diseases and disorders / edited by Brayden Burton.
    p. cm.
Includes bibliographical references and index.
ISBN 979-8-88740-622-0
1. Eye--Diseases--Diagnosis. 2. Eye--Diseases--Treatment. 3. Eye--Abnormalities.
4. Eye--Care and hygiene. I. Burton, Brayden.
RE46 .D53 2023
617.7--dc23

American Medical Publishers,
41 Flatbush Avenue,
1st Floor, New York,
NY 11217, USA

ISBN 979-8-88740-622-0 (Hardback)

# Contents

**Permissions**

**List of Contributors**

**Index**

# Preface

Eye diseases and disorders encompass a wide range of conditions that can affect the health and function of the eyes. These conditions can vary in severity and may impact vision to different degrees. Some common eye diseases and disorders are refractive errors, cataracts and glaucoma. Refractive errors, including myopia, hyperopia, astigmatism and presbyopia, result in blurry vision due to an abnormality in the way light is focused on the retina. Cataracts occur when the clear lens of the eye becomes clouded, leading to blurry vision, sensitivity to light, and difficulty seeing at night. Glaucoma is a group of eye conditions characterized by damage to the optic nerve, often caused by increased intraocular pressure. It can lead to gradual vision loss and even permanent blindness. The book aims to shed light on some of the unexplored aspects of eye diseases and disorders, and the recent researches in this field. It will provide comprehensive knowledge to the readers.

After months of intensive research and writing, this book is the end result of all who devoted their time and efforts in the initiation and progress of this book. It will surely be a source of reference in enhancing the required knowledge of the new developments in the area. During the course of developing this book, certain measures such as accuracy, authenticity and research focused analytical studies were given preference in order to produce a comprehensive book in the area of study.

This book would not have been possible without the efforts of the authors and the publisher. I extend my sincere thanks to them. Secondly, I express my gratitude to my family and well-wishers. And most importantly, I thank my students for constantly expressing their willingness and curiosity in enhancing their knowledge in the field, which encourages me to take up further research projects for the advancement of the area.

**Editor**

# Progression of Subclinical Pachychoroid Neovasculopathy to an Active Neovascularization in the Presence of Acquired Vitelliform Lesions

**Manoj Soman,**[1,2] **Sameer Iqbal,**[1] **Jay U. Sheth** ⓘ**,**[1,2] **Padmanaban Meleth,**[1] **and Unnikrishnan Nair**[1,2]

[1]*Vitreoretinal Services, Chaithanya Eye Hospital and Research Institute, Trivandrum, India*
[2]*Chaithanya Innovation in Technology and Eyecare (Research), Trivandrum, India*

Correspondence should be addressed to Jay U. Sheth; drjay009@gmail.com

Academic Editor: Maurizio Battaglia Parodi

We describe a unique case of bilateral acquired vitelliform lesions in a 67-year-old-female with pachychoroid associated with subretinal fluid in the right eye (OD) and a nonexudative choroidal neovascular membrane (CNVM) in the left eye (OS). Multimodal imaging performed at baseline and over the ensuing two years showed an increase in the OS vitelliform lesions with a concurrent transformation of quiescent CNVM to an exudative form. Further studies are warranted to gain better insight into the etiopathogenesis of these vitelliform lesions in pachychoroid and their potential role in instigating CNVM activation.

## 1. Introduction

Acquired vitelliform lesions (AVL) are a focal or multifocal subretinal accumulation of autofluorescent material reported in various dystrophic, degenerative, paraneoplastic, toxic, and vitreoretinal interface disorders involving the macula [1]. The natural course of these lesions is often a gradual decrease in size with fragmentation and slow resorption, resulting in photoreceptor disruption and eventual atrophy [2]. In this case report, we demonstrate that these acquired vitelliform deposits herald the transformation of a nonexudative choroidal neovascular membrane (CNVM) to an exudative one in a patient with pachychoroid.

## 2. Case Report

A 67-year-old lady with a history of hypertension, dyslipidemia, and ischemic heart disease presented to us with complaints of diminution of vision in the right eye for 1.5 years. Her best-corrected visual acuity (BCVA) was 20/40 in the right eye (OD) and 20/20 in the left eye (OS). OU

anterior segment was normal. Fundus examination showed patterned retinal pigment epithelial (RPE) alterations in OD and nonspecific RPE changes in OS, seen better on multicolor imaging (Figures 1(a) and 1(b)). Vitelliform-like deposits were also seen in OU (Figures 1(a) and 1(b)). Spectral-domain optical coherence tomography (SD-OCT) revealed pachychoroid features with hyperreflective lesions in subretinal space and a shallow pigment epithelial detachment (PED) in OD (Figures 1(c) and 1(d)) and similar hyperreflective material extending into outer retinal layers and a focal extra-foveal double-layer sign (DLS; Figure 1(e)) in OS. Blue peak autofluorescence (BAF) imaging revealed increased autofluorescence from vitelliform deposits in both eyes (Figures 2(a) and 2(b)), while infrared images showed corresponding increased reflectance (Figures 2(c) and 2(d)). Combined fundus fluorescein angiography (FFA) and indocyanine green angiography (ICGA) showed window defects with foci of blocked fluorescence corresponding to the vitelliform lesions without any evidence of neovascularization (Figures 3(a)–3(h)). OCT angiography (OCTA) however revealed a nonexudative CNVM in OS corresponding to the

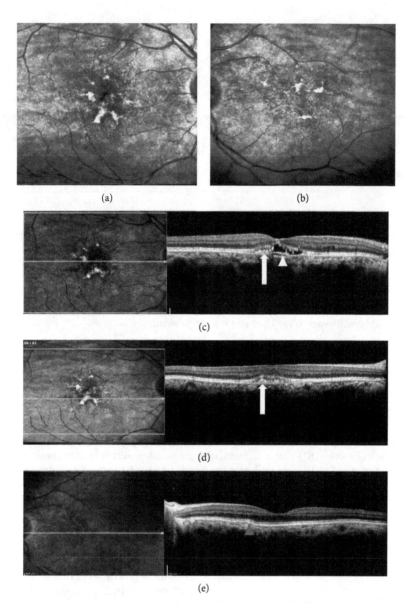

FIGURE 1: (a) and (b) Multicolour images (a) showing retinal pigment epithelial (RPE) alterations with vitelliform deposits in both macula simulating pattern dystrophy. Spectral-domain optical coherence tomography (SD-OCT) showing hyperreflective lesions in subretinal space ((c), (d)—arrows) with a shallow PED in the subfoveal region of the right eye ((c)—arrowhead) and similar deposition in the left eye (e) and focal extrafoveal DLS ((e) red arrowhead). Note the pachychoroid features in both eyes.

focal DLS (Figure 3(i)). The patient was managed conservatively with scheduled follow-up visits.

Serial infrared reflectance (IR; Figure 4) and SD-OCT (Figure 5) imaging over the next two years showed a gradual flattening of the PED with central migration of the vitelliform deposits and absorption in OD. The vision was maintained at 20/40 at all the visits in OD. In OS, the vitelliform deposits initially decreased only to reappear at different locations (Figure 4) with the onset of subretinal fluid (SRF; Figure 5). On colocalizing the vitelliform deposits with OCTA, we noted an abnormal network in the avascular slabs with dilated vessel complex in choroidal slabs suggestive of pachychoroid neovasculopathy (PNV; Figure 6). The size of the network had increased marginally as compared to baseline (Figure 7). Since the patient was symptomatic in OS with a

decrease in BCVA to 20/40, she received two monthly doses of intravitreal ranibizumab injection and subsequently had complete resolution of SRF with BCVA improving to 20/20 (Figure 8).

## 3. Discussion

The purpose of this case report was to highlight the conversion of quiescent PNV to an exudative network with progressive deposition of AVL. We also illustrate the role of OCTA in detecting quiescent networks that are likely to be missed on dye-based angiography and for their periodic noninvasive monitoring. Additionally, intravitreal ranibizumab monotherapy can be successfully used to treat PNV in the presence of AVL.

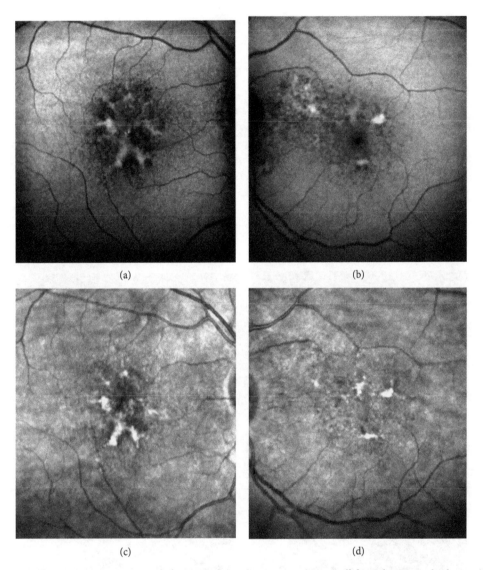

(a)

(b)

(c)

(d)

FIGURE 2: Blue peak autofluorescence imaging revealed increased autofluorescence from vitelliform deposits in both eyes ((a) and (b)) while infrared images showed corresponding increased reflectance ((c) and (d)).

In the current case, there was presence of bilateral pachychoroidopathy with AVL deposition. One eye showed spontaneous resolution of the deposits while the other eye having PNV demonstrated recurrent deposition with the onset of exudation. Freund et al. had reported features of AVL eyes demonstrating the natural history and imaging characteristics of these lesions [1]. 2.2% of the eyes in their series had CSCR and associated vitelliform lesions. Although these eyes could have associated pachychoroid features, this feature was not highlighted in the series. The presence of chronic SRF leads to loss of apposition between the photoreceptor tips and the RPE which can interfere with the phagocytosis of shed outer segments resulting in vitelliform deposition in these eyes [1, 3, 4]. In our case, the deposition seemed to appear along with or before the occurrence of SRF, especially in OS and was additionally associated with a neovascular network.

Agawa et al. [5] recently reported findings in eyes with PNV but did not comment on such observations in the AF/IR imaging.

We believe that in pachychoroid eyes, the dilated outer choroidal vessels with a resultant choriocapillaris compression led to a primary RPE dysfunction. This can alter the physiological homeostasis of the RPE and neurosensory retina causing poor phagocytosis of the shed outer segments that can accumulate over time as the vitelliform lesions. Spontaneous resolution may occur when there has been sufficient photoreceptor loss to allow for the normal mechanisms of photoreceptor outer segment turnover to "catch up," whereby RPE phagocytosis of the abnormal subretinal material may occur [1]. This phenomenon was demonstrable in the right eye of our case. However, the prevalent underlying choroidal neovascularization with episodes of activity in the left eye could have contributed to recurrent

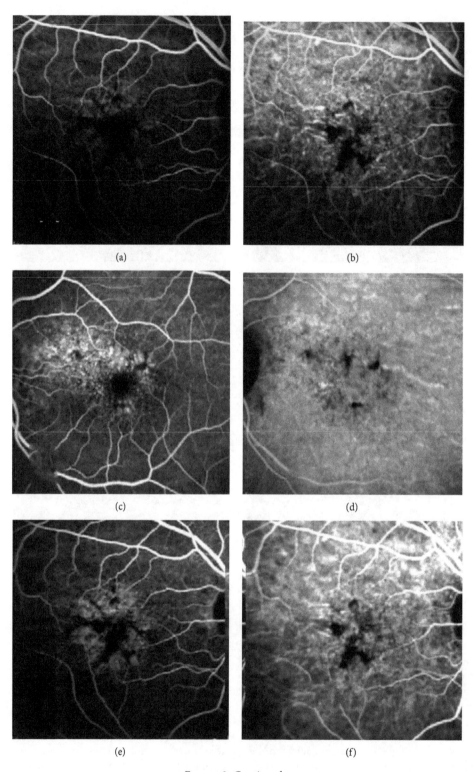

(a)

(b)

(c)

(d)

(e)

(f)

Figure 3: Continued.

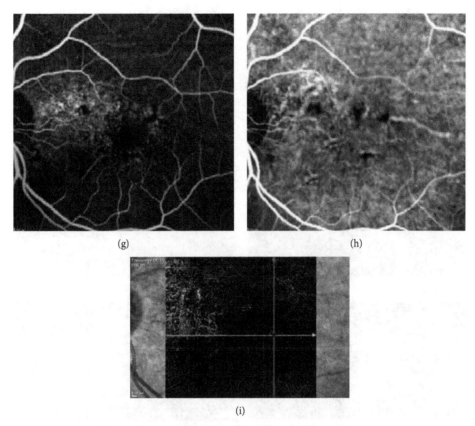

FIGURE 3: (a)–(h) Early and late phase combined fundus fluorescein angiography (FFA) and indocyanine green angiography (ICGA) showing window defects and blocked fluorescence corresponding to vitelliform deposits with no evidence of neovascularization network. Note the abnormal network evident on OCTA (i) in the left eye suggestive of nonexudative choroidal neovascular membrane (CNVM).

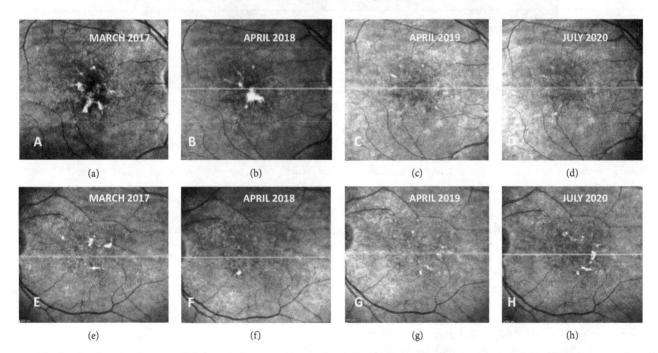

FIGURE 4: Serial infrared reflectance (IR) images demonstrating in the right eye (first row) central migration and gradual disappearance of vitelliform lesions and the left eye (bottom row) even though lesions disappeared initially, it reappeared at different locations in the macula.

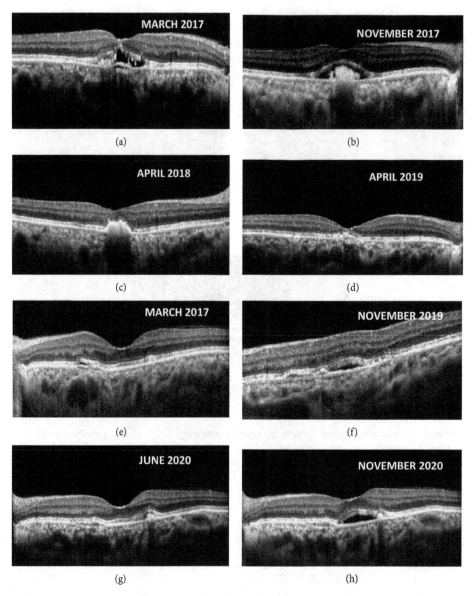

FIGURE 5: Serial spectral-domain optical coherence tomography (SD-OCT) images of right eye revealing flattening of pigment epithelial detachment (PED) (a) and central clumping of vitelliform deposits (b) and later resorption ((c) and (d)) while the left eye revealed focal double-layer sign (DLS; (e)) and development of extrafoveal fluid (f) managed conservatively and later new vitelliform deposition (g) followed by submacular fluid (h) necessitating treatment. Note that these new hyperreflective lesions appear before the onset of exudation (g).

accumulation as seen in the left eye. Thus, unlike other causes of AVL, pachychoroid eyes could have recurrent vitelliform deposits. Also, the presence of vitelliform lesions reflective on near-infrared reflectance (nIR) reflectance suggests a high content of melanin, supporting a possible origin from the RPE monolayer in the form of RPE hyperplasia or macrophages containing large amounts of melanolipofuscin granules [6, 7]. Freund et al. [1] imaged some AVL eyes simultaneously with SD-OCT, autofluorescence, and nIR imaging and demonstrated near-infrared hyperreflectivity corresponding to presumed collections of vitelliform deposits, an observation also seen in our case.

Although many eyes having primary pattern dystrophy with vitelliform deposits are misdiagnosed as age-related macular degeneration (AMD), central serous chorioretino-

pathy (CSCR), or nonspecific RPE changes [8], the converse may also be a possibility. Entities such as pachychoroidopathy could present findings simulating pattern dystrophy [9]. The older age of the patient, absence of family history, asymmetrical features [10], appearances of recurrent new deposition, typical choroidal OCT features, and central migration of the deposits as seen in our case could differentiate this from primary pattern dystrophy.

In conclusion, our case highlights the presence of vitelliform lesions in pachychoroid eyes. We noted the transformation of a subclinical PNV to an exudative one with progressive deposition of vitelliform lesions. To the best of our knowledge, this is the first case report to describe the simultaneous occurrence of these two pathologies, namely, PNV and AVL. More research is needed to ascertain

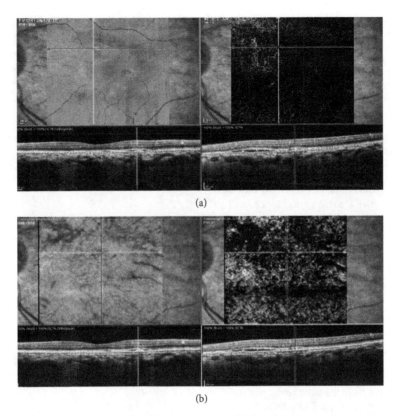

FIGURE 6: Optical coherence tomography angiography (OCTA) images of left eye corresponding to hyperreflective spot on infrared reflectance (IR) image showing an abnormal network in avascular layer and presence of prominent underlying and adjoining large dilated choroidal vascular complex.

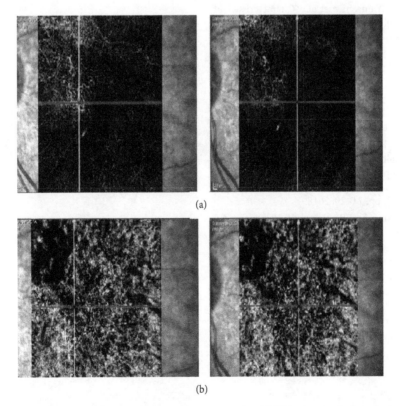

FIGURE 7: Comparison of baseline optical coherence tomography angiography (OCTA; nonexudative state) and OCTA at the time of submacular fluid (exudative state). Note the slight increase in the size of the vascular network in avascular slabs and the appearance of new dilated vessels in choroidal slabs.

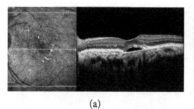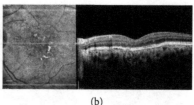

(a)                                                    (b)

FIGURE 8: Pre- and posttreatment spectral-domain optical coherence tomography (SD-OCT) images ((a) and (b)) showing resolution of subretinal fluid and persistent reflective deposits on infrared reflectance (IR) imaging.

whether the simultaneous occurrence of these two pathologies is linked to each other or is a mere coincidence.

## References

[1] K. B. Freund, K. Laud, L. H. Lima, R. F. Spaide, S. Zweifel, and L. A. Yannuzzi, "Acquired vitelliform lesions," *Retina*, vol. 31, no. 1, pp. 13–25, 2011.

[2] G. Querques, R. Forte, L. Querques, N. Massamba, and E. H. Souied, "Natural Course of Adult-Onset Foveomacular Vitelliform Dystrophy: A Spectral- Domain Optical Coherence Tomography Analysis," *American Journal of Ophthalmology*, vol. 152, no. 2, pp. 304–313, 2011.

[3] R. Spaide, "Autofluorescence from the outer retina and subretinal SPACE," *Retina*, vol. 28, no. 1, pp. 5–35, 2008.

[4] K. Laud, S. Visaetsilpanonta, L. A. Yannuzzi, and R. F. Spaide, "Autofluorescence imaging of optic pit maculopathy," *Retina*, vol. 27, no. 1, pp. 116–119, 2007.

[5] M. Tagawa, S. Ooto, K. Yamashiro et al., "Characteristics of pachychoroid neovasculopathy," *Scientific Reports*, vol. 10, no. 1, article 16248, 2020.

[6] J. J. Arnold, J. P. Sarks, M. C. Killingsworth, E. K. Kettle, and S. H. Sarks, "Adult vitelliform macular degeneration: a clinicopathological study," *Eye*, vol. 17, no. 6, pp. 717–726, 2003.

[7] G. T. Frangieh, W. R. Green, and S. L. Fine, "A histopathologic study of Best's macular dystrophy," *Archives of Ophthalmology*, vol. 100, no. 7, pp. 1115–1121, 1982.

[8] A. Ozkaya, R. Garip, H. Nur Tarakcioglu, Z. Alkin, and M. Taskapili, "Les resultats cliniques et d'imagerie des sous-types de pattern-dystrophies ; les erreurs diagnostiques et les traitements inutiles dans la vie reelle," *Journal Français d'Ophtalmologie*, vol. 41, no. 1, pp. 21–29, 2018.

[9] D. J. Warrow, Q. V. Hoang, and K. B. Freund, "Pachychoroid pigment epitheliopathy," *Retina*, vol. 33, no. 8, pp. 1659–1672, 2013.

[10] A. M. Hanif, J. Yan, and N. Jain, "Pattern dystrophy: an imprecise diagnosis in the age of precision medicine," *International Ophthalmology Clinics*, vol. 59, no. 1, pp. 173–194, 2019.

# Endogenous *Clostridium perfringens* Panophthalmitis with Potential Entry Port from Diverticulitis Exacerbated by Proliferative Diabetic Retinopathy

**Vamsee Neerukonda,**[1] **Anny M. S. Cheng,**[2] **Swetha Dhanireddy** ⓘ,[1] **Samuel Alpert,**[1] **and Han Y. Yin** ⓘ [1,2]

[1]*SUNY Upstate Medical University, Department of Ophthalmology, Syracuse, NY, USA*
[2]*Florida International University, Herbert Wertheim College of Medicine, Miami, FL, USA*

Correspondence should be addressed to Han Y. Yin; hhyin003@gmail.com

Academic Editor: Kevin J. Blinder

*Purpose.* To report a rapid endogenous fulminating panophthalmitis from *Clostridium perfringens* in a patient with diverticulitis and proliferative diabetic retinopathy. *Methods.* A 61-year-old female with poorly controlled diabetes mellitus, active proliferative diabetic retinopathy, and recent diverticulitis presented with conjunctival injection, ocular discharge, and sudden onset of painful vision loss of the left eye. Patient denied history of ocular trauma, intraocular surgery, or intravenous drug abuse. Examination revealed an erythematous, proptotic eye with restricted extraocular movements, mucopurulent discharge, diffuse corneal edema, and vitreous haze and cell. Orbital computed tomography (CT) confirmed no retained intraocular foreign body. *Results.* Despite 48 hours of treatment with systemic broad spectrum antimicrobial therapy (vancomycin, meropenem, and amphotericin B), patient underwent enucleation due to declined condition and progressive infection. Patient's culture revealed gram-positive bacillus microbes (*Clostridium perfringens*). Patient's subsequent CT abdomen showed resolved diverticulitis after antimicrobial therapy. *Conclusion.* Although rare, *Clostridium perfringens* infection can be a cause of rapid loss of vision from fulminate endogenous panophthalmitis. Urgent extensive systemic work-up to identify potential port of entry from visceral pathology and rapid removal of source of infection are pivotal to avoid high rate of mortality.

## 1. Introduction

*Clostridium perfringens* endophthalmitis is a rare but vision threatening infection. The source *Clostridium perfringens* is usually exogenous [1–6], and there is limited literature regarding an endogenous source. Endogenous *Clostridium perfringens* endophthalmitis can pose serious threats to both vision and is associated with high mortality [7, 8]. Previous reports demonstrated an underlying inflamed gallbladder [9], biliary infection [7], and acute abdomen [8] as causative sources. Herein, we report a case of endogenous *Clostridium perfringens* panophthalmitis in a patient with diverticulitis and proliferative diabetic retinopathy (PDR).

## 2. Case Report

A 61-year-old female with poorly controlled diabetes mellitus with severe bilateral PDR presented to the emergency department at Upstate University Medical Center. Initially, the patient presented to an outside emergency room with conjunctival injection, copious purulent discharge and associated painful vision loss to no light perception (NLP) in the left eye. Patient was then transferred to Upstate University Medical Center for higher level care and was evaluated by the ophthalmology service 18 hours after symptom onset. She underwent lateral canthotomy and cantholysis at the outside hospital 6 hours prior to arrival, due to severe pain and concern for orbital compartment syndrome; however patient

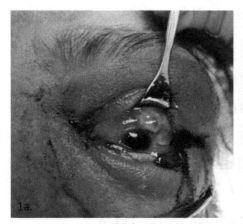

(a) Edematous, erythematous, and proptotic eye with severe restricted extraocular movements

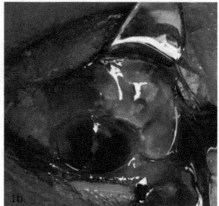

(b) Diffuse conjunctival injection and dense mucopurulent collection of the superotemporal quadrant

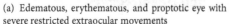

FIGURE 1: Panophthalmitis of the left eye.

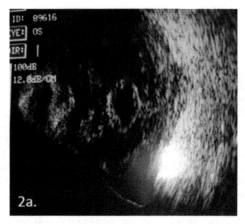

(a) Ultrasonography illustrating dense vitritis with subluxed lens of the left eye

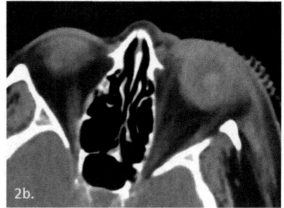

(b) Computer tomography of the orbit showing no retained intraocular foreign body or occult penetrating injury, in the left eye

FIGURE 2

endorsed complete loss of vision 12 hours prior in her left eye. She had no ocular trauma or history of intravenous drug abuse. However, she noted to have a two-month history of intermittent left abdominal pain and diarrhea, along with an abdominal computed tomography (CT) reporting diverticulitis. On presentation, examination revealed an edematous, erythematous, and proptotic left eye with severely restricted extraocular movements (Figure 1(a)). The anterior segment exam revealed diffuse conjunctival injection, mucopurulent discharge from superotemporal globe (Figure 1(b)), diffuse corneal edema and haze, and extensive fibrin in the anterior chamber. The dilated exam was limited due to corneal edema, diffuse anterior chamber reaction, and dense vitritis. Ophthalmic ultrasonography revealed a subluxed lens with diffuse vitritis (Figure 2(a)). Orbital CT confirmed no retained intraocular foreign body (Figure 2(b)) or occult penetrating injury.

Upon admission, patient's blood and specimens from ocular mucopurulent discharge were sent for gram stain and

culture. The gram stain revealed gram-positive bacillus. The patient was admitted and started on intravenous (IV) broad spectrum antimicrobial therapy (vancomycin, meropenem, and amphotericin B). Due to progressive clinical decline with associated leukocytosis and encephalopathy 48 hours after initiating systemic antimicrobial treatment and gram stain results, she underwent enucleation of the left eye. Postoperatively, the patient completed a full course of IV vancomycin and meropenem.

Reflex anaerobic culture from the mucopurulent collection grew *Clostridium perfringens* and gross specimen from the enucleation revealed numerous gram-positive bacillus microbes. Anaerobic microbes seen on staining and samples were inoculated onto prereduced anaerobically sterilized Brucella blood agar, phenylethyl alcohol blood agar, kanamycin-vancomycin laked blood agar, and Bacteroides bile esculin agar (Oxyrase, Inc., Mansfield, OH). The inoculated plates were incubated at 35 degrees C anaerobically using the AnaeroPack-Anaero Anaerobic Gas Generator

(Mitsubishi Gas Chemical America, New York, NY). After 48 hours of incubation, 2+ growth of a gram-positive bacillus was noted on the Brucella blood agar. These colonies were identified as *Clostridium perfringens* by Matrix-Assisted Laser Desorption Ionization-Time of Flight Mass Spectrometry (Vitek MS, bioMerieux, Inc., Durham, NC). No other growth was observed.

Amphotericin B was discontinued once fungal etiology was excluded. Subsequently, both the periorbital edema and erythema resolved. Additionally, the patient regained consciousness, as her encephalopathy and infection improved. She was subsequently transferred to local rehabilitation facility. A repeat CT abdomen demonstrated the previous inflammation had resolved, likely due to the aggressive inpatient broad spectrum antibiotics. No comorbid occult distal gastrointestinal malignancies were found.

## 3. Discussion

*Clostridium perfringens* is a rare ocular infection that results in devastating panophthalmitis with poor visual prognosis. The source of *Clostridium perfringens* is usually exogenous. The first report was described in a large series of 54 cases [1]. In that study, the authors noted that rapid painful visual loss developed within 12 hours; however all subjects had penetrating injuries. Since then, similar findings have been reported in isolated case reports after trauma [5], intravitreal injection [4], penetrating keratoplasty [3], cataract surgery [6], and among IV drug abusers [2]. Although the lateral canthotomy and cantholysis is a potential exogenous source of infection, this is much less likely in our patient, given the endogenous infection resulted in vision loss occurred 6 hours prior to the lateral canthotomy and cantholysis was performed.

There is limited literature regarding an endogenous source. To our knowledge, this is the fourth case of endogenous source of panophthalmitis resulting from *Clostridium perfringens*. The first case, described in 1974, showed a 68-year-old patient with endogenous endophthalmitis secondary to a biliary infection [7]. The gallbladder perforated despite surgical management and systemic IV antibiotics. The patient suffered associated rapid vision loss and the patient subsequently passed away from *Clostridium septicemia*. The second case, reported in 1992, was a patient with endogenous *Clostridium perfringens* endophthalmitis in setting of acute cholecystitis [9]. Despite surviving after surgical and IV interventions the patient's vision decreased to NLP vision within 24 hours of the globe perforating. The third case, reported in 2005, was acute painful loss of vision within 12 hours of developing an acute abdomen. The patient subsequently passed away from multiorgan failure from clostridial septicemia [8]. These 3 cases illustrate that endogenous *Clostridium perfringens* endophthalmitis can result in rapid complete loss of vision, and 2 out of 3 patients had fulminant systemic illnesses that resulted in mortality.

The clinical presentation of endogenous *Clostridium perfringens* endophthalmitis is a rare ocular manifestation. Although the portal of entry into the bloodstream in endogenous *Clostridium perfringens* infection remains unknown,

studies have suggested that another Clostridium species, *Clostridium septicum*, has a strong association with diverticulosis, diabetes mellitus, severe arteriosclerotic disease, and occult visceral malignancy [10–12]. This patient had distal diverticulitis based on the abdominal CT two months prior to her ocular presentation. We propose that it is possible that the portal of entry into the bloodstream is from the distal sigmoid region. Our patient also had a history of poorly controlled diabetes with PDR changes affecting the inner blood retinal barrier. In addition to immunocompromised state in diabetes, PDR disrupts the inner blood retinal barrier by causing increased vascular permeability, loss of tight junctions [13], and a potential route for clostridial bacteremia to spread intraocularly. Further, given the immunocompromised state from diabetes, retinal neovascularization, and recent history of diverticulitis, our case highlights the importance of considering *Clostridium perfringens* as a cause of endogenous ocular dissemination. Further studies are needed to determine whether diverticulitis and PDR increase the risk of endogenous eye spreading in *Clostridium perfringens* infection.

In the setting of rapid painful loss of vision due to fulminate endophthalmitis, though it is rare, *Clostridium perfringens* must be considered as the endogenous infection may be associated with a life-threatening condition. Exogenous causes such as occult penetrating injury, intravenous drug use, and postsurgical procedures complications should be ruled out first. As this condition is rare, it is difficult to identify risk factors to alert an ophthalmologist to consider *Clostridium perfringens* as a possible etiology for orbital infection. Nevertheless, if endogenous endophthalmitis is suspected after excluding exogenous causes, a multidisciplinary systemic work-up with special emphasis on identifying the port of entry and promptly initiating appropriate broad spectrum antimicrobial coverage are warranted to avoid mortality.

## Acknowledgments

The pathology study was performed by the Department of Ophthalmology at Upstate Medical Center. Special acknowledgements for Dr. Maria Del Valle Estopinal for the preparation of pathology slides and Dr. Scott W. Riddell for preparation of microbiology study. This study was approved by the Institutional Review of Department of Center for Vision Care, Syracuse, NY.

## References

[1] R. B. Leavelle, "Gas gangrene panophthalmitis," *JAMA Ophthalmology*, vol. 53, no. 5, pp. 634–642, 1955.

[2] A. Shwe-Tin, T. Ung, C. Madhavan, and T. Yasen, "A case of endogenous clostridium perfringens endophthalmitis in an intravenous drug abuser," *Eye*, vol. 21, no. 11, pp. 1427-1428, 2007.

[3] J. H. Hou, A. Tannan, J. B. Rubenstein et al., "Clostridium perfringens endophthalmitis after penetrating keratoplasty with contaminated corneal allografts: A case series," *Cornea*, vol. 34, no. 1, pp. 23–27, 2015.

[4] S. Kancherla, A. Ross, S. T. Stefko, and J. N. Martel, "Clostridium perfringens panophthalmitis after intravitreal anti-vascular

endothelial growth factor injection," *Retinal cases & Brief Reports*, 2017.

[5] G. Guedira, N. Taright, H. Blin et al., "Clostridium perfringens panophthalmitis and orbital cellulitis: a case report," *BMC Ophthalmology*, vol. 18, no. 1, p. 88, 2018.

[6] D. P. Romsaiton and C. M. Grasso, "Clostridium perfringens endophthalmitis following cataract surgery," *Arch Ophthalmol*, vol. 117, no. 7, pp. 978-979, 1999.

[7] J. F. Frantz, M. A. Lemp, R. L. Font, R. Stone, and E. Eisner, "Acute endogenous panophthalmitis caused by Clostridium perfringens," *American Journal of Ophthalmology*, vol. 78, no. 2, pp. 295–303, 1974.

[8] A. K. Lauer, K. Riley, J. Wentzien, and S. W. Marsal, "Acute painful vision loss and acute abdomen: a case of endogenous clostridium perfringens endophthalmitis," *Canadian Journal of Ophthalmology*, vol. 40, no. 2, pp. 208–210, 2005.

[9] V. Nangia and C. Hutchinson, "Metastatic endophthalmitis caused by clostridium perfringens," *British Journal of Ophthalmology*, vol. 76, no. 4, pp. 252-253, 1992.

[10] J. R. Koransky, M. D. Stargel, and V. Dowell, "Clostridium septicum bacteremia and its clinical significance," *American Journal of Medicine*, vol. 66, no. 1, pp. 63–66, 1979.

[11] L. Slagsvold and J. E. Slagsvold, "Binocular endogenous Clostridium septicum endophthalmitis," *Acta Ophthalmologica Scandinavica*, vol. 85, no. 2, pp. 232–234, 2007.

[12] J. L. Eisenrich, A. M. Herro, M. Schmutz, and K. S. Nagi, "Clostridium septicum endophalmitis associated with colon adenocarcinoma," *Digital journal of ophthalmology : DJO*, vol. 20, no. 3, pp. 41-42, 2014.

[13] S. Kusuhara, Y. Fukushima, S. Ogura, N. Inoue, and A. Uemura, "Pathophysiology of diabetic retinopathy: the old and the new," *Diabetes & Metabolism Journal*, vol. 42, no. 5, pp. 364–376, 2018.

# 3

# Cytomegalovirus Retinitis Associated with Lenalidomide use for Multiple Myeloma in an Immunocompetent Patient

**Matthew K. Adams and Christina Y. Weng**(ID)

*Department of Ophthalmology, Baylor College of Medicine, 6565 Fannin Street, NC-205, Houston, TX 77030, USA*

Correspondence should be addressed to Christina Y. Weng; christina.weng@bcm.edu

Academic Editor: Alexander A. Bialasiewicz

*Purpose.* The aim of this report is to present a case of cytomegalovirus (CMV) retinitis in an immunocompetent patient using lenalidomide. *Methods.* Case report with fundus photography, spectral-domain optical coherence tomography, and fluorescein angiography imaging. *Results.* A 55-year-old male with history of multiple myeloma treated with lenalidomide presented with blurriness and floaters in his right eye and was found to have vitreous biopsy-confirmed CMV retinitis. The patient was treated with pars plana vitrectomy, oral valganciclovir, and intravitreal foscarnet. More than one year later, the patient was doing well with visual acuity of 20/25 and no recurrence of retinitis. *Conclusion.* This represents the second report of CMV retinitis associated with lenalidomide therapy. It suggests that even immunocompetent patients can be affected by CMV retinitis in the context of lenalidomide treatment. It is critical that patients being treated with lenalidomide receive prompt evaluation if they develop ophthalmic symptoms.

## 1. Introduction

Cytomegalovirus (CMV) infection typically occurs in immunocompromised patients and can present as a primary infection, reinfection, or reactivation. While generally asymptomatic in immunocompetent individuals, CMV can lead to serious pathology in those who are immunocompromised, such as transplant recipients, patients with immunodeficiency disorders, and those on immunosuppressive treatment [1].

Lenalidomide (Revlimid®; Celgene, Summit, NJ), an analogue of thalidomide, is an FDA-approved treatment for multiple myeloma, myelodysplastic syndrome, and mantle cell lymphoma. Its mechanism of action is complex and includes immunomodulation, antiangiogenic effects, and direct cytotoxic activity [2, 3]. While it is thought to have a more favorable side-effect profile than its parent drug, thalidomide, it still has potential serious adverse effects that include birth defects, neutropenia, and thrombocytopenia [4].

CMV retinitis is most commonly seen in AIDS patients with a CD4+ count < 50 cells/$\mu$L; it is less commonly seen in patients with other causes of immunosuppression [5]. However, it has been reported once before in an immunocompetent multiple myeloma patient following lenalidomide therapy [6]. Here, we present the second reported case of CMV retinitis in a similar patient who was treated with lenalidomide; differences in management between the first reported case and ours are discussed.

## 2. Case Report

A 55-year-old male with multiple myeloma on his eighth cycle of chemotherapy with bortezomib, lenalidomide (recently decreased to 10 mg po daily from 25 mg po daily), and dexamethasone presented with a two-week history of worsening blurriness and floaters in his right eye. An outside provider noted panuveitis and retinal whitening on examination. Anterior chamber paracentesis was negative for CMV, HSV-1, HSV-2, VZV, and Toxoplasmosis. Oral valacyclovir and topical steroids and cycloplegics were started for presumed acute retinal necrosis, and the patient was referred to our institution for further diagnostic work-up and management. Of note, recent serum laboratory values revealed a normal

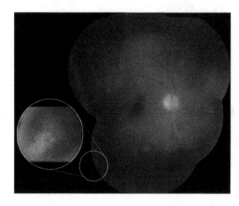

FIGURE 1: Color fundus photograph of the right eye shows vitreous haze, vascular sheathing, and granular retinal whitening in the inferotemporal periphery (inset).

white blood cell count (9.41 k/$\mu$L; range 4.5–11 k/$\mu$L) and neutrophilic profile (71.0%; range 39–69%) with negative CMV antigen and aerobic blood culture; lambda light chain immunoglobulins were significantly elevated (67.29 mg/L, range 5.7–26.3 mg/L) and alpha-2 globulin proteins were abnormally high on serum electrophoresis (0.93 g/dL, range 0.58–0.84 g/dL) as expected given his disease.

Best-corrected visual acuity (BCVA) was 20/60 in the right eye, 20/20 in the left. Pupils and intraocular pressures were normal. Slit lamp examination of the right eye revealed mild anterior chamber flare without cell, mild cataract, and 3+ cell in the anterior vitreous. Dilated funduscopic examination revealed vitreous haze, diffuse vascular sheathing, and a poorly-defined area of inferotemporal retinal whitening without associated hemorrhage (Figure 1). The left eye was normal. Spectral-domain optical coherence tomography of the right eye showed no significant abnormalities aside from overlying hyperreflective vitreous debris (Figure 2). Fluorescein angiography demonstrated irregular vascular filling and blockage from vitreous debris (Figure 3).

Given the previous negative anterior chamber tap, worsening clinical exam, and high suspicion for infectious retinitis, the decision was made to proceed with a diagnostic vitrectomy. Diluted and undiluted vitreous biopsy were obtained via a 23-gauge pars plana vitrectomy. Intraoperatively, extensive retinal whitening and granular necrosis were observed along with diffuse vascular sheathing and perivascular inflammatory aggregates (Figure 4). Endolaser was placed 360 degrees prophylactically. The vitreous biopsy was sent for gram stain, cytology (to rule out malignant infiltration), fungal culture, Toxoplasmosis, AFB, VZV, EBV, CMV, HSV-1, HSV-2, and RPR testing.

On postoperative day 2, the vitreous PCR returned positive for CMV; all other tests were negative. The patient was switched from oral valacyclovir to valganciclovir 900 mg po twice daily. By postoperative day 3, the patient's visual acuity declined to 20/200 and there was an increase in anterior chamber cell. Hence, intravitreal foscarnet (2.4 mg/0.1 cc) was injected. At the postoperative week 1 visit, visual acuity had not improved, but the area of retinitis appeared less active (Figure 5). Repeat intravitreal foscarnet

was given. Improvement continued over the first month with complete resolution of the patient's uveitis, vasculitis, and retinitis. By postoperative month 2, BCVA had improved to 20/63 without evidence of active disease. Five months after the vitreous biopsy, the patient remained without signs of intraocular infection with BCVA 20/50, mostly limited by cataract. Following cataract extraction one year later, his visual acuity was 20/25 with stable fundus findings (Figure 6).

## 3. Discussion

Cytomegalovirus retinitis is thought to result from reactivation of a latent infection and is typically only seen in those with a compromised immune system. Multiple myeloma itself, although capable of causing an immunocompromised state by affecting cellular immunity, has never been reported to cause CMV retinitis [7]. Given that our patient was essentially immunocompetent (by definition of a normal white blood cell count and differential) along with the fact that lenalidomide-associated CMV retinitis has been previously reported, it is reasonable to assume that lenalidomide played a role in this patient's development of CMV retinitis. Notably, none of his other medications have been associated with this condition.

The first case of CMV retinitis following lenalidomide treatment was presented by Lim et al. in 2013 [6]. Similar to this case, CMV retinitis presented in their patient with multiple myeloma, on lenalidomide therapy, and in the absence of detectable systemic CMV titers. Lenalidomide can cause myelosuppression, but, like the previously-reported patient, our patient had a normal white blood cell count without neutropenia [4]. Our patient also received multiple blood draws during his treatment period and never had detectable CMV antigen. This lends itself to the likelihood that lenalidomide crosses the blood-retinal barrier to alter local intraocular immunity which can lead to CMV reactivation [8]. While no consensus exists, there is some evidence to support that the drug can modulate the blood-retinal barrier which typically protects the eye from bloodstream pathogens [9].

Some differences between the diagnostic work-up and management of these two cases exist. Unlike the case presented by Lim and colleagues, our patient first received an anterior chamber paracentesis which was negative. Vitreous sample was obtained surgically via pars plana vitrectomy as opposed to a vitreous tap. Although both approaches were successful in identifying a causative organism, our approach allowed for concurrent removal of vitreous debris and placement of prophylactic endolaser to the necrotic retina. This may prevent future retinal detachment, a devastating sequela of CMV retinitis that occurs in upwards of 30% of patients [10]. Our patient was treated only with oral valganciclovir versus intravenous ganciclovir. Both patients did well with a good visual outcome and no recurrence. We continued our patient on a maintenance dose of oral valganciclovir 900 mg po daily for the duration of his lenalidomide therapy.

This case represents the second report of CMV retinitis associated with lenalidomide, a relatively new drug that received FDA approval in 2013. Lenalidomide is a derivative

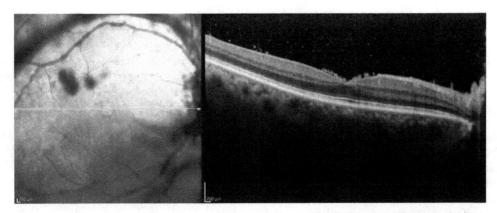

FIGURE 2: Spectral-domain OCT of the right eye demonstrates vitreous debris overlying a well-preserved foveal contour.

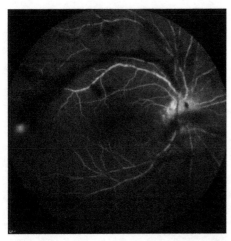

FIGURE 3: Fluorescein angiography of the right eye reveals irregular filling defects and blockage from overlying vitreous debris; of note, the inferotemporal area of retinal whitening is not captured in this image.

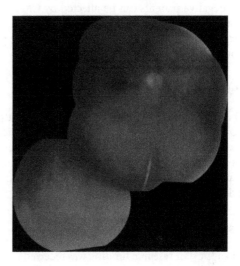

FIGURE 5: Fundus photograph from postoperative week 1 demonstrates improving vasculitis and retinitis.

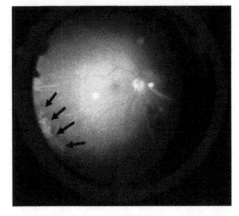

FIGURE 4: Intraoperative image of fundus reveals diffuse vascular sheathing with perivascular inflammatory aggregates and an area of granular retinal necrosis and whitening (arrows) involving the inferotemporal periphery.

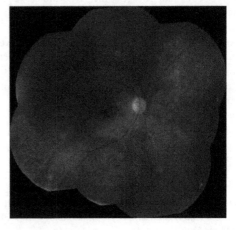

FIGURE 6: Fundus photograph more than one year following initial presentation shows resolution of retinitis with laser scars in the periphery.

of thalidomide and works by modulating the substrate specificity of the CRL4$^{\text{CRBN}}$E3 ubiquitin ligase which leads to subsequent proteasomal degradation of certain transcription factors that kills multiple myeloma cells. It is more appropriate to consider lenalidomide an immunomodulator rather than an immunosuppressant because its use actually stimulates certain immunogenic cell lines (IL-2 production in T lymphocytes, natural killer cells). Its use in diseases like myelodysplastic syndromes and mantle cell lymphoma is growing, and it is possible that cases such as this one will be seen more frequently in upcoming years. Although CMV retinitis often carries a poor visual prognosis, its course can be halted with early diagnosis and treatment. Because CMV retinitis classically affects AIDS patients, providers may fail to consider this diagnosis in the types of patients treated with lenalidomide. However, it seems that even immunocompetent HIV-negative patients can be affected by CMV retinitis in the context of lenalidomide treatment. Thus, it is critical that patients being treated with lenalidomide receive prompt evaluation if they develop ophthalmic symptoms.

## Additional Points

*Summary Statement.* A relatively immunocompetent patient with multiple myeloma being treated with lenalidomide presented with cytomegalovirus (CMV) retinitis. This report supports an association between lenalidomide and CMV retinitis and offers a different management approach from the one previously reported in a similar case.

## Disclosure

No grant support or research funding was received in relation to this study. The authors alone are responsible for the content and writing of the manuscript.

## References

[1] J. G. P. Sissons and A. J. Carmichael, "Clinical aspects and management of cytomegalovirus infection," *Infection*, vol. 44, no. 2, pp. 78–83, 2002.

[2] M. Arora, S. Gowda, and J. Tuscano, "A comprehensive review of lenalidomide in B-cell non-Hodgkin lymphoma," *Therapeutic Advances in Hematology*, vol. 7, no. 4, pp. 209–221, 2016.

[3] V. Kotla, S. Goel, S. Nischal et al., "Mechanism of action of lenalidomide in hematological malignancies," *Journal of Hematology & Oncology*, vol. 2, no. 12, article 36, 2009.

[4] J. Zeldis, R. Knight, C. Jacques et al., "Lenalidomide in multiple myeloma: current role and future directions," *Expert Opinion on Pharmacotherapy*, vol. 11, no. 5, pp. 829–842, 2011.

[5] I. C. Kuo, J. H. Kempen, J. P. Dunn, G. Vogelsang, and D. A. Jabs, "Clinical characteristics and outcomes of cytomegalovirus retinitis in persons without human immunodeficiency virus infection," *American Journal of Ophthalmology*, vol. 138, no. 3, pp. 338–346, 2004.

[6] H. Y. Lim, D. Francis, J. Yeoh, and L. L. Lim, "Cytomegalovirus retinitis after treatment with lenalidomide for multiple myeloma," *Retinal Cases and Brief Reports*, vol. 7, no. 2, pp. 172–175, 2013.

[7] M. Nucci and E. Anaissie, "Infections in patients with multiple myeloma in the era of high-dose therapy and novel agents," *Clinical Infectious Diseases*, vol. 49, no. 8, pp. 1211–1225, 2009.

[8] M. Zhang, H. Xin, and S. S. Atherton, "Murine cytomegalovirus (MCMV) spreads to and replicates in the retina after endotoxin-induced disruption of the blood-retinal barrier of immunosuppressed BALB/c mice," *Journal of NeuroVirology*, vol. 11, no. 4, pp. 365–375, 2005.

[9] M. C. Cox, G. Mannino, L. Lionetto, V. Naso, M. Simmaco, and M. A. A. Spiriti, "Lenalidomide for aggressive B-cell lymphoma involving the central nervous system?" *American Journal of Hematology*, vol. 86, no. 11, pp. 957-957, 2011.

[10] G. N. Holland, "AIDS and ophthalmology: the first quarter century," *American Journal of Ophthalmology*, vol. 145, no. 3, pp. 397–408, 2008.

# 4

# A Case of Chorioretinitis with Retinal Angiomatous Proliferation

**Yanru Chen**[ID],[1,2] **Mingyan Wei,**[3,4,5,6] **Qian Chen**[ID],[3,4,5,6] **and Minghan Li**[ID][1,2]

[1]*Xiamen University Affiliated Xiamen Eye Center, Xiamen, Fujian 36100, China*
[2]*Fujian Key Laboratory of Ocular Surface and Corneal Diseases, Xiamen, Fujian 36100, China*
[3]*Department of Ophthalmology, Xiang'an Hospital of Xiamen University, Xiamen, Fujian 36102, China*
[4]*Fujian Provincial Key Laboratory of Ophthalmology and Visual Science, Xiamen, Fujian 36102, China*
[5]*Eye Institute of Xiamen University, Xiamen, Fujian 36102, China*
[6]*School of Medicine, Xiamen University, Xiamen, Fujian 36102, China*

Correspondence should be addressed to Qian Chen; qchen2@xmu.edu.cn and Minghan Li; 740118340@qq.com

Academic Editor: Stephen G. Schwartz

A 48-year-old woman had an acute blurred vision in the right eye immediately after drainage of liver abscess. Her best corrected visual acuity (BCVA) was 8/400; fundus photography suggested the diagnosis of endogenous endophthalmitis with chorioretinitis and vitritis. Due to the bad systemic condition, a systemic antibiotic combined with periocular triamcinolone (TA) was carried out first. Inflammatory cells in the vitreous cavity were decreased after treatment; however, fundus fluorescein angiography (FFA) showed abnormal dilation and leakage of the capillaries and retinal-choroidal anastomose, supporting that there was retinal angiomatous proliferation (RAP). Vitreous interleukin-6 (IL-6) was only slightly elevated; the ratio of interleukin-10 (IL-10) and IL-6 was less than 1, and the etiological test was negative. After receiving intravitreal vancomycin injection combined with periocular TA injection, the patient's BCVA was improved from 16/400 to 20/400 with a reduction in vitreous inflammatory cells. However, the patient's RAP was progressed and her BCVA was dramatically decreased to count finger/30 cm. After intravitreal injection of ranibizumab, the patient's BCVA was 5/400 with a significant shrink in lesions and absorption of hemorrhage, exudation, and fluid. Thus, we suggest that early anti-inflammatory treatment in conjunction with anti-VEGF may achieve a better prognosis in patients with inflammatory retinal angiomatous proliferation (RAP).

## 1. Introduction

Chorioretinitis is a type of posterior uveitis. According to the etiology, it can be divided into noninfectious and infectious chorioretinitis [1]. Early recognition with prompt treatment is fundamental to prevent severe loss of vision. Infectious chorioretinitis can be caused by blood-borne pathogens, such as fungi, viruses, bacteria, and endogenous parasites; endophthalmitis can be the reason [2]. Klebsiella pneumoniae is the main pathogen of liver abscess [3]. Among the extrahepatic invasive manifestations, organs such as the lung, brain, and eye are the most common invasive sites [4]. Pathogenic detection is the gold standard for diagnosis, but medical history and empirical therapy are also important when the diagnosis is ambiguous. Early combination therapy has great value for the patients who have endophthalmitis along with retinal angiomatous proliferation (RAP).

## 2. Case Report

A 48-year-old female complained of defective vision in the right eye immediately after drainage of liver abscess. Her best corrected visual acuity was 8/400 in the right eye and 20/20 in the left eye. There was no evidence of anterior chamber cells or keratic precipitates, and the intraocular pressure was normal. Dense vitreous opacities obscured the visualization of fundus of the right eye. Chorioretinitis with exudation and hemorrhage were present in the macular and inferonasal peripheral retina (Figures 1(a) and 1(b)). The fundus of the left eye is normal (Figure 1(c)). Optical coherence tomography (OCT) showed epiretinal membrane on the inner retinal surface of macular foveal and pigment epithelial detachment (PED) (Figures 1(d) and 1(e)). The patient's blood culture was positive for Klebsiella pneumoniae. Rheumatoid factor (RF), antistreptolysin antibody

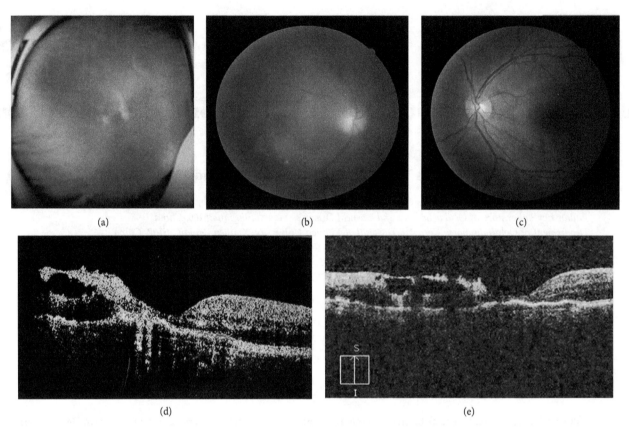

FIGURE 1: Inflammation was present in the right eye. (a) The fundus was opaque, and exudation and hemorrhage could be seen in the macular and inferonasal peripheral retina. (b) Dense vitreous opacities obscured the visualization of the fundus of the right eye. Chorioretinitis with exudation and hemorrhage was seen in the macular. (c) Normal fundus of left eye. (d, e) OCT showed an epiretinal membrane above the inner retinal surface of macular fovea and pigment epithelial detachment (PED).

(ASO), human immunodeficiency virus (HIV), TP particle agglutination assay, and purified protein derivative (PPD) tuberculin skin test were all negative. The possibility of endogenous endophthalmitis was considered in ophthalmologic consultation. Taking into account the patient's poor general condition, systemic cephalosporin therapy combined with periocular triamcinolone injection was given to her.

Four months later, the patient returned to the ophthalmology department with stable condition after the antibiotic therapy. Her BCVA was 16/400 and vitreous inflammatory cells in the right eye were decreased; flaky yellowish-white elevated lesions surrounded by hemorrhages can be visualized in the macular and inferonasal peripheral retina. The crooked retinal arterioles and retinal venules extended into the outer nuclear layers of the macula of the right eye (Figure 2(a)). OCT showed that a dense epiretinal membrane was attached in the inner surface of the retina, hyperreflective materials were located at the level of the outer retinal layers, and vascularized PED was found in the macular fovea of the right eye (Figures 2(b) and 2(c)). Optical coherence tomography angiography (OCTA) detected abnormal vascular networks in the superficial, deep retinal capillary plexus/inner retina, outer retina, and choroidal layers (Figures 2(d)–2(f)). Fundus fluorescein angiography (FFA) showed that an intraretinal vascular complex was formed by retinal artery and retinal vein anastomosis in the macular, and a hyperfluorescent lesion was detected at the

inferonasal peripheral retina of the right eye (Figures 2(g)–2(j)). During the course of the fluorescein angiography, the vascular complex, abnormal dilation of the capillaries, and hyperfluorescent lesion had progressively increased levels of leaked dye. Vitreous humor testing was performed, and the results showed that interleukin-6 (IL-6) was 33 mg/ml, which was slightly higher than normal, suggesting that intraocular inflammation was present. However, polymerase chain reaction (PCR) showed that the pathogen was negative. The ratio of interleukin-10 (IL-10) and IL-6 was less than 1, indicating that the diagnosis of lymphoma was not supportive. Based on the symptoms and clinic tests, the clinical diagnosis was endophthalmitis with RAP. Considering that the patient had an infection history and presented chorioretinitis, empirical treatments such as intravitreal vancomycin injection combined with periocular triamcinolone injection were recommended. After treatment, her vitreous inflammatory cells of the right eye were decreased; the patient's BCVA was improved to 20/400.

Five months later, the inflammation was under control (Figure 3(a)), but her RAP was progressed and resulted in serious damage in her central vision. Her BCVA was decreased to count finger (CF/30 cm). OCT showed that intra- and subretinal fluids were increased (Figures 3(b) and 3(c)). Areas of abnormal vascular network on OCTA were enlarged (Figures 3(d)–3(f)). Anti-VEGF therapy was given to her. After three intravitreal injections of ranibizumab (once a

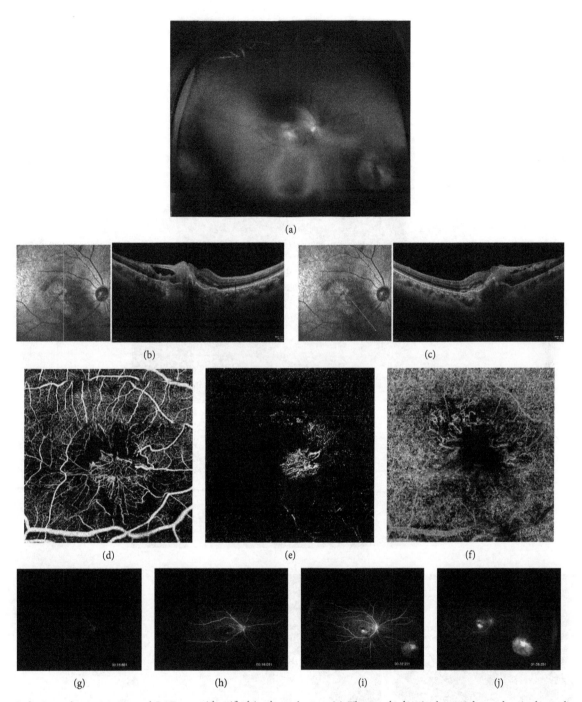

Figure 2: Infectious chorioretinitis and RAP were identified in the right eye. (a) The crooked retinal arterioles and retinal venules extend into deeper layers in the macula. (b, c) OCT showed a thickened epiretinal membrane, hyperreflective material located at the level of the outer retinal layers, and vascularized PED in macular fovea of the right eye. (d–f) OCTA detected abnormal vascular networks in the superficial retinal capillary plexus (d), deep retinal capillary plexus (e), and choroid layers (f). (g–j) Fundus fluorescein angiography (FFA) of the patient: (g) a central, intraretinal hyperfluorescent lesion was visible, which is probably fed by the retinal arteriolar vessel at 2 o'clock; (h) progressive filling of the venous circulation, connected to the hyperfluorescent lesion; (i) the central, intraretinal vascular complex was clearly recognizable in macular, and a round hyperfluorescent lesion was detected at inferonasal peripheral retina; (j) leakage of fluorescent dye from the vascular complex, abnormal dilation of the capillaries, and the hyperfluorescent lesion.

month), the lesions shrunk compared to before the VEGF treatment (Figures 4(a) and 4(b)). OCT revealed that sub- and intraretinal fluids were partly absorbed than before in the right eye (Figures 4(c) and 4(d)). The patient's BCVA was improved to 5/400.

## 3. Discussion

In this case, the patient had blurred vision immediately after drainage of liver abscess; Klebsiella pneumoniae was positive in blood culture, so endogenous infectious endophthalmitis

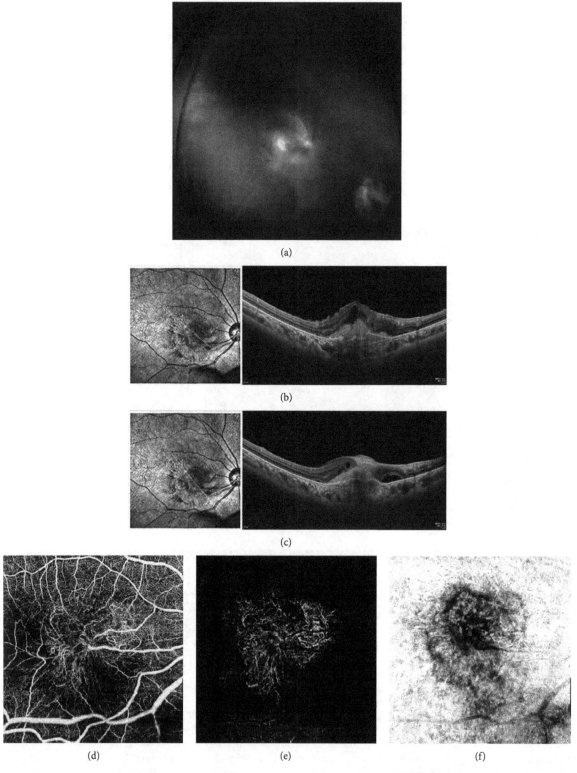

FIGURE 3: The deterioration of RAP in the right eye. (a) Inflammatory cells in the vitreous cavity disappeared and fundus can be seen clearly. (b) The central retinal thickness increased; intra- and subretinal fluid produced. (c) OCTA showed the area of abnormal vascular network in the inner retina (d) and outer retina (e), and choroid layers (f) were enlarged.

was assumed at the initial diagnosis. Considering the poor systemic condition of the patient, systemic antibiotic therapy combined with periocular TA was carried out first [5]. Four months later, the patient's systemic condition was stable,

and inflammatory cells in the vitreous were decreased. However, FFA showed abnormal dilation and leakage of the capillaries, suggesting that inflammatory activity was still present. Vitreous humor testing showed that IL-6 was only

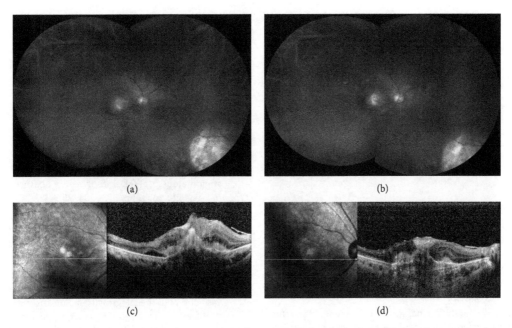

(a)                                                    (b)

(c)                                                    (d)

FIGURE 4: Comparison of lesions before and after the treatment of anti-VEGF. (a, b) The color fundus photograph of the right eye before and after treatment. (a) The lesions have obscure boundaries and are surrounded with hemorrhages. (b) The yellow-white lesions in the macular and inferonasal peripheral retina. Retina were well-demarcated and shrunk, hemorrhage was absorbed, and exudation around the optic nerve reduced significantly. (c, d) The OCT images of RAP before and after treatment: (c) intra- and subretinal fluids were increased; (d) sub- and intraretinal fluids were partly absorbed, and central retinal thickness was reduced from 841 $\mu$m to 690 $\mu$m.

slightly elevated, and the etiological test was negative. It may be explained as the following reasons: (1) the patient has received treatments for liver abscess, and the information is under control; (2) although the positive rate of PCR detection can be more than 90% [6–9], there may be still false negatives; (3) the patient actually has noninfectious chorioretinitis due to the hypoimmunity caused by liver abscess and surgery. Considering that the patient had a confirmed infection history, she was treated by the empirical intravitreal injection of vancomycin combined with periocular TA injection [10]. After the treatment, the vitreous inflammatory cells reduced, suggesting the inflammation was controlled, which supported our primary diagnosis as infectious endophthalmitis.

In inflammatory eye diseases, inflammatory factors promote the upregulation of vascular endothelial growth factor (VEGF), accelerate the development of abnormal angiogenesis, and often result in concurrent inflammatory CNV [11, 12]. RAP is a special subtype of neovascular lesion occurring in age-related macular degeneration (AMD), which is also referred to as type 3 neovascularization. Although its origin is controversial [13–16], it is characterized by detecting chorioretinal anastomosis as neovascularization. Chorioretinitis with RAP is not common, and attention should be paid to distinguish it from inflammatory CNV. In this patient, FFA showed large areas of capillary dilation; leakages of fluorescent dye were present in macular and inferonasal peripheral retinal lesions, retinal arterioles and venules extended into the avascular photoreceptor layers, and the choroid vessels also extended through the disrupted retinal pigment epithelial, suggesting the formation of retinal-choroidal anastomoses (RCA). OCTA

detected abnormal vascular network in superficial, retina, and choroidal layers. All of the evidence supported the diagnosis of chorioretinitis and RAP.

Most of documented studies have recommended the application of intravitreal injection of anti-VEGF drug for treating RAP, which was considered as a form of exudative AMD [17–19]. Since inflammation was involved in the pathogenesis of RAP, recent research studies have shown the efficacy of intravitreal or periocular TA injection in the treatment of RAP [20, 21]. In this case, the patient only received antibiotic and triamcinolone therapy in the early stage due to the severe systemic inflammatory reactions. Several months later, her inflammation was under control, but her RAP was progressed and her visual function suffered serious damage. Anti-VEGF drugs can reduce inflammation, which has been widely demonstrated in studies of inflammatory CNV [22, 23], and has a high efficacy in RAP with uveitis. In a case report, Haq et al. demonstrated a successful treatment for RAP with combined intravitreal ranibizumab and intravitreal TA [24]. After combined treatment with intravitreal ranibizumab, the fundus lesions significantly shrunk, and the hemorrhage, exudation, and fluid significantly were absorbed, suggesting that the anti-VEGF treatment was effective. Therefore, we concluded that early anti-inflammatory treatment combined with anti-VEGF may achieve a better prognosis in patients with RAP and inflammation.

## 4. Conclusion

RAP with endophthalmitis is rare; early anti-inflammatory and anti-VEGF treatments were effective in this case. When vitreous humor and laboratory results are ambiguous to distinguish infectious from noninfectious inflammation, the history and clinical signs may help to support the primary diagnosis and experimental treatment.

## Authors' Contributions

Yanru Chen and Mingyan Wei contributed equally to this work.

## References

[1] J. Deschenes, P. I. Murray, N. A. Rao, and R. B. Nussenblatt, "International Uveitis Study Group (IUSG): clinical classification of uveitis," *Ocular Immunology and Inflammation*, vol. 16, no. 1-2, pp. 1-2, 2008.

[2] N. Relhan, R. K. Forster, and H. W. Flynn Jr., "Endophthalmitis: then and now," *American Journal of Ophthalmology*, vol. 187, pp. xx–xxvii, 2018.

[3] F. Tsai, Y. T. Huang, L. Y. Chang, and J. T. Wang, "Pyogenic liver abscess as endemic Disease, Taiwan," *Emerging Infectious Diseases*, vol. 14, no. 10, pp. 1592–1600, 2008.

[4] S. Lee, Y. S. Chen, H. C. Tsai et al., "Predictors of septic metastatic infection and mortality among patients with Klebsiella pneumoniae liver abscess," *Clinical Infectious Diseases*, vol. 47, no. 5, pp. 642–650, 2008.

[5] J. Davis, "Diagnostic dilemmas in retinitis and endophthalmitis," *Eye*, vol. 26, no. 2, pp. 194–201, 2012.

[6] D. Seal, U. Reischl, A. Behr et al., "Laboratory diagnosis of endophthalmitis: comparison of microbiology and molecular methods in the European Society of Cataract & Refractive Surgeons multicenter study and susceptibility testing," *Journal of Cataract and Refractive Surgery*, vol. 34, no. 9, pp. 1439–1450, 2008.

[7] P. Bispo, G. B. de Melo, A. L. Hofling-Lima, and A. C. C. Pignatari, "Detection and gram discrimination of bacterial pathogens from aqueous and vitreous humor using real-time PCR assays," *Investigative Ophthalmology & Visual Science*, vol. 52, no. 2, pp. 873–881, 2011.

[8] P. Sowmya and H. Madhavan, "Diagnostic utility of polymerase chain reaction on intraocular specimens to establish the etiology of infectious endophthalmitis," *European Journal of Ophthalmology*, vol. 19, no. 5, pp. 812–817, 2009.

[9] A. Oahalou, P. A. W. J. F. Schellekens, J. D. de Groot-Mijnes, and A. Rothova, "Diagnostic pars plana vitrectomy and aqueous analyses in patients with uveitis of unknown cause," *Retina*, vol. 34, no. 1, pp. 108–114, 2014.

[10] A. Sallam, K. A. Kirkland, R. Barry, M. K. Soliman, T. K. Ali, and S. Lightman, "A review of antimicrobial therapy for infectious uveitis of the posterior segment," *Medical Hypothesis, Discovery & Innovation in Ophthalmology*, vol. 7, no. 4, pp. 140–155, 2018.

[11] N. Gulati, F. Forooghian, R. Lieberman, and D. A. Jabs, "Vascular endothelial growth factor inhibition in uveitis: a systematic review," *The British Journal of Ophthalmology*, vol. 95, no. 2, pp. 162–165, 2011.

[12] N. Ferrara, H. Gerber, and J. LeCouter, "The biology of VEGF and its receptors," *Nature Medicine*, vol. 9, no. 6, pp. 669–676, 2003.

[13] L. A. Yannuzzi, S. Negrão, T. Iida et al., "Retinal angiomatous proliferation in age-related macular degeneration," *Retina*, vol. 21, no. 5, pp. 416–434, 2001.

[14] J. D. M. Gass, A. Agarwal, A. M. Lavina, and K. A. Tawansy, "Focal inner retinal hemorrhages in patients with drusen: an early sign of occult choroidal neovascularization and chorioretinal anastomosis," *Retina*, vol. 23, no. 6, pp. 741–751, 2003.

[15] K. B. Freund, I. van Ho, I. A. Barbazetto et al., "Type 3 NEOVASCULARIZATION," *Retina*, vol. 28, no. 2, pp. 201–211, 2008.

[16] L. Yannuzzi, K. Freund, and B. Takahashi, "Review of retinal angiomatous proliferation or type 3 neovascularization," *Retina*, vol. 28, no. 3, pp. 375–384, 2008.

[17] J. Maaß, D. Sandner, and E. Matthé, "Intravitreal ranibizumab for the treatment of retinal angiomatous proliferation," *Der Ophthalmologe: Zeitschrift der Deutschen Ophthalmologischen Gesellschaft*, vol. 114, no. 6, pp. 534–542, 2017.

[18] M. Gharbiya, F. Parisi, F. Cruciani, F. Bozzoni-Pantaleoni, F. Pranno, and S. Abdolrahimzadeh, "Intravitreal antivascular endothelial growth factor for retinal angiomatous proliferation in treatment-naive eyes: long-term functional and anatomical results using a modified PrONTO-style regimen," *Retina*, vol. 34, no. 2, pp. 298–305, 2014.

[19] K. Tsaousis, V. E. Konidaris, S. Banerjee, and T. Empeslidis, "Intravitreal aflibercept treatment of retinal angiomatous proliferation: a pilot study and short-term efficacy," *Graefe's archive for clinical and experimental ophthalmology = Albrecht von Graefes Archiv fur klinische und experimentelle Ophthalmologie*, vol. 253, no. 4, pp. 663–665, 2015.

[20] A. A. Rouvas, T. D. Papakostas, D. Vavvas et al., "Intravitreal ranibizumab, intravitreal ranibizumab with PDT, and intravitreal triamcinolone with PDT for the treatment of retinal angiomatous proliferation: a prospective study," *Retina*, vol. 29, no. 4, pp. 536–544, 2009.

[21] S. Honda, Nakano, H. Ou, M. Kita, and Akira Negi, "Effect of photodynamic therapy (PDT), posterior subtenon injection of triamcinolone acetonide with PDT, and intravitreal injection of ranibizumab with PDT for retinal angiomatous proliferation," *Clinical Ophthalmology*, vol. 6, pp. 277–282, 2012.

[22] R. Agrawal, S. B. B. Tun, P. K. Balne, H. Y. Zhu, N. Khandelwal, and V. A. Barathi, "Fluorescein labeled leukocytes forin vivoImaging of retinal vascular inflammation and infiltrating leukocytes in laser-induced choroidal neovascularization model," *Ocular Immunology and Inflammation*, vol. 28, no. 1, pp. 7–13, 2020.

[23] M. N. Lott, J. C. Schiffman, and J. L. Davis, "Bevacizumab in inflammatory eye disease," *American Journal of Ophthalmology*, vol. 148, no. 5, pp. 711–717.e2, 2009.

[24] A. Haq, B. Kapoor, M. Logendran, and G. Reddy, "Successful treatment of retinal angiomatous proliferation with intravitreal triamcinolone and ranibizumab injections in a 67-year-old male," *Case Reports in Ophthalmology*, vol. 5, no. 3, pp. 392–399, 2014.

# Sudden Vision Loss Secondary to Optic Nerve Infiltration as a Presenting Symptom of Metastatic Lung Adenocarcinoma

**M. M. Shamim** ⓘD,[1] **M. Whaley** ⓘD,[1] **H. Rana** ⓘD,[2] **S. K. Jeffus** ⓘD,[3] **S. Bhatti** ⓘD,[4] and **A. B. Sallam** ⓘD[1]

[1]Department of Ophthalmology, Harvey and Bernice Jones Eye Institute, University of Arkansas for Medical Sciences (UAMS) Medical Center, Little Rock, Arkansas, USA
[2]Hospitalist, UAMS Medical Center, Little Rock, Arkansas, USA
[3]Department of Pathology, UAMS Medical Center, Little Rock, Arkansas, USA
[4]Department of Oncology, Winthrop P. Rockefeller Cancer Institute, UAMS Medical Center, Little Rock, Arkansas, USA

Correspondence should be addressed to A. B. Sallam; ahmedsallam11@yahoo.com

Academic Editor: J. Fernando Arevalo

*Purpose.* To report a rare case of left-sided metastatic optic nerve infiltration and right-sided choroidal mass with exudative retinal detachment caused by EGFR exon 19 deletion positive non-small-cell lung adenocarcinoma that responded to targeted therapy with osimertinib (EGFR-TKI). Our patient demonstrated an excellent response with reduced size of the metastatic choroidal mass of the right orbit and improved visual acuity, in addition to systemic disease control. *Case.* A 66-year-old male patient with a history of diabetes mellitus, hypertension, and tobacco use presented with sudden vision loss in the left eye secondary to optic nerve infiltration and subacute vision loss in the right eye secondary to exudative retinal detachment from a choroidal metastasis. He was found to have a right lung mass, multiple metastatic pulmonary nodules, and liver and bone metastases. Biopsy from a mediastinal lymph node confirmed the diagnosis of metastatic lung adenocarcinoma. He was found to have exon 19 deletion on next-generation sequencing. We treated him with local radiation therapy to the left eye and systemic osimertinib (EGFR-TKI). *Conclusion.* To our knowledge, our case is the first report of a patient who initially presented with acute vision loss and was found to have metastatic retrobulbar optic nerve infiltration in one eye and metastatic choroidal lesion with exudative retinal detachment in the fellow eye secondary to lung adenocarcinoma. Due to the rarity of this condition, literature regarding effective treatment is scarce. Our patient demonstrated significant improvement in visual acuity and resolution of exudative retinal detachment in the right eye following osimertinib treatment and radiation therapy to the left eye. Further investigation into the role of tyrosine kinase inhibitors and radiation therapy in treating intraocular metastasis involving the optic nerve is needed.

## 1. Introduction

Intraocular metastases are commonly asymptomatic and rarely the initial presentation of a primary tumor [1]. When intraocular metastases cause vision loss, it is typically progressive rather than acute [2]. Intraocular metastasis portends a poor visual prognosis, and the majority of cases do not resolve with chemotherapy [3]. Most of the ocular metastases cases in the literature involve the uvea, orbit, or central nervous system [4]. Optic nerve infiltration secondary to metastatic lung adenocarcinoma is rare. We present a case of bilateral vision loss as the presenting symptom of lung adenocarcinoma. Our patient had choroidal

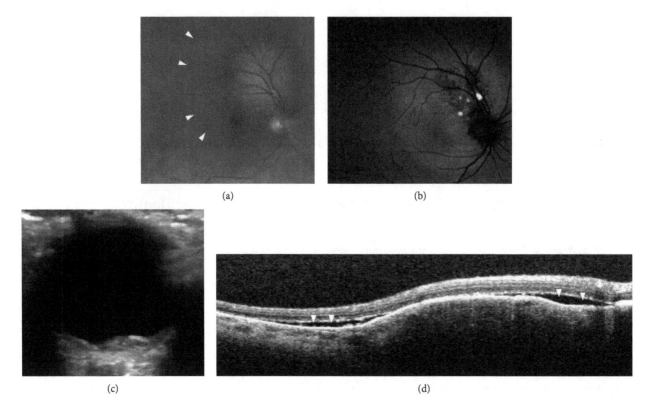

FIGURE 1: Right eye at presentation. (a) Fundus photograph showing choroidal mass and subretinal fluid (arrowheads) with (b) corresponding autofluorescence image; (c) B-scan and (d) optical coherence tomography demonstrate exudative retinal detachment (arrowheads).

metastasis with an exudative retinal detachment of the macula in one eye and a metastatic infiltration of the optic nerve without other central nervous system involvement in the fellow eye.

## 2. Case Presentation

A 66-year-old male with a history of diabetes mellitus, hypertension, and tobacco use presented to the emergency department with acute vision loss in the left eye and progressively decreased vision in the right eye. Visual acuity was 20/200 in the right eye and light perception (LP) in the left eye. He had a relative afferent pupillary defect (RAPD) in the left eye. Slit lamp examination of the anterior segment was unrevealing. A fundus examination showed a choroidal mass measuring approximately 6 mm × 6 mm superior to the optic nerve with an exudative retinal detachment of the right macula. Fundus examination of the left eye was unremarkable. Fundus autofluorescence revealed hyperautofluorescent specks overlying the choroidal mass in the right eye (Figure 1). Optical coherence tomography (OCT) of the retina and B-scan ultrasonography (Figure 1) confirmed a choroidal mass and exudative retinal detachment in the right eye.

He was admitted to the hospital for further workup. CT angiogram of the head and neck revealed an incidental finding of a cavitating mass in the right upper lobe. Follow-up CT chest imaging (Figure 2) showed a large right upper lobe cavitary mass, mediastinal adenopathy, and bilateral pulmonary nodules. A diagnostic bronchoscopy was performed with a biopsy of the lung mass. The biopsy revealed lung adenocarcinoma (Figure 2).

MRI of the brain and orbits with and without contrast demonstrated thickening in the right posterior globe and optic nerve changes on the left side. After discharge from the hospital, the patient had PET–CT performed demonstrating PET-avid RUL lung mass with extensive pulmonary, nodal, liver, and osseous metastatic disease consistent with the clinical staging of IVB (cT3, cN2, and pM1c). A blood next-generation sequencing test was positive for an EGFR exon 19 deletion. Subsequently, he was started on osimertinib, an oral third-generation irreversible EGFR tyrosine kinase inhibitor, at a dose of 80 mg daily. The patient underwent radiation therapy to the left orbit × 3 for a total of 2400 cGy. At the patient's one-month follow-up appointment, the right eye showed complete resolution of subretinal fluid, shrinking of the right choroidal mass, and improved visual acuity in the right eye (20/30) (Figure 3).

The left eye vision did not improve, and disc pallor was noted. A posttreatment CT of the chest, abdomen, and pelvis with contrast demonstrated significant interval improvement of right upper lobe mass, improvement in mediastinal and right hilar lymphadenopathy, and improvement in metastatic liver lesions. The patient is continuing follow-up with both ophthalmology and oncology services.

## 3. Discussion

Our patient's presentation was unorthodox, with vision loss from a metastatic choroidal mass with exudative retinal detachment in the right eye and optic nerve involvement in

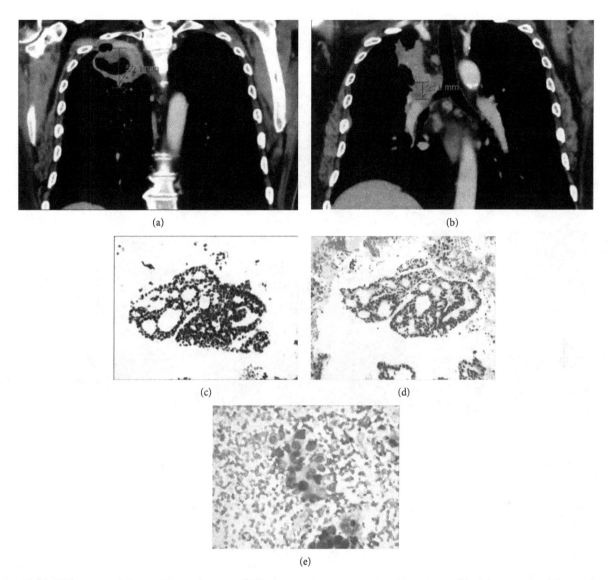

FIGURE 2: (a) Right upper lobe cavitary pulmonary lesion measuring up to $6.0 \times 6.3 \times 5.0$ cm; (b) right superior hilar/mediastinal heterogeneously enhancing mass measuring up to $3.7 \times 4.8 \times 2.1$ cm; (c) smear (Diff-Quik-stained slide, $400 \times$ magnification) showing cohesive malignant cells characterized by enlarged nuclei with pleomorphism and moderate cytoplasm, consistent with metastatic non-small-cell carcinoma; (d) cell block (H&E stain, $200 \times$ magnification) showing tumor cells that are arranged in a cribriforming growth pattern consistent with metastatic adenocarcinoma. This growth pattern has been associated with aggressive behavior; (e) immunohistochemical stain (TTF − 1, $200 \times$ magnification) shows that the tumor cells are strongly and diffusely positive for TTF-1 (nuclear staining). This supports the diagnosis of metastasis from a lung primary (in the setting of a lung mass).

the left. Metastases from other primary sites are the most frequent intraocular tumor in adults, with the choroid being the most common intraocular site for metastases due to its high vascular supply [5]. However, metastases to the optic nerve were shown to be extremely rare. A publication by Shields et al. with 660 cases of intraocular metastases reported a prevalence of 4.5% for optic nerve involvement [6]. Shields et al. characterized optic disc metastases as a unilateral creamy-looking infiltrate which can be associated with peripapillary hemorrhages and cotton wool spots [6]. Unique to our case is the absence of optic nerve edema in the left eye and the unremarkable appearance of the fundus despite the left RAPD indicating retrobulbar involvement of the optic nerve. Another important feature of the presented case is how the patient's subretinal fluid in the right eye resolved completely

after systemic osimertinib therapy. Only the left orbit was irradiated; no irradiation was applied to the right orbit. In the FLAURA trial, osimertinib (EGFR-TKI) was shown to be beneficial for untreated, EGFR mutant advanced non-small-cell lung carcinoma, showing superior efficacy compared to earlier generation EGFR-tyrosine kinase inhibitors [7]. Osimertinib also has better CNS penetration leading to favorable CNS overall response rates and CNS progression-free survival and has previously been shown to successfully treat choroidal metastasis in a patient with EGFR-mutated lung adenocarcinoma [8].

In summary, this is the first report to our knowledge of a patient who presented with metastatic choroidal lesion with exudative retinal detachment in one eye and retrobulbar optic nerve infiltration in the fellow eye. He demonstrated significant

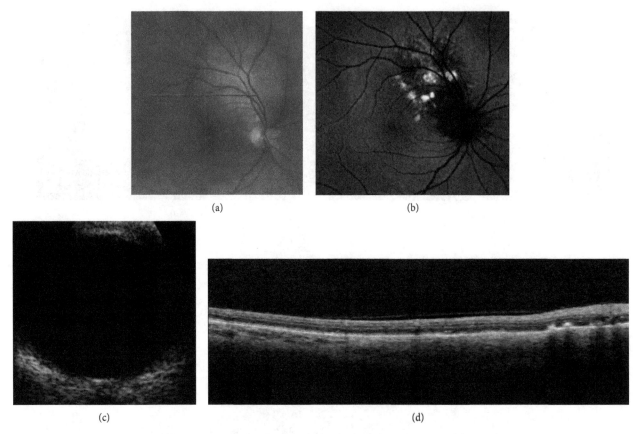

(a)

(b)

(c)

(d)

FIGURE 3: Right eye at one-month follow-up. (a) Fundus photograph showing resolution of choroidal mass with disappearance of subretinal fluid around the lesion (b) corresponding autofluorescence image; (c) B-scan showing reduction in lesion thickness and (d) optical coherence tomography demonstrating resolution of exudative retinal detachment.

improvement in visual acuity with resolution of exudative retinal detachment in the right eye following osimertinib therapy. Additional studies are warranted to further understand the role of tyrosine kinase inhibitors in the treatment of intraocular metastases.

## Consent

Written consent to publish this case has not been obtained. This report does not contain any personal identifiable information.

## Acknowledgments

Funding for the publication of this work was provided by the Harvey and Bernice Jones Eye Institute of the University of Arkansas for Medical Sciences.

## References

[1] C. Porrello, R. Gullo, C. M. Gagliardo et al., "Choroidal metastasis from lung adenocarcinoma: a rare case report," *Il Giornale di Chirurgia-Journal of the Italian Surgical Association*, vol. 40, no. 2, pp. 137–140, 2019.

[2] S. Salah, J. Khader, Y. Yousef, A. Salem, M. Al-Hussaini, and R. Al-Asady, "Choroidal metastases as the sole initial presentation of metastatic lung cancer: case report and review of literature," *Nepalese Journal of Ophthalmology*, vol. 4, no. 2, pp. 339–342, 2012.

[3] P. Martín Martorell, J. F. Marí Cotino, and A. Insa, "Choroidal metastases from lung adenocarcinoma," *Clinical & Translational Oncology*, vol. 11, no. 10, pp. 694–697, 2009.

[4] G. L. Kanthan, J. Jayamohan, D. Yip, and R. M. Conway, "Management of metastatic carcinoma of the uveal tract: an evidence-based analysis," *Clinical & Experimental Ophthalmology*, vol. 35, no. 6, pp. 553–565, 2007.

[5] K. M. Kreusel, T. Wiegel, M. Stange, N. Bornfeld, W. Hinkelbein, and M. H. Foerster, "Choroidal metastasis in disseminated lung cancer: frequency and risk factors," *American Journal of Ophthalmology*, vol. 134, no. 3, pp. 445–447, 2002.

[6] J. A. Shields, C. L. Shields, and A. D. Singh, "Metastatic neoplasms in the optic Disc," *Archives of Ophthalmology*, vol. 118, no. 2, pp. 217–224, 2000.

[7] J.-C. Soria, Y. Ohe, J. Vansteenkiste et al., "Osimertinib in UntreatedEGFR-Mutated Advanced Non–Small-Cell Lung Cancer," *New England Journal of Medicine*, vol. 378, no. 2, pp. 113–125, 2018.

[8] M. G. Field, H. C. Boldt, T. A. Hejleh, and E. M. Binkley, "Successful response to first-line treatment with osimertinib for choroidal metastasis from EGFR-mutated non-small-cell lung cancer," *American Journal of Ophthalmology Case Reports*, vol. 26, article 101459, 2022.

# Congenital Microphthalmia with Intraorbital Cyst: A Rare Case Report

**Bishow Raj Timalsina ⓘ, Gulshan Bahadur Shrestha, and Madhu Thapa**

*Department of Ophthalmology, B.P. Koirala Lions Centre for Ophthalmic Studies, Kathmandu, Nepal*

Correspondence should be addressed to Bishow Raj Timalsina; rajbishow@gmail.com

Academic Editor: Cristiano Giusti

Microphthalmia is considered to be the most common congenital malformation of the eye after congenital cataract. However, its association with intraorbital cyst is considered to be very rare. Most of the lesions are still misdiagnosed as orbital tumor and teratomas as there is a general paucity of data reported in literature. Herein, we report a rare case of congenital microphthalmia with intraorbital cyst in an eight-month-old male patient.

## 1. Introduction

Congenital microphthalmia with intraorbital cyst is a rare condition occurring due to defective closure of the embryonic fissure as well as over-growth of the inner layer of the optic cup [1]. The fissures begin to close at about 11 mm stage and is completed by 18 mm stage. As the inner layer of the optic cup develops faster, the margins of the fissures becomes slightly everted. Presence of a fully formed retina at the margins of the fissure prevents the closure of the optic cup leading to the formation of a typical coloboma without overlying the retina [2]. Microphthalmia is characterized by a small but recognizable eye with the eye elements such as the lens, choroid, and retina [3]. In contrast to this, anophthalmia is characterized by the complete absence of the eye due to the lack of development or arrest of differentiation of the optic vesicles in early stage of development [4]. The prevalence rate of microphthalmia is found to be 1.4–3.5 per 10,000 births [5]. Microphthalmia with orbital cyst is considered to be extremely rare with no agreed prevalence rate [1].

Cysts associated with microphthalmia and anophthalmia represent two points on the spectrum of the colobomatous eye disorder and may create difficulty in clinical distinction [5].

## 2. Case Report

An eight-month-old male was presented by the parents with the chief complaints of inability to open the right eye since birth and gradual progressive swelling underneath the right lower lid for three months.

The past medical history revealed that the patient was taken to the local eye hospital one week after birth with the chief complaints of inability to open the right eye (RE) since birth. The medical reports revealed that the right globe was not visible and the left eye (LE) was normal with no developmental anomalies at that time. The USG A+B scan showed chorioretinal coloboma with cystic (hyperechoic) space behind the chorioretinal surface and a small optic nerve stump on the RE with normal LE findings.

Three months later, cystic swelling appeared from the inferior orbit that was gradually increasing in size and was more prominent during coughing. This lead to the right lower lid ectropion and exposure of the palpebral conjunctiva associated with redness and occasional discharge. Swelling gradually increased in size with mild keratinization of the exposed surface (Figure 1). The LE showed inferior key hole iris (coloboma) with chorioretinal coloboma on indirect ophthalmoscopy. The USG A+B scan showed no identifiable RE structures while LE showed chorioretinal coloboma.

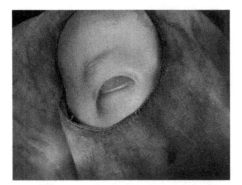

FIGURE 1: Preoperative view of right eye.

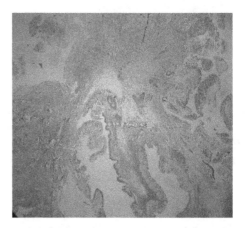

FIGURE 3: Glial tissue with cystic component 200x.

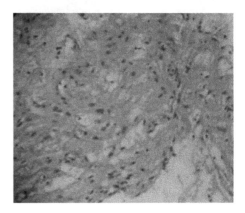

FIGURE 4: Higher power view of Glial tissue 400x.

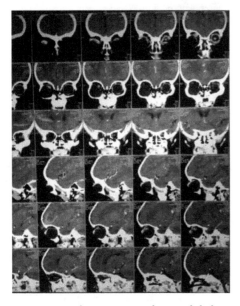

FIGURE 2: MDCT showing cyst and microphthalmic eye.

At eight months, when the child was brought to our center, multidetector computed tomography (MDCT) was advised which showed non enhancing right intraorbital cyst with small right globe and dysplastic optic nerve (Figure 2). There was no intracranial communication or extension. Findings were suggestive of colobomatous cyst. Right orbitotomy with right eye enucleation and cyst excision was performed under general anesthesia and the specimen was sent for histopathological examination. Histopathology revealed heterotopic glial tissue with cystic component in the orbit consistent with choriostomatous cyst (Figures 3 and 4). The eyeball was found to be atrophic. Based on these findings, the diagnosis of the right eye microphthalmos with intraorbital cyst and left eye complete coloboma was confirmed.

## 3. Discussion

Microphthalmia is considered to be the most common congenital malformation of the eye after congenital cataract. Its association with the intraorbital cyst is considered as a rare developmental anomaly of the globe that can affect one or both the eyes [6]. Studies have shown that unilateral cases are more common than bilateral cases. Out of 150 cases reported in literature, only one third of them were bilateral [7].

The detection of microphthalmia can be done in early neonatal period. It typically presents as a protruding mass in the inferior orbit associated with microphthalmic eye. The globe may be completely surrounded by the cyst in some cases, while others may present with very rudimentary displaced microphthalmic eye, thus creating difficulty in identifying the eye clinically as in our case [2]. In some cases, cysts associated with microphthalmia can be diagnosed clinically, whereas in others, it can be doubtful. Studies have shown that additional imaging can be valuable in these cases. Orbital ultrasound A+B scan is of great importance in identifying orbital cysts [5]. In our case too, orbital ultrasound A+B scan along with MDCT proved to be valuable in diagnosing the condition. These imaging modalities are not only useful in diagnosis, but can also be very helpful in identifying other abnormalities such as of the brain. Systemic defects such as the cleft lip, basal encephalocele, mid brain deformity, microcephalus, agenesis of corpus callosum, and saddle nose have been found to be associated with the condition mostly with bilateral cases. In such cases, preoperative imaging could be of great importance [4]. In our case, it was an isolated malformation without any systemic defects.

Although it is clearly a defined entity, sometimes it becomes difficult to differentiate it from some lesions such as congenital cystic eye, meningocele, arachnoid cyst, primary optic nerve sheath cysts, and teratomas of the orbit. Lieb et al. has mentioned the importance of imaging techniques in ruling out these differentials [2].

Histopathologically, cyst in a microphthalmic eye is similar to the congenital cystic eye. Nevertheless in congenital cystic globes, the cyst is located centrally or slightly upward in the orbit and histologically it lacks normal ocular structures and shows the presence of the cyst lined with neuroglial tissue. However, in microphthalmos with cyst, there is bulging of the lower eyelid as the cyst is attached to the inferior portion of the globe along with evidence of ocular development in conjunction with a small cornea, iris, ciliary body, lens, vitreous cavity, retina, and choroid [6].

The treatment strategy for patients with microphthalmos and orbital cyst depends on several factors such as visual potential, age at presentation, and volume of the orbital content [5]. Clinical assessment of the orbital volume can be done by Duke-Elder classification [8]. Patients with poor orbital volume, if treated early with implant and conformers can show good cosmetic results. Studies have shown that enucleation during childhood compromises the orbital growth especially when no orbital implant is used [9, 10]. Not only that, small cyst helps to stimulate orbital expansion much more effectively than an artificial implant [5]. However, individualized interventions are utmost to improve esthetic outcomes [11]. Chaudhry et al. have proposed the treatment protocol for congenital microphthalmos and orbital cyst. In case of mild microphthalmia, if the cyst is small, cyst aspiration, and observation is recommended, whereas if it is large affecting cosmesis, excision of the cyst should be performed. In case of severe microphthalmia, both the cyst and globe should be excised with replacement of volume [6]. In our case, as the cyst was large and rudimentary microphthalmic eye was presented, enucleation, and cyst excision was used as the treatment option. Repeated follow up should be kept in consideration to prevent recurrence and development of neoplasia [7].

## 4. Conclusion

In this case report, we tried to report a rare case of congenital microphthalmia with intraorbital cyst. Several studies are still required to understand the spectrum of this complex condition, which is considered as one of the cause for childhood blindness. Advanced ultrasound technology using three dimensional image and computed tomography can be helpful in early diagnosis of the lesion which in turn provide great help in counseling the parents and provide appropriate treatment options in early neonatal life.

## Consent

Informed consent was obtained from the parents for publication of the case.

## References

[1] Y. Cui, Y. Zhang, Q. Chang, J. Xian, Z. Hou, and D. Li, "Digital evaluation of orbital cyst associated with microphthalmos: characteristics and their relationship with orbital volume," *PLoS One*, vol. 11, no. 6, pp. 1–17, 2016.

[2] W. Lieb, R. Rochels, and U. Gronemeyer, "Microphthalmos with colobomatous orbital cyst: clinical, histological, immunohistological, and electronmicroscopic findings," *British Journal of Ophthalmology*, vol. 74, no. 1, pp. 59–62, 1990.

[3] A. K. Khurana, I. Khurana, A. K. Khurana, and B. Khurana, *Anatomy and Physiology of Eye*, CBS Publishers & Distributors Pvt Limited, Chennai, 2017.

[4] T. Stahnke, A. Erbersdobler, S. Knappe, R. F. Guthoff, and N. J. Kilangalanga, "Management of congenital clinical anophthalmos with orbital cyst: a Kinshasa case report," *Case Reports in Ophthalmological Medicine*, vol. 2018, pp. 1–6, 2018.

[5] C. J. McLean, N. K. Ragge, R. B. Jones, and J. R. O. Collin, "The management of orbital cysts associated with congenital microphthalmos and anophthalmos," *British Journal of Ophthalmology*, vol. 87, no. 7, pp. 860–863, 2003.

[6] I. A. Chaudhry, Y. O. Arat, F. A. Shamsi, and M. Boniuk, "Congenital microphthalmos with orbital cysts: distinct diagnostic features and management," *Ophthalmic Plastic & Reconstructive Surgery*, vol. 20, no. 6, pp. 452–457, 2004.

[7] D. Hamal, P. A. Kafle, P. Poudyal, R. Saiju, H. Kc, and S. Kafle, "Congenital microphthalmia with orbital cyst: a case series," *Journal of Nepal Medical Association*, vol. 57, no. 217, pp. 193–197, 2019.

[8] S. Duke-Elder, "Normal and abnormal development; congenital deformities," *System of Ophthalmology*, vol. 3, pp. 648–650, 1964.

[9] L. Apt and S. Isenberg, "Changes in orbital dimensions following enucleation," *Archives of Ophthalmology*, vol. 90, no. 5, pp. 393–395, 1973.

[10] C. Hintschich, F. Zonneveld, L. Baldeschi, C. Bunce, and L. Koornneef, "Bony orbital development after early enucleation in humans," *British Journal of Ophthalmology*, vol. 85, no. 2, pp. 205–208, 2001.

[11] Y. Cui, Y. Li, Z. Hou et al., "Management of congenital microphthalmos and anophthalmos with orbital cyst," *Journal of American Association for Pediatric Ophthalmology and Strabismus*, vol. 23, pp. 92.e1–92.e6, 2019.

# Contralateral Effect following Intravitreal Brolucizumab Injection in Diabetic Macular Edema

## Somnath Chakraborty[1] and Jay Umed Sheth[2]

[1]Retina Institute of Bengal, Siliguri, India
[2]Surya Eye Institute and Research Center, Mumbai, India

Correspondence should be addressed to Somnath Chakraborty; somnathboom@gmail.com

Academic Editor: Claudio Campa

The authors describe a novel case of a 48-year-old male with bilateral diabetic macular edema (DME) who underwent intravitreal injection (IVI) of brolucizumab in the left eye. At four weeks, the patient demonstrated a bilateral response by way of improvement in the best-corrected visual acuity (BCVA) and reduction in the central macular thickness (CMT) in both eyes. Further studies on the ocular and systemic assays of the brolucizumab molecule are warranted to evaluate its systemic escape and to better understand the pharmacokinetics behind the bilateral effect.

## 1. Introduction

Antivascular endothelial growth factor (anti-VEGF) therapy has become the treatment of choice for retinal vascular disorders such as diabetic macular edema (DME) [1, 2]. Pegaptanib sodium (Macugen®, Eyetech/OSI Pharmaceuticals, New York, NY, USA), ranibizumab (Lucentis®; Genentech, S. San Francisco, CA/Roche, Basel, Switzerland), aflibercept (Eylea®, Regeneron, Tarrytown, NY), and brolucizumab (Beovu®; Novartis, Basel, Switzerland) are four antivascular endothelial growth factor (anti-VEGF) agents that the US Food and Drug Administration (FDA) has approved for intraocular usage [3–5]. Amongst them, brolucizumab is the latest to receive approval for neovascular age-related macular disorders (nAMD). In the case of DME, two phase 3 clinical studies, KESTREL and KITE, are underway to assess the role of brolucizumab, while its off-label usage in eyes with recalcitrant DME has already been described [6, 7].

The contralateral effect of intravitreal injections, including ranibizumab, bevacizumab, aflibercept, triamcinolone acetonide, and dexamethasone implant, has been described [8–12]. In our case report, we demonstrate the bilateral response following unilateral intravitreal injection (IVI) of brolucizumab in a patient with DME, which remains unreported in the literature.

## 2. Case Report

A 48-year-old male patient with non-insulin-dependent diabetes mellitus (NIDDM) for 10 years presented with diminution of vision in both eyes (OU) for three months. His best-corrected visual acuity (BCVA) was 20/60 in the right eye (OD) and 20/120 in the left eye (OS). OU anterior segment was normal. Based on fundus examination, he was diagnosed with OU severe nonproliferative diabetic retinopathy (NPDR) with clinically significant macular edema (CSME) involving the OS more than the OD (Figures 1(a) and 1(b)). The presence of CSME was confirmed on the spectral-domain optical coherence tomography (SD-OCT) with a central subfield thickness (CST) of $321\,\mu m$ in OD and $637\,\mu m$ in OS (Figures 2(a) and 2(b)).

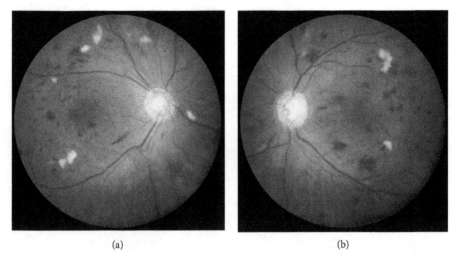

(a)                                                              (b)

FIGURE 1: Fundus photographs of both the eyes demonstrating severe nonproliferative diabetic retinopathy (NPDR) with clinically significant macular edema (CSME) (a, b).

At baseline, his HbA1c levels were 6.8% with normal renal parameters (blood urea: 20 mg/dL, serum creatinine: 0.9 mg/dL). For economic constraints, the patient underwent IVI brolucizumab only in the OD, while OS was observed. At one month, the patient had bilateral improvement in the visual acuity (OU: 20/40) with a reduction in the CSME, although only the OS was injected. On SD-OCT, the CST reduced to 272 $\mu$m in the OD and 248 $\mu$m in the OS, i.e., a quantitative decrease of 15.26% and 61.07% in the OD and the OS, respectively (Figures 2(c) and 2(d)). There were no ocular or systemic adverse events after the brolucizumab therapy.

## 3. Discussion

Diabetic macular edema is a leading cause of vision impairment on a global scale [13]. The extensive use of intravitreal anti-VEGF therapy has transformed DME care. Newer molecules such as aflibercept and brolucizumab have a longer half-life and durability, thus having the capability of reducing the overall treatment burden [7]. Prospective phase 3 studies (KITE and KESTREL) are being conducted to investigate IVI brolucizumab's role in the management of DME, based on the encouraging results of phase 3 trials testing it in the treatment of nAMD [6, 7]. Brolucizumab was found to be noninferior to aflibercept in terms of mean change in visual acuity at one year in the interim results of the KITE and KESTREL studies, which were reported at the end of 2020 [7]. Chakraborty et al. have demonstrated excellent anatomical and visual improvement with brolucizumab in eyes with recalcitrant DME [7]. Based on these encouraging results, our patient was offered treatment with IVI brolucizumab.

To the best of our knowledge, no reports of intravitreal brolucizumab affecting the contralateral eye have been published. Furthermore, the exact mechanism by which it may occur has yet to be determined. Other anti-VEGF medications

have occasionally been shown to produce similar contralateral effects [8–12]. The most universally recognized hypothesis is the systemic escape of the molecule which can then lead to a contralateral effect [9]. Microvascular permeability and molecule size have been shown to be inversely related in studies [14]. For this reason, the brolucizumab molecule, which has the lowest weight amongst all anti-VEGF agents (brolucizumab (26 kDa) versus bevacizumab (149 kDa) versus ranibizumab (48 kDa) versus aflibercept (110 kDa)), can easily enter the systemic circulation and have a contralateral effect. Additionally, diabetic retinopathy is associated with altered inner blood-retinal barrier and increased vascular permeability [2]. These dysfunctional retinal vascular changes may also influence the systemic absorption of intravitreally administered medications.

One drawback of our case is that we did not get drug quantification assays from the aqueous, vitreous, and serum samples. Moreover, improvements in SD-OCT parameters and BCVA in the contralateral eye may be due to the disease's natural progression. However, in our case, the patient's systemic parameters, including the glycemic status and the renal profile, were well controlled at baseline. As a result, a reduction in the quantum of macular edema in the contralateral eye of up to 16% is extremely unlikely due to systemic parameter management. Thus, this contralateral effect in all probability is secondary to a systemic crossover of the brolucizumab molecule. While this systemic crossover proved beneficial in our situation, it is crucial to remember that it can also be associated with harmful systemic side effects. This demands extensive investigation into the pharmacokinetics of the brolucizumab molecule, which guards against unanticipated ocular and systemic adverse effects.

In conclusion, our case report highlights the bilateral response after IVI brolucizumab therapy in a single eye most probably due to the systemic escape phenomenon. More research on the ocular and systemic assays of the

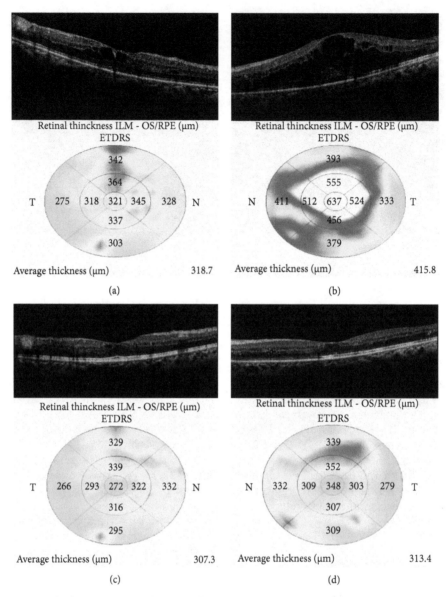

FIGURE 2: Spectral-domain optical coherence tomography scans of both the eyes (OU) showing the presence of cystoid macular edema (CME) at baseline (a, b). One month after intravitreal brolucizumab therapy, the patient demonstrated a bilateral reduction in the CME (c, d).

brolucizumab molecule is needed to assess its systemic escape and better understand the pharmacokinetics of the bilateral action.

## References

[1] D. Yorston, "Anti-VEGF drugs in the prevention of blindness," *Community Eye Health*, vol. 27, no. 87, pp. 44–46, 2014.

[2] N. Gupta, S. Mansoor, A. Sharma, A. Sapkal, J. Sheth, and P. Falatoonzadeh, "Diabetic retinopathy and VEGF," *The Open Ophthalmology Journal*, vol. 7, pp. 4–10, 2013.

[3] E. Li, S. Donati, K. B. Lindsley, M. G. Krzystolik, and G. Virgili, "Treatment regimens for administration of anti-vascular endothelial growth factor agents for neovascular age-related macular degeneration," *Cochrane Database of Systematic Reviews*, vol. 5, no. 5, 2016.

[4] C. Campa, G. Alivernini, E. Bolletta, M. B. Parodi, and P. Perri, "Anti-VEGF therapy for retinal vein occlusions," *Current Drug Targets*, vol. 17, no. 3, pp. 328–336, 2016.

[5] S. E. Mansour, D. J. Browning, K. Wong, H. W. Flynn Jr., and A. R. Bhavsar, "The evolving treatment of diabetic retinopathy," *Clinical Ophthalmology*, vol. Volume 14, pp. 653–678, 2020.

[6] J. G. Garweg, "A randomized, double-masked, multicenter, phase III study assessing the efficacy and safety of brolucizumab versus aflibercept in patients with visual impairment due to diabetic macular edema (KITE)," *Klinische Monatsblätter für Augenheilkunde*, vol. 237, no. 4, pp. 450–453, 2020.

[7] D. Chakraborty, J. U. Sheth, S. Boral, and T. K. Sinha, "Off-label intravitreal brolucizumab for recalcitrant diabetic macular edema: a real-world case series," *American Journal of Ophthalmology Case Reports*, vol. 24, 2021.

[8] H. Al-Dhibi and A. O. Khan, "Bilateral response following unilateral intravitreal bevacizumab injection in a child with uveitic cystoid macular edema," *Journal of AAPOS*, vol. 13, pp. 400–402, 2009.

[9]   Z. Wu and S. R. Sadda, "Effects on the contralateral eye after intravitreal bevacizumab and ranibizumab injections: a case report," *Annals of the Academy of Medicine, Singapore* vol. 37, p. 591, 2008.

[10]  M. Shimura, T. Nakazawa, K. Yasuda et al., "Comparative Therapy Evaluation of Intravitreal Bevacizumab and Triamcinolone Acetonide on Persistent Diffuse Diabetic Macular Edema," *American Journal of Ophthalmology*, vol. 145, no. 5, pp. 854–861.e3, 2008.

[11]  A. Sharma, J. Sheth, R. J. Madhusudan, and S. K. Sundaramoorthy, "Effect of intravitreal dexamethasone implant on the contralateral eye: a case report," *Retinal Cases and Brief Reports*, vol. 7, no. 3, pp. 217–219, 2013.

[12]  R. Campos Polo and S. C. Rubio, "Anti-VEGF and its impact on the outer retina: retinal pigment epithelium tear after an injection of aflibercept in contralateral eye," *Archivos de la Sociedad Española de Oftalmología*, vol. 91, no. 5, pp. 245–249, 2016.

[13]  E. Prokofyeva and E. Zrenner, "Epidemiology of major eye diseases leading to blindness in Europe: a literature review," *Ophthalmic Research*, vol. 47, no. 4, pp. 171–188, 2012.

[14]  R. L. Avery, A. A. Castellarin, N. C. Steinle et al., "Systemic pharmacokinetics following intravitreal injections of ranibizumab, bevacizumab or aflibercept in patients with neovascular AMD," *The British Journal of Ophthalmology*, vol. 98, no. 12, pp. 1636–1641, 2014.

# Managing a Case of a Congenital Cystic Eyeball: Case Report with Review of Literature

Aashish Raj Pant◐,[1] Rinkal Suwal◐,[2] Purushottam Joshi◐,[3] and Santosh Chaudhary◐[4]

[1]Department of Oculofacial Plastic Surgery, Mechi Eye Hospital, Jhapa, Nepal
[2]Department of Optometry, B.P. Eye Foundation, Hospital for Children, Eye, ENT and Rehabilitation Services (CHEERS), Bhaktapur, Nepal
[3]Department of Vitreo-Retina, Mechi Eye Hospital, Jhapa, Nepal
[4]Department of Ophthalmology, B.P. Koirala Institute of Health Sciences, Dharan, Nepal

Correspondence should be addressed to Aashish Raj Pant; aashish.raj.pant@gmail.com

Academic Editor: Kamal Kishore

A congenital cystic eyeball is an extremely rare condition, with only 52 cases reported in the literature to date. An orbital cyst replaces the eyeball which occurs due to the complete or partial failure in invagination of the primary optic vesicle during the fourth week of gestation. We discuss a case of a congenital cystic eyeball in a 14-year-old female who presented to us for a cosmetic blemish due to a large swelling in the right eyelid with the absence of a right eyeball since birth. She underwent removal of the cyst followed by an orbital implant and later prosthesis. Diagnosis of the congenital cystic eyeball was made based on the clinical and ultrasound B-scan features, intraoperative findings, and histopathology report. This article adds one more case to the existing literature on the congenital cystic eyeball. Orbital implant with prosthesis after excision of the cyst provided definitive diagnosis and a good cosmetic outcome in our case.

## 1. Introduction

The congenital cystic eyeball (CCE) was first reported by Taylor and Collins in 1906 [1] and later explained in detail by Mann in 1939 [2]. Mann also coined the term "anophthalmos with cyst" for the congenital cystic eyeball [3]. A complete or partial failure in invagination of primary optic vesicle leads to the development of congenital cystic eyeball [4, 5]. Noninvagination of the optic vesicle takes place in the middle of 2 mm and 7 mm phases of the embryonic development which usually occurs during the fourth week of gestation. The cyst which replaces the eye is formed due to the failure of the anterior primary optic vesicle to involute. It should be differentiated from microphthalmos with cyst which occurs due to the failure of fetal fissure closure at 7-14 mm phase, presents as a cyst in the anterior and inferior part of the orbital cavity, and is associated with a microphthalmic colobomatous eye. Cases of CCE are remarkably rare. To date, only 52 cases of congenital cystic

eyeball have been reported in the literature [5–12]. We discuss a case of a congenital cystic eyeball in a 14-year female and also describe the clinical features, diagnostic tools, differentials, and the management approach for such cases through an extensive literature review.

## 2. Case Presentation

A 14-year female presented with a complaint of cosmetic disfigurement caused by a large swelling in the right eye (RE) since birth which was gradually increasing with her age. The patient was aware of no vision from that eye. There was no history of perinatal complications or consanguineous marriage. On examination, the vision in RE was no perception of light (NPL) whereas the vision in the left eye (LE) was 1/60 on the Snellen distant visual acuity chart. RE examination revealed a large cystic swelling predominantly in the lower eyelid but no visible eyeball in the palpebral aperture (Figure 1). The swelling was single, soft, smooth, bluish-

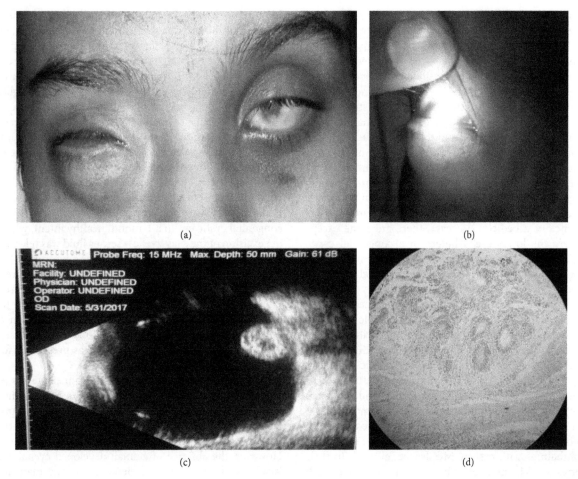

(a)

(b)

(c)

(d)

FIGURE 1: (a) RE congenital cystic eyeball in a 14-year female: LE microcornea with inferior scar. (b) Cyst shows a positive transillumination test. (c) B-scan USG of the RE showing a stump of optic nerve-like structure in the posterior aspect of a large cyst. (d) Histopathology of the excised cyst showing cyst lined by neuroglial tissue. No specific remnants of the eye could be identified.

tinged, nontender, nonpulsatile, and brilliantly transilluminating (Figure 1(b)). The bony orbital rim was normal. Examination of the LE suggested a microcornea, inferior corneal scar, iris coloboma, and chorioretinal coloboma involving the optic disc and macula (Figure 1). The patient underwent B-scan ultrasonography (USG) which demonstrated a large cyst in the right bony orbit with no evidence of a well-formed eyeball. Typically, a stump of the optic nerve-like structure was seen in the posterior aspect of the cyst (Figure 1(c)). A provisional diagnosis of CCE was made based on the clinical and radiological findings. Pediatrician consultation was done, and neuroimaging was performed to rule out systemic associations especially intracranial abnormalities, which was normal. The patient and her parents were counseled regarding the nil visual prognosis and were advised for surgery. The patient had the cyst removed and an orbital ball implant and a conformer placed, and inferior fornix was reconstructed using sutures. The cyst was sent for histopathological examination which revealed an irregular cyst lined externally by a connective tissue layer and internally by glial tissues (Figure 1(d)) without a histologically identifiable eyeball, which confirmed the diagnosis of the congenital cystic eyeball. She was prescribed an ocular prosthesis after 6 weeks of surgery.

## 3. Discussion

A congenital cystic eyeball occurs because of a developmental anomaly occurring during the third week of embryogenesis. An arrest in the invagination of the primary optic vesicles during the 2 mm-7 mm stage is attributed to this rare congenital anomaly [5]. Though the etiology of CCE is unknown, some authors have related it to an inflammatory cause due to the presence of inflammatory cells in the histopathological picture of the cystic eyeball [5].

Cases are usually unilateral, although few bilateral cases have been described in the literature. A case of bilateral congenital cystic eyeball was reported by Sacks and Linderberg. In two cases reported by Hayashi et al., one had bilateral involvement although the nature of the lesion was not established [13]. The patients usually present with a swelling in the eyelid of the involved eye since birth. However, the cyst may not be evident at birth in some cases. Such patients present with an absence of the eyeball and later with a cystic swelling when the cyst progressively enlarges due to the continuous production of fluid into the cyst probably from the neuroglial tissues. This fluid can be dark viscous, serosanguineous, or proteinaceous [13, 14], but the fluids usually have similar biochemical properties as the serum [15].

Diagnostic workup for a case of CCE starts from the examination of the eyes and orbits and extends to the whole body to rule out systemic associations which may be life-threatening. In infants, the cyst can be examined properly using eyelid retractors, such as Desmarre's, to look for the presence of a microphthalmic eye which is the most important differential diagnosis. Where congenital cystic eyeballs have the complete absence of a globe, microphthalmos with cyst usually has a small eyeball and the cyst is attached to the sclera or choroid [11, 16]. Incomplete closure of the fetal cleft leads to microphthalmos with cyst which often has coloboma of uveal tissue, lens, and retina. Cysts are generally placed in the inferior orbit. Inversely, a congenital cystic eyeball typically causes the upper eyelid to bulge, and there is the presence of a pedicle. However, there are some exceptions where the lower eyelid bulges in a congenital cystic eyeball [13, 17]. In our case, the cyst was located in the inferior part of the orbital cavity presenting as a swelling in the lower eyelid.

The fellow eye in our case had microcornea with an inferior corneal scar and, iris, and fundal coloboma. As anophthalmos and microphthalmos (with or without cyst) and uveal coloboma—all are congenital abnormalities occurring due to the failure of invagination of optic vesicle at various stages of development of ocular structures, these are often found in association. Tucker et al. found abnormal second eye in 21% cases of unilateral anophthalmos without a cyst [18]. Although the data with anophthalmos with cyst is limited, we can take reference from the largest case series of anophthalmos with cyst by McClean et al. [19]. In their case series of 34 cases of orbital cysts associated with anophthalmos or microphthalmos, they have described 14 cases of anophthalmos with cyst wherein 5 cases were unilateral with fellow eye normal, 3 cases had microphthalmos in fellow eye with or without uveal coloboma, 3 cases had anophthalmos without a cyst in fellow eye, and the remaining 3 had bilateral anophthalmos with cyst. There were 2 cases described in the case series where the fellow eye had both microphthalmos and uveal coloboma similar to our case. Similarly, Hayashi et al. [13] reported a case of congenital cystic eyeball with microphthalmos in the fellow eye. Hence, our case report is rarer in view of involvement of fellow eye with microphthalmos and uveal coloboma.

Radiological investigations such as B-scan ultrasonography (USG), computed tomography (CT) scan, or magnetic resonance imaging (MRI) form the logical next step in the diagnosis of CCE. B-scan USG is usually readily available at the ophthalmology outpatient department and gives valuable information about the cyst, absence or presence of an eyeball, and an associated optic nerve-like stump. Cysts may be replaced partially or even completely by neuroglial tissues [20]. Baghdassarian et al. found a 2 mm round structure posteriorly, resembling an optic nerve at the posterior aspect of a cyst [21]. We also found a small round stump of an optic nerve-like structure at the posterior part of the cyst in our case on B-scan USG. Studies have revealed the presence of patent optic stalk [22]; however, there have been reports of nonpatent [23] or even absence of a posterior stalk

[13]. Reports with CT scan or MRI frequently reveals a cystic mass in the orbital cavity which might be unilateral [24] or bilateral [20, 25]. Microphthalmos and any optic nerve stalks will also be evident on CT or MRI. Usually, extraocular muscles are absent and cystic mass probably has a soft tissue component depending upon the amount of glial proliferation [4, 25].

The mainstay of management of the congenital cystic eyeball is excision of the cyst followed by an orbital implant. Morselli et al. reported a case of the congenital cystic eyeball where they followed up the case serially from 20 weeks of gestation till birth [26]. The case was managed by a multidisciplinary team of ophthalmologists, plastic surgeons, pediatricians, and neurosurgeons. Guthoff et al. reported a congenital cystic eye in a 1-month healthy infant, where during excision of the mass, yellow serous fluid was released [27]. A spherical silicone orbital implant was inserted. The optic nerve was not identified in this study. Holland et al. removed the cyst in a case of the congenital cystic eyeball and replaced it with a bioceramic implant [12]. Our case, an early teenage girl, underwent excision of the orbital cyst with an orbital implant and conformer by an oculofacial plastic surgeon. After 6 weeks, an ocular prosthesis was prescribed for cosmetic rehabilitation.

An irregularly shaped cyst with a connective tissue layer externally and an inner neuroglial tissue layer is the common histopathological picture in CCE. There is no presence of epithelial linings of cysts in the CCE and microphthalmos with cyst, and thus, they are similar in histopathology [28]. However, the absence of a small developed eyeball and the lack of surface ectodermal elements are the main features for differentiating CCE from microphthalmos with a cyst. Our case had features suggestive of CCE without an identifiable eyeball on histopathology.

Although CCE usually does not have associated nonocular abnormalities, some bilateral congenital cystic eyes [17, 29] and unilateral congenital cystic eye [28] with nonocular anomalies have also been reported. Some of these may have intracranial abnormalities such as agenesis of the corpus callosum, midbrain deformity, and basal encephalocele [4, 13]. Furthermore, grey matter heterotopias with corpus callosum agenesis have also been illustrated in MRI [7]. Studies have described the presence of intracranial abnormalities in CCE which required ventriculoperitoneal shunting [4, 11, 25, 29, 30]. Hence, cases of microphthalmia and anophthalmia with or without a cyst need radiological investigation especially neuroimaging to rule out systemic associations such as intracranial abnormalities. Ragge et al. in their review of management of anophthalmia and microphthalmia have described the frequent association with ocular abnormalities and infrequently with nonocular abnormalities such as CHARGE syndrome [31]. Similarly, Das et al. have recently reported a case of congenital cystic eyeball with associated intracranial abnormalities in a 15-day-old girl [32]. A full list of cases reported till date is shown in Table 1 which demonstrates the frequency and the type of the ocular and systemic associations. Our case was reviewed by a pediatrician before the surgery which revealed no neurological abnormality. Studies to date have

TABLE 1: A table of all 52 cases reported till date with ocular and systemic associations.

| S no | Author | Title | Year of publication | No. of cases | Age of onset | Affected eye | Findings | | Systemic association |
|---|---|---|---|---|---|---|---|---|---|
| | | | | | | | RE | LE | |
| 1 | Rice et al. [33] | Case of congenital cystic Eye and accessory limb of the lower eyelid | 1966 | One | Eight months | LE | Normal | Cystic swelling which distended the upper lid, while projecting from the left lower lid was a rudimentary accessory limb | Multiple dermal appendages on the face inferotemporal to the left orbit, anterior to the tragus of the ear and an appendage present on the upper part of the neck |
| 2 | Dollfus et al. [28] | Congenital cystic eyeball | 1968 | One | At birth | LE | Normal | A plum sized mass in the left orbit distending the upper lid and projecting between the eyelids). | Malformation of the left nostril and small cutaneous tumors of the left upper lid. |
| 3 | Sacks and Lindenberg [29] | Efferent nerve fibers in the anterior visual pathways In bilateral congenital cystic eyeballs | 1969 | One | 6 years | BE | Somewhat firm, spherical mass measuring approximately 10 mm in diameter | Somewhat firm, spherical mass measuring approximately 10 mm in diameter | Severely retarded and had other congenital anomalies consisting of saddle nose, harelip, cleft palate, and bifid left thumb |
| 4 | Helveston et al. [23] | Congenital cystic eye | 1970 | One | One day old | LE | Normal | Mass protruding between the left eye lids | — |
| 5 | Baghdassarian et al. [21] | Congenital cystic eye | 1973 | One | Ten days old | LE | Normal | Cystic mass in the left orbit, bulging forward, stretching the upper eyelid, and displacing the lower eyelid downward | — |
| 6 | Waring et al. [30] | Clinicopathologic correlation of microphthalmos with cyst | 1976 | One | New born | RE | RE cystic eyeball | Normal | Mild microcephaly, severe bilateral cleft lip and palate with absent philtrum; microphallus with left hydrocele; decreased neurologic tone; and hyperconvex fingernails on short stubby fingers |
| 7 | Pillai and Sambasivan [25] | Congenital cystic eye-a case report with CT scan | 1987 | One | Two months | RE | Cystic eye | Normal | — |
| 8 | Gupta et al. [34] | Congenital cystic eyeball | 1990 | One | One day old | LE | Normal | Large cystic mass bulging forwards stretching the upper lid | Microcephaly |

TABLE 1: Continued.

| S no | Author | Title | Year of publication | No. of cases | Age of onset | Affected eye | RE | Findings LE | Systemic association |
|---|---|---|---|---|---|---|---|---|---|
| 9 | Pasquale et al. [4] | Congenital cystic eye with multiple ocular and intracranial anomalies | 1991 | One | New born | LE | Persistent hyperplastic primary vitreous | Left orbital mass protruding through the palpebral fissure | Cerebrocutaneous abnormalities consisting of agenesis of the corpus callosum, midbrain deformity, malformed sphenoid bone, right upper eyelid coloboma, and a left periocular hamartoma |
| 10 | Goldberg et al. [17] | Bilateral congenital ocular cysts* | 1991 | One | One month old | BE | Cystic eye | Cystic eye | Mild facial clefting (median cleft lip and cleft palate) and basal cephalocele |
| 11 | Mansour and Li [15] | Congenital cystic eye | 1996 | One | One day old | RE | Congenital cystic eye | Normal | Holoprosencephaly and tetralogy of Fallot |
| 12 | Albernaz et al. [16] | Imaging findings in patients with clinical anophthalmos | 1997 | One | — | — | Congenital cystic eye | Anophthalmos | 1 case out of reported 8 cases had congenital cystic eyeball. Systemic association noted in bilateral anophthalmos cases |
| 12 | Hayashi et al. [13] | Congenital cystic eye: report of two cases and review of the literature | 1999 | Two | Case 1: 13 months Case 2: 2 weeks | Case 1: LE Case 2: LE | Microphthalmos Normal | Cystic eye Cystic eye | — |
| 13 | Gupta et al. [20] | Congenital cystic eye with multiple dermal appendages: a case report | 2003 | One | One day old | LE | Normal | Large orbital mass in the left orbit that bulged forwards and stretched the eyelids | — |
| 14 | McClean et al. [19] | The management of orbital cysts associated with congenital microphthalmos and anophthalmos | 2003 | Fourteen | — | RE: 5 LE: 6 BE: 3 | 24-month female, left eye cyst right eye microphthalmos, systemically associated with oculo-cerebro-cutaneous syndrome 30-month female, patient had unilateral right eye cyst, no systemic associations 12-month male with both eye cyst and no systemic associations 11-month male with left eye cyst with no systemic association 50-month female with left eye cyst, right microphthalmos with colobomatous iris and retina and developmental delay 3-month female with left eye cyst with no systemic associations 1-month female right eye cyst with cleft lip and palate, atrial septal defect, and choanal atresia 6-month male left eye with no systemic associations 2-month female with right eye cyst and left eye retinal coloboma and no systemic associations 204-month male left eye cyst and right congenital nystagmus 2-month female both eyes cyst with congenital hip dislocation 2 months male both eye cyst with no systemic association 1-month male right eye with fistula-in-ano 2-month male right eye with no systemic association | | |

TABLE 1: Continued.

| S no | Author | Title | Year of publication | No. of cases | Age of onset | Affected eye | Findings RE | Findings LE | Systemic association |
|---|---|---|---|---|---|---|---|---|---|
| 15 | Robb and Anthony [14] | Congenital cystic eye: recurrence after initial surgical removal | 2003 | One | Six weeks | RE | Large right orbital cyst, which pushed the upper eyelid forward and filled the interpalpebral space | Normal | — |
| 16 | Guthof et al. [27] | Congenital cystic eye | 2004 | One | 4 years | RE | Presented with complete ptotic right upper lid without levator function and displacement of the prosthesis due to the enlarged cystic mass | Normal | — |
| 17 | Chaudhry et al. [11] | Congenital cystic eye with intracranial anomalies: a clinicopathologic study | 2007 | Two | Case 1: 15 days Case 2: six months | Case 1: RE Case 2: LE | Case 1: RE cyst Case 2: high myopia in RE | LE anophthalmic socket without cyst LE cyst | Both cases had intracranial abnormalities requiring ventroperitoneal shunt and one case had hemifacial ipsilateral hypotony |
| 18 | Gupta et al. [7] | Congenital cystic eye: Features on MRI | 2007 | One | 5 years | LE | Normal | Presented with a left orbital mass | — |
| 19 | Quintyn-Ranty et al. [35] | Congenital cystic eye | 2007 | One | Neonatal | LE | Normal | Tomodensitometry revealed a solid, cystic orbital mass, with no calcification or bone lysis | — |
| 20 | Kavanagh et al. [8] | Detection of a congenital cystic eyeball by prenatal ultrasound in a newborn with Turner's syndrome | 2007 | One | At birth | RE | Presented with RE anophthalmos with cyst | Normal | Turner syndrome |
| 21 | Subramaniam et al. [36] | Prepucial skin graft for forniceal and socket reconstruction in complete cryptophthalmos with congenital cystic eye | 2008 | One | 23 days old | RE | Complete cryptophthalmos and congenital cystic eye | Normal | — |
| 22 | Gangadhar et al. [6] | Congenital cystic eye with meningocele | 2009 | One | 2 years s | RE | RE cyst | Normal | Meningocoele |

TABLE 1: Continued.

| S no | Author | Title | Year of publication | No. of cases | Age of onset | Affected eye | RE | Findings LE | Systemic association |
|------|--------|-------|---------------------|--------------|--------------|--------------|-----|-------------|----------------------|
| 23 | Mehta et al. [37] | Congenital cystic eye: a clinicopathologic study | 2010 | One | 13 years | LE | Normal | A mass bulging through the ptotic left upper eyelid On opening the palpebral aperture, a white sclera like structure could be seen beneath the conjunctiva with absence of other anterior segment structures | Associated with ectopic glial tissue in the brain |
| 24 | Tsitouridis et al. [10] | Congenital cystic eye with multiple dermal appendages and intracranial congenital anomalies | 2010 | One | 3 months | LE | Normal | Mass in the left orbit and the dermal appendages on the ipsilateral side of the face | — |
| 25 | Morselli et al. [26] | Congenital cystic eye: from prenatal diagnosis to therapeutic management and surgical treatment | 2011 | One | 20-week gestation female fetus | RE | Congenital cystic eye | Coloboma and corneal dermoid | Left brachycephaly |
| 26 | Pinto et al. [38] | Congenital cystic eye with corpus callosum hypoplasia: MRI findings | 2011 | One | 3 months | LE | Normal | Cystic eye | Corpus callosum hypoplasia |
| 27 | Doganay et al. [39] | Bilateral congenital cystic eye posterior to the lower eyelid: case report | 2012 | One | One day old | BE | Cystic eye | Cystic eye | — |
| 28 | Singer et al. [9] | Congenital cystic eye in utero: novel prenatal magnetic resonance imaging findings | 2013 | One | 26-week gestation | LE | Normal | Cystic eye | Left frontal dysplasia, colpocephaly, and agenesis of the corpus callosum and septum pellucidum discovered in utero via ultrasonography |

TABLE 1: Continued.

| S no | Author | Title | Year of publication | No. of cases | Age of onset | Affected eye | Findings RE | Findings LE | Systemic association |
|---|---|---|---|---|---|---|---|---|---|
| 29 | Cefalo et al. [40] | Congenital cystic eye associated with a low-grade cerebellar lesion that spontaneously regressed | 2014 | One | 6 month old | LE | Normal | Cystic eye | Cerebellar lesion accidentally detected at magnetic resonance imaging |
| 30 | Holland et al. [12] | Congenital cystic eye with optic nerve | 2015 | One | 3 days old | RE | Cystic eye | Normal | — |
| 31 | Souhail et al. [41] | Congenital cyst eye, one clinical case | 2015 | One | 7 years | RE | Fleshy mass in the right eye, the upper lid appeared ballooned and a reddish pink mass was bulging out | Normal | — |
| 32 | Yan et al. [42] | Rare orbital cystic lesions in children | 2015 | One | 6 months | LE | Normal | Ptosis and protrusion of left upper eyelid. A large well-defined soft mass | Complete agenesis of the corpus callosum, hydrocephaly, and asymmetry of the ventricular system |
| 33 | Musa et al. [43] | Congenital cystic eye: a clinicopathological review | 2018 | One | 7 months | RE | Cystic eye | Normal | — |
| 34 | Stahnke et al. [44] | Management of congenital clinical anophthalmos with orbital cyst: a Kinshasa case report | 2018 | One | 14 months | LE | Normal | A transilluminating cyst protruding out of the left orbit | — |
| 35 | Harakuni et al. [45] | A rare case of left sided anophthalmos with congenital cystic eyeball with right sided microphthalmos | 2019 | One | 19 years | LE | Microphthalmos, with horizontal nystagmus and healed perforated corneal ulcer | Anophthalmos | — |
| 36 | Das et al. [32] | Congenital cystic eyeball with intracranial anomalies: a rare entity | 2021 | One | 15 days | LE | Normal | Cystic eye | Dysgenesis of corpus callosum with dorsal interhemispheric cyst communicating with the third ventricle |

not demonstrated any hereditary associations or chromosomal defects for the congenital cystic eyeball [4, 13, 17, 30].

Clinical assessment and radiological investigations aid in the confirmation of the diagnosis of CCE. However, a definitive diagnosis can only be made through histopathology. Removal of the cyst followed by an orbital implant, conformer, and later on ocular prosthesis seems to be the appropriate management approach for CCE.

## Consent

Written informed consent was obtained from the patient's legal guardian for the publication of this case report and any accompanying images. A copy of the written consent is available for review by the editor-in-chief of this journal.

## References

[1] S. J. Taylor and E. T. Collins, "Congenitally malformed cystic eye, causing extensive protrusion of upper eyelid, and complete extrusion of conjunctival sac through the palpebral fissure," *Ophthalmological Society of the United Kingdom*, 1906.

[2] I. Mann, "A case of congenital cystic eye," *Transactions of the Ophthalmological Society Of Australia*, vol. 1, pp. 120–124, 1939.

[3] I. Mann, "Developmental abnormalities of the eye," *CUP Archive*, vol. 1, 1957.

[4] L. R. Pasquale, N. Romayananda, J. Kubacki, M. H. Johnson, and G. H. Chan, "Congenital cystic eye with multiple ocular and intracranial anomalies," *Archives of Ophthalmology*, vol. 109, no. 7, pp. 985–987, 1991.

[5] S. Duke-Elder, "System of ophthalmology, congenital deformities, vol 35, pt 2. St Louis," *CV Mosby Co, London*, vol. 35, pp. 606–610, 1963.

[6] J. L. Gangadhar, B. Indiradevi, and V. C. Prabhakaran, "Congenital cystic eye with meningocele," *Journal of Pediatric Neurosciences*, vol. 4, no. 2, pp. 136–138, 2009.

[7] R. Gupta, A. Seith, B. Guglani, and T. Jain, "Congenital cystic eye: features on MRI," *The British Journal of Radiology*, vol. 80, no. 955, pp. e137–e140, 2007.

[8] M. C. Kavanagh, D. Tam, J. J. Diehn, A. Agadzi, E. L. Howes, and D. R. Fredrick, "Detection of a congenital cystic eyeball by prenatal ultrasound in a newborn with turner's syndrome," *British Journal of Ophthalmology*, vol. 91, no. 4, pp. 559-560, 2007.

[9] J. R. Singer, P. J. Droste, and A. S. Hassan, "Congenital cystic eye in utero," *JAMA Ophthalmology*, vol. 131, no. 8, pp. 1092-1095, 2013.

[10] I. Tsitouridis, M. Michaelides, C. Tsantiridis, S. Spyridi, M. Arvanity, and I. Efstratiou, "Congenital cystic eye with multiple dermal appendages and intracranial congenital anomalies," *Diagnostic and Interventional Radiology*, vol. 16, no. 2, pp. 116–121, 2010.

[11] I. A. Chaudhry, F. A. Shamsi, E. Elzaridi, Y. O. Arat, and F. C. Riley, "Congenital cystic eye with intracranial anomalies: a clinicopathologic study," *International ophthalmology*, vol. 27, no. 4, pp. 223–233, 2007.

[12] L. Holland, A. Haridas, G. Phillips, and T. Sullivan, "Congenital cystic eye with optic nerve," *Case Reports*, vol. 2015, article bcr2015210717, 2015.

[13] N. Hayashi, M. X. Repka, H. Ueno, N. T. Iliff, and W. R. Green, "Congenital cystic eye: report of two cases and review of the literature," *Survey of Ophthalmology*, vol. 44, no. 2, pp. 173–179, 1999.

[14] R. M. Robb and D. C. Anthony, "Congenital cystic eye: recurrence after initial surgical removal," *Ophthalmic Genetics*, vol. 24, no. 2, pp. 117–123, 2003.

[15] A. Mansour and H. K. Li, "Congenital cystic eye," *Ophthalmic Plastic and Reconstructive Surgery*, vol. 12, no. 2, pp. 104–107, 1996.

[16] V. S. Albernaz, M. Castillo, P. A. Hudgins, and S. K. Mukherji, "Imaging findings in patients with clinical anophthalmos," *American Journal of Neuroradiology*, vol. 18, no. 3, pp. 555–561, 1997.

[17] S. H. Goldberg, M. G. Farber, J. D. Bullock, K. R. Crone, and W. S. Ball, "Bilateral congenital ocular cysts," *Ophthalmic Paediatrics and Genetics*, vol. 12, no. 1, pp. 31–38, 1991.

[18] S. Tucker, B. Jones, and R. Collin, "Systemic anomalies in 77 patients with congenital anophthalmos or microphthalmos," *Eye*, vol. 10, no. 3, pp. 310–314, 1996.

[19] C. J. McLean, N. K. Ragge, R. B. Jones, and J. R. Collin, "The management of orbital cysts associated with congenital microphthalmos and anophthalmos," *British Journal of Ophthalmology*, vol. 87, no. 7, pp. 860–863, 2003.

[20] P. Gupta, K. P. S. Malik, and R. Goel, "Congenital cystic eye with multiple dermal appendages: a case report," *BMC Ophthalmology*, vol. 3, no. 1, pp. 1–5, 2003.

[21] S. A. Baghdassarian, K. F. Tabbara, and C. S. Matta, "Congenital cystic eye," *American Journal of Ophthalmology*, vol. 76, no. 2, pp. 269–275, 1973.

[22] S. Duke-Elder, "Normal and abnormal development; congenital deformities," *System of Ophthalmology*, vol. 3, pp. 648–650, 1964.

[23] E. M. Helveston, E. Malone, and M. H. Lashmet, "Congenital cystic eye," *Archives of Ophthalmology*, vol. 84, no. 5, pp. 622–624, 1970.

[24] U. K. Raina, D. Tuli, R. Arora, D. K. Mehta, and R. Bansal, "Congenital cystic eyeball," *Ophthalmic Surgery and Lasers*, vol. 33, no. 3, pp. 262-263, 2002.

[25] A. M. Pillai and M. Sambasivan, "Congenital cystic eye–a case report with CT scan," *Indian Journal of Ophthalmology*, vol. 35, no. 2, pp. 88–91, 1987.

[26] P. G. Morselli, A. Morellini, R. Sgarzani, T. Ghi, and E. Galassi, "Congenital cystic eye," *Journal of Craniofacial Surgery*, vol. 22, no. 1, pp. 360–363, 2011.

[27] R. Guthoff, R. Klein, and W. E. Lieb, "Congenital cystic eye," *Graefe's Archive for Clinical and Experimental Ophthalmology*, vol. 242, no. 3, pp. 268–271, 2004.

[28] M. Dollfus, P. Marx, J. Langlois, J. Clement, and J. Forthomme, "Congenital cystic eyeball," *American Journal of Ophthalmology*, vol. 66, no. 3, pp. 504–509, 1968.

[29] J. G. Sacks and R. Lindenberg, "Efferent nerve fibers in the anterior visual pathways in bilateral congenital cystic eyeballs," *American Journal of Ophthalmology*, vol. 68, no. 4, pp. 691–695, 1969.

[30] G. O. Waring, A. M. Roth, and M. M. Rodrigues, "Clinicopathologic correlation of microphthalmos with cyst," *American Journal of Ophthalmology*, vol. 82, no. 5, pp. 714–721, 1976.

[31] N. K. Ragge, I. D. Subak-Sharpe, and J. R. Collin, "A practical guide to the management of anophthalmia and microphthalmia," *Eye*, vol. 21, no. 10, pp. 1290–1300, 2007.

[32] D. Das, M. S. Bajaj, S. Gupta, and S. Agrawal, "Congenital cystic eyeball with intracranial anomalies: a rare entity," *Indian Journal of Ophthalmology-Case Reports*, vol. 1, no. 4, article 885, 2021.

[33] N. S. Rice, S. P. Minwalla, and J. H. Wania, "Case of congenital cystic eye and accessory limb of the lower eyelid," *The British Journal of Ophthalmology*, vol. 50, no. 7, pp. 409–413, 1966.

[34] V. P. Gupta, K. U. Chaturvedi, D. K. Sen, and K. K. Govekar, "Congenital cystic eyeball," *Indian Journal of Ophthalmology*, vol. 38, no. 4, pp. 205-206, 1990.

[35] M. L. Quintyn-Ranty, J. C. Quintyn, C. Mazerolles, S. Moalic, and M. B. Deslisle, "Congenital cystic eye," *Investigative Ophthalmology & Visual Science*, vol. 48, no. 13, article 3599, 2007.

[36] N. Subramaniam, P. Udhay, and L. Mahesh, "Prepucial skin graft for forniceal and socket reconstruction in complete cryptophthalmos with congenital cystic eye," *Ophthalmic Plastic & Reconstructive Surgery*, vol. 24, no. 3, pp. 227–229, 2008.

[37] M. Mehta, N. Pushker, S. Sen et al., "Congenital cystic eye: a clinicopathologic study," *Journal of Pediatric Ophthalmology and Strabismus*, vol. 1, article e1, 2010.

[38] P. S. Pinto, V. Ribeiro, and B. Moreira, "Congenital cystic eye with corpus callosum hypoplasia: MRI findings," *The Neuroradiology Journal*, vol. 24, no. 3, pp. 452–455, 2011.

[39] S. Doganay, A. Alkan, C. Cankaya, and P. Firat, "Bilateral congenital cystic eye posterior to the lower eyelid: case report," *Case Report. Turkiye Klinikleri Tip Bilimleri Dergisi*, vol. 32, no. 4, pp. 1118–1121, 2012.

[40] M. G. Cefalo, G. S. Colafati, A. Romanzo, A. Modugno, R. De Vito, and A. Mastronuzzi, "Congenital cystic eye associated with a low-grade cerebellar lesion that spontaneously regressed," *BMC Ophthalmology*, vol. 14, no. 1, pp. 1–6, 2014.

[41] H. Souhail, S. Ifrkhas, and A. Laktaoui, "Congenital cyst eye, one clinical case," *Journal of Surgery*, vol. 3, no. 3, pp. 18–20, 2015.

[42] J. Yan, Y. Li, Q. Chen, X. Ye, and J. Li, "Rare orbital cystic lesions in children," *Journal of Cranio-Maxillofacial Surgery*, vol. 43, no. 2, pp. 238–243, 2015.

[43] Z. Y. Musa, B. H. Askira, and A. B. Zarami, "Congenital cystic eye: a clinicopathological review," *Borno Medical Journal*, vol. 15, no. 1, pp. 103–106, 2015.

[44] T. Stahnke, A. Erbersdobler, S. Knappe, R. F. Guthoff, and N. J. Kilangalanga, "Management of congenital clinical anophthalmos with orbital cyst: a Kinshasa case report," *Case Reports in Ophthalmological Medicine*, vol. 2018, Article ID 5010915, 6 pages, 2018.

[45] U. Harakuni, K. S. Smitha, N. Chougule, M. Patil, P. Sudhakaran, and M. S. Linda, "A rare case of left sided anophthalmos with congenital cystic eyeball with right sided microphthalmos," *The Official Scientific Journal of Delhi Ophthalmological Society*, vol. 29, no. 3, pp. 86–88, 2019.

# 9

# Sustained Control of Serpiginous Choroiditis with the Fluocinolone Acetonide 0.18 mg Intravitreal Implant

**Yousuf Siddiqui,[1] Olufemi E. Adams ⓓ,[2] Michael A. Simmons,[2] Justin Yamanuha,[2] and Dara D. Koozekanani[2]**

[1]University of Minnesota Medical School, University of Minnesota, 420 Delaware St SE, Minneapolis, MN 55455, USA
[2]Department of Ophthalmology and Visual Neurosciences, University of Minnesota, 516 Delaware Street SE, Minneapolis, MN 55455, USA

Correspondence should be addressed to Olufemi E. Adams; adams977@umn.edu

Academic Editor: Kevin J. Blinder

*Purpose.* To describe an alternative treatment for a patient with serpiginous choroiditis (SC) who was not tolerant to systemic therapies. *Methods.* Case report of a patient with serpiginous choroiditis with their clinical course followed with ophthalmic examinations and multimodal imaging overtime. *Patients and Results.* A 57-year-old female with serpiginous choroiditis was treated for seven years with numerous therapies including systemic steroids, immunosuppressive agents, and repeated dexamethasone intravitreal implants. The patient was intolerant of systemic therapies and would flare if dexamethasone injections were performed less frequently than every 8 weeks, making a viable long-term treatment plan problematic. Following one injection of the fluocinolone acetonide 0.18 mg intravitreal implant, she has experienced sustained control for 20 months. *Discussion and Conclusions.* Real-world treatment of SC is complex as long-term control is necessary, and associated side effects of the therapies provided may limit sustained use. The fluocinolone acetonide implant lasts 36 months and may be an alternative long-term management option, especially in the setting of systemic medication intolerance for some patients with SC.

## 1. Introduction

Serpiginous Choroiditis (SC) is a rare inflammatory condition that usually occurs bilaterally and is a cyclically progressive disease characterized by periods of dormancy requiring continued treatment to control inflammation and prevent severe vision loss from complications such as macular scarring and choroidal neovascular membranes [1]. Management of SC usually requires ongoing systemic immunomodulatory agents [2, 3]; however, these can have serious adverse systemic effects.

YUTIQ (EyePoint Pharmaceuticals, Inc., MA, USA) is a sustained-release, 0.18 mg fluocinolone acetonide intravitreal implant that has demonstrated success in treating noninfectious uveitis [4, 5]. To our knowledge, no data exists in the literature on the efficacy of the fluocinolone acetonide intravitreal implant in managing SC. Herein, we present a case of SC that has now been controlled for 20 months following a single injection of the fluocinolone acetonide intravitreal implant in one eye.

## 2. Case Report

This is a case report of a 57-year-old female who presented to our institution with serpiginous choroiditis in both eyes (worse in the left than the right). She had originally been diagnosed 20 years prior, with prior treatment including oral prednisone and subtenon's triamcinolone acetonide injections. She presented with a visual acuity of 20/70 right eye (OD) and hand-motion left eye (OS). Dilated funduscopic examination was remarkable for chorioretinal scars in the posterior pole with an active area of fovea-threatening choroiditis in the right eye. The left eye had extensive chorioretinal scars in the posterior pole contiguous with the optic nerve head and a fibrotic subfoveal scar with subretinal fluid and blood.

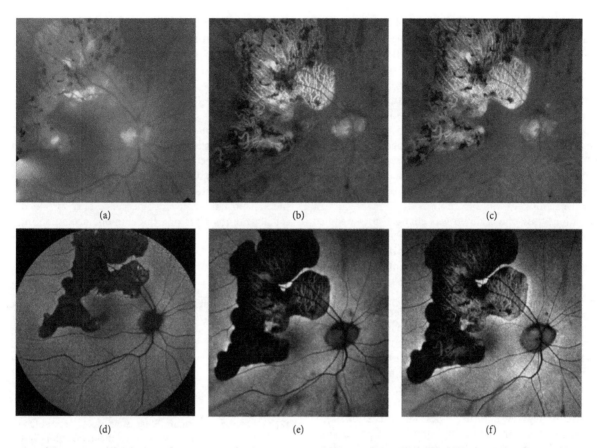

FIGURE 1: Fundus image and fundus autofluorescence of right eye on initial presentation (a, d), right eye 6 years later—prior to fluocinolone acetonide intravitreal implant—(b, e), and right eye 15 months after fluocinolone acetonide intravitreal implant (c, f).

Fundus autofluorescence (FAF) depicted hypofluorescent serpentine-like lesions, with a hyperautofluorescent edge in close proximity to the fovea OD (Figure 1). Optical coherence tomography (OCT) revealed temporal outer retinal atrophic changes without fluid OD (Figure 2). On fluorescein angiography, these lesions exhibited early hypofluorescence with late staining at the edges in both eyes. Laboratory testing for tuberculosis, syphilis, sarcoidosis, and toxoplasmosis were negative.

The SC was initially treated with a combination of oral prednisone, azathioprine, and cyclosporine. Despite treatment, the inflammation persisted, and after three months, immunosuppressive therapy was escalated to include a 3-month course of intravenous cyclophosphamide and intravitreal triamcinolone acetonide (IVTA). The patient was unable to tolerate side effects from this regimen and thus was changed to mycophenolate with oral prednisone after another 3 months. She was unable to tolerate this either, and ultimately stopped further treatment nine months after her initial presentation. She also developed a juxtafoveal choroidal neovascular membrane (CNVM) requiring intravitreal bevacizumab (IVB) twice. The SC remained in remission for two years without treatment other than a preventative IVTA and oral steroid burst given at the time of cataract surgery with intraocular lens implantation during this time period. She also required occasional IVB for the CNVM.

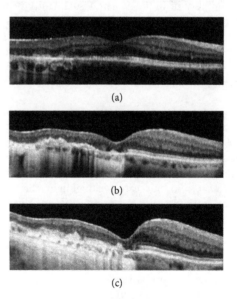

FIGURE 2: Optical coherence tomography (OCT) of the right eye on initial presentation (a), right eye 6 years later—prior to fluocinolone acetonide intravitreal implant—(b), and right eye 15 months after fluocinolone acetonide intravitreal implant (c).

After 2 years, she returned with vision complaints from a reactivation of the SC and CNVM. Her visual acuity was still 20/60 in her right eye. At this point, she resumed systemic therapy and initiated a new course of cyclophosphamide and oral prednisone. She also received IVB for her CNVM. However after 3 months, she again stopped further systemic treatment due to intolerable side effects. At that time, visual acuity was reduced to 20/200 in the right eye.

Within 4 months of stopping treatment, she had recurrent inflammation again. To avoid further systemic side effects, a local steroid treatment regimen was initiated with repeated IVTA that was then transitioned to dexamethasone 0.7 mg intravitreal implants (Ozurdex, Allergan) on a pro re nata (PRN) basis. She also received ranibizumab PRN for the CNVM. She repeatedly required dexamethasone implant injections every 2-4 months to treat recurrent inflammation; thus, the regimen was changed to scheduled dexamethasone implant injections every 8 weeks. During the following 3 years, after receiving 4 ranibizumab intravitreal injections and 14 dexamethasone implant injections, her visual acuity was 20/400 and intraocular pressure was stable with anti-ocular hypertensive drops.

In an effort to reduce the treatment burden from frequent injections, an attempt was made to reinitiate mycophenolate, but she was intolerant to therapy within 2 months. Fluocinolone acetonide intravitreal implant was then provided to the right eye. This was placed 6 weeks after the last dexamethasone implant, and since then, no further intravitreal or systemic treatments have been required. The patient has undergone regular monitoring with clinical exams and multimodal imaging, including OCT and FAF. Upon evaluation 15 months after fluocinolone acetonide implant placement, there was no recurrence of inflammation evident (Figures 1 and 2), and repeat assessment at 20 months revealed stability of findings. The visual acuity in the right eye remained stable at 20/300. Her intraocular pressure has been stable without the need for additional therapy. Through this entire course, her left eye has been stable at a visual acuity of hand motion and no additional therapies have been performed.

## 3. Discussion

The gold standard of treatment for SC is the use of immunosuppressants in combination with steroids, as this has been shown to shorten the duration of acute attacks and prevent recurrences [6]. In our case we highlight the real-world experience of the complex treatment course of a patient with SC. Over the course of seven years, our patient tried multiple systemic immunosuppressive therapies to control the SC. She was intolerant to all the systemic therapies she tried, however, and experienced several recurrences which led to disease progression and vision loss.

She was ultimately able to achieve disease stability with local treatment using scheduled dexamethasone intravitreal implants every 8 weeks. However, this created a significant treatment burden for her. With the introduction of the fluocinolone acetonide intravitreal implant, the patient experienced rapid stabilization of her vision and has remained quiescent for fifteen months without the need for additional systemic or local treatment and without any significant adverse effects. We propose that the fluocinolone acetonide

0.18 mg intravitreal implant may be considered as an alternative long-term management option for serpiginous choroiditis for some patients, especially those unable to tolerate systemic medications.

## Additional Points

*Summary Statement.* Serpiginous choroiditis is a progressive, chronic inflammatory uveitic condition which often requires systemic immunomodulatory agents. We present a case of a 57-year-old female with serpiginous choroiditis intolerant of systemic therapies during seven years of treatment, who has achieved quiescence and sustained control for 20 months after one fluocinolone acetonide intravitreal implant.

## Disclosure

All authors attest that they meet the current ICMJE criteria for authorship.

## References

[1] W. K. Lim, R. R. Buggage, and R. B. Nussenblatt, "Serpiginous choroiditis," *Survey of Ophthalmology*, vol. 50, no. 3, pp. 231–244, 2005.

[2] A. Samy, S. Lightman, F. Ismetova, L. Talat, and O. Tomkins-Netzer, "Role of autofluorescence in inflammatory/infective diseases of the retina and choroid," *Journal of Ophthalmology*, vol. 2014, Article ID 418193, 9 pages, 2014.

[3] E. K. Akpek, D. A. Jabs, H. H. Tessler, B. C. Joondeph, and C. S. Foster, "Successful treatment of serpiginous choroiditis with alkylating agents," *Ophthalmology*, vol. 109, no. 8, pp. 1506–1513, 2002.

[4] C. Pavesio and C. Heinz, "Non-infectious uveitis affecting the posterior segment treated with fluocinolone acetonide intravitreal implant: 3-year fellow eye analysis," *Eye*, vol. 36, no. 6, pp. 1231–1237, 2022.

[5] G. J. Jaffe and C. E. Pavesio, "Effect of a fluocinolone acetonide insert on recurrence rates in noninfectious intermediate, posterior, or panuveitis: three-year results," *Ophthalmology*, vol. 127, no. 10, pp. 1395–1404, 2020.

[6] R. N. Vianna, P. C. Ozdal, J. Deschênes, and M. N. Burnier Jr., "Combination of azathioprine and corticosteroids in the treatment of serpiginous choroiditis," *Canadian Journal of Ophthalmology*, vol. 41, no. 2, pp. 183–189, 2006.

# 10

# Bilateral Granulomatous Iridocyclitis Associated with Early-Onset Juvenile Psoriatic Arthritis

Christian Nieves-Ríos [1] Guillermo A. Requejo Figueroa,[2] Sofía C. Ayala Rodríguez [2] Alejandra Santiago-Díaz,[2] Eduardo J. Rodriguez-Garcia [2] Alejandro L. Perez,[2] Erick Rivera-Grana,[2] Adriana C. Figueroa-Díaz,[3] Rafael Martín-García,[3] and Armando L. Oliver [2]

[1]Ponce Health Sciences University, Department of Surgery, Ponce, PR, USA
[2]University of Puerto Rico School of Medicine, Department of Ophthalmology, Medical Sciences Campus, San Juan, PR, USA
[3]University of Puerto Rico School of Medicine, Department of Dermatology, Medical Sciences Campus, San Juan, PR, USA

Correspondence should be addressed to Armando L. Oliver; armando.oliver@upr.edu

Academic Editor: Takaaki Hayashi

*Purpose.* The purpose of this study is to report on a case of bilateral granulomatous iridocyclitis in a patient with early-onset juvenile psoriatic arthritis (JPsA). *Methods.* The method used is an observational case report. *Observations.* A 3-year-old Hispanic girl was sent to our uveitis service for further evaluation of her granulomatous uveitis. The initial ophthalmologic examination revealed bilateral band keratopathy, large mutton-fat keratic precipitates, multiple posterior synechiae, and 4+ anterior chamber cells. The physical exam was notable for left knee edema and right axillary rash. Laboratory testing was remarkable for an erythrocyte sedimentation rate of 80 mm/h, positive antinuclear antibodies (1:1, 280), and negative human leukocyte antigen B27. A cutaneous biopsy was obtained, which confirmed the diagnosis of a psoriatic rash. Treatment with oral prednisolone and topical prednisolone acetate with atropine sulfate resulted in the complete resolution of the uveitis. *Conclusion and Importance.* Bilateral granulomatous iridocyclitis may be a rare presentation of ocular involvement in patients with early-onset JPsA.

## 1. Introduction

Uveitis has been documented as one of the most common extra-articular manifestations in patients with psoriatic arthritis (PsA) [1–4]. In the pediatric population, it has been shown that juvenile PsA (JPsA) is more frequently associated with uveitis than other subgroups of juvenile idiopathic arthritis (JIA) [5], with an estimated prevalence between 7 to 21% [3, 5–8]. Moreover, the characterization of uveitis in children with PsA indicates that it has noticeable distinctions from the uveitis seen in adults with PsA [9].

JPsA can be divided into 2 clinical subgroups that are based on age at disease onset [3, 6, 9]. Patients with early-onset JPsA are more likely to be female and express antinuclear antibodies (ANAs) [6, 10], and they are at a higher risk for ocular involvement [3, 10]. Uveitis in this subgroup is currently characterized as bilateral, chronic, anterior, and/or intermediate [2, 9]. However, a detailed description of uveitis in JPsA is limited due to its rarity [2].

Most of the previously reported cases of JPsA-associated uveitis have been clinically described as nongranulomatous [2, 3, 7–9, 11–18]. However, for JIA-associated uveitis in general, recent studies have shown that granulomatous uveitis may be more common than previously thought [19, 20]. Along those lines, we present a rare case of bilateral granulomatous iridocyclitis associated with early-onset JPsA.

## 2. Case Presentation

A 3-year-old Hispanic girl with no prior history of systemic disease was sent for a consultation to our uveitis service for the further evaluation of her bilateral granulomatous uveitis. Her family history was remarkable for PsA in her father and uncle. The review of systems revealed that she had a 3-month history of a skin eruption and left knee arthralgia.

Upon a comprehensive examination, her best-corrected visual acuity (BCVA) was 20/60 in both eyes. The intraocular pressure was 13 mmHg in the right eye (OD) and 14 mmHg in the left eye (OS). A slit-lamp exam revealed bilateral band keratopathy, large mutton-fat keratic precipitates (KPs), multiple posterior synechiae (Figures 1(a)–1(d)), and 4+ anterior chamber cells. The fundus view was very poor for both eyes due to the presence of band keratopathy and limited pupillary dilation. A B-scan ultrasound was unremarkable, with no evidence of vitreous opacity.

The physical examination was remarkable for left knee edema and a right axillary nonpruritic eruption consisting of irregularly shaped erythematous papules and plaques with thin scale (Figure 2(a)). No dactylitis, enthesitis, or nail changes were identified. As the differential diagnosis of granulomatous iridocyclitis includes infectious and noninfectious etiologies, a diagnostic work-up was ordered, and the patient was started on hourly topical prednisolone acetate 1% and atropine sulfate 1%, the latter, twice a day.

The radiological images were remarkable only for left knee effusion. The girl's chest X-ray was normal, with no lymphadenopathy, opacities, or cavitations. Routine laboratory tests revealed an erythrocyte sedimentation rate of 80 mm/h and an unremarkable complete metabolic panel (CMP) (Na: 141 mEq/L, K: 3.7 mEq/L, Cl: 103 mEq/L, blood urea nitrogen: 9.00 mg/dL, and serum creatinine: 0.25 mg/dL) and urinalysis (negative for glucose, protein, red blood cells, white blood cells, and casts). Her immunology work-up was remarkable for a positive ANA test (1 : 1,280), with a homogenous pattern and negative anti-double-stranded DNA antibody, anti-Smith antibody, rheumatoid factor (<10 IU/mL), and cyclic citrullinated peptide IgG. Fluorescent treponemal antibody absorption (FTA-ABS), venereal disease research laboratory (VDRL), and tuberculosis interferon-gamma release assay (IGRA) tests were negative. Serological tests for the human leukocyte antigen B27 haplotype, HIV, hepatitis A IgM, hepatitis B core IgG, and the hepatitis C antibody were negative.

A punch biopsy of a skin lesion revealed psoriasiform acanthosis, thin supra-papillary plates, neutrophils in the stratum corneum, and superficial perivascular lymphocytic infiltrate (Figure 2(b)). Based on these results, the uveitis specialist concluded a diagnosis of bilateral granulomatous iridocyclitis associated with early-onset JPsA.

After establishing a tissue diagnosis of JPsA, oral prednisolone (1 mg/kg) was added to her therapy. Following 2 weeks of treatment, her uveitis was inactive, bilaterally. The BCVA improved to 20/40 in OD and remained stable at 20/60 in OS. At the 2-month follow-up visit, her uveitis remained inactive, and her BCVA improved to 20/30 in OD and 20/40 in OS. At this visit, a standardized prednisolone tapering protocol was begun, and she was started on subcutaneous methotrexate (0.2 mg/kg/week) as a corticosteroid-sparing therapy.

## 3. Discussion

To the best of our knowledge, as of the writing of this manuscript, this case represents the first report of early-onset JPsA associated with bilateral granulomatous iridocyclitis. In addition, our findings are in agreement with those of an increasing number of reports revealing the presence of granulomatous manifestations in JIA-related uveitis (with reported prevalences ranging from 7 to 32%) [19–21].

Uveitis in adults with PsA has been studied extensively; however, much less is known about its presentation in JPsA [3, 9]. A case series from Salek et al. was the first article to characterize uveitis in childhood PsA [9]. Although the sample size was small, Salek and his team described uveitis in children with early-onset (6 years old or younger) JPsA as being bilateral, chronic, anterior, and/or intermediate [9]. In their study, 5 of the 10 affected eyes developed band keratopathy [9], a complication typically associated with chronic intraocular inflammation [22]. In a recent study by Baquet-Walscheid et al. on JPsA, most of the participating patients presented with insidious, anterior uveitis that could be either unilateral or bilateral [3]. However, ophthalmological descriptions were available for only 18% of the patients with JPsA-related uveitis and were not stratified by the age of onset. Moreover, none of these studies specified whether the ocular findings were consistent with granulomatous or nongranulomatous uveitis.

Juvenile psoriatic arthritis exhibits a biphasic age of onset, in which distinguishing clinical differences can be identified between both age groups [3, 6, 10]. Previous studies noted that patients with early-onset JPsA were more often female and ANA positive [6], had a higher risk for uveitis, and were less frequently diagnosed with psoriasis [3, 10]. With its relatively smaller plaques and thinner scales, childhood psoriasis may present more subtly than does adult plaque psoriasis. Involvement of the scalp, face, and flexural areas is also more characteristic of childhood-onset psoriasis [17, 23].

According to a study that examined systemic manifestations of sarcoidosis in patients with ocular sarcoid uveitis, cutaneous sarcoid was the second most common systemic manifestation [24]. In that line, we considered obtaining a punch biopsy of the patient's rash to rule out conditions including sarcoidosis (which can be associated with granulomatous uveitis) [24, 25]. As the histological analysis results were consistent with psoriasis, we concluded a diagnosis of granulomatous iridocyclitis associated with JPsA. On the other hand, given the clinical presentation, the unremarkable chest X-ray (without bilateral adenopathy or opacities), and the patient's young age (3-year-old), we did not order a chest CT scan to limit the patient's radiation exposure. Moreover, previous studies have shown that sarcoid arthritis is an uncommon manifestation of systemic sarcoidosis, typically reported in 5% or less [24, 26], making it less likely to be the cause in our case.

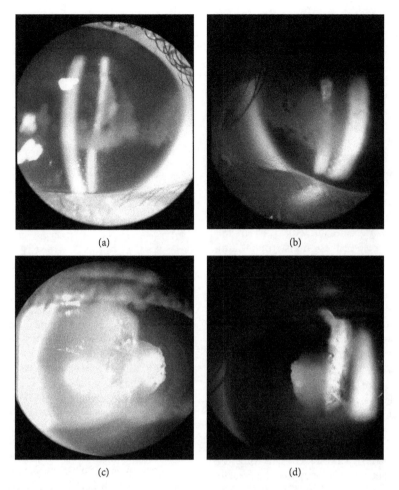

(a)

(b)

(c)

(d)

FIGURE 1: Color photographs (obtained upon presentation) showing granulomatous (mutton-fat) KPs, band keratopathies (a and b), and multiple posterior synechiae (c and d); OD and OS, respectively.

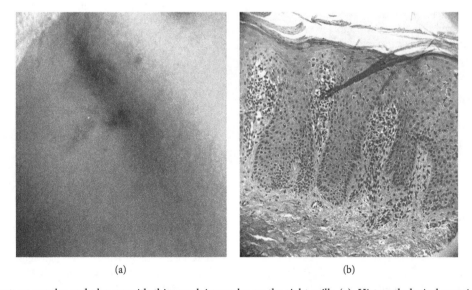

(a)

(b)

FIGURE 2: Erythematous papules and plaques with thin overlying scales on the right axilla (a). Histopathological examination (H&E stain, 200X) demonstrates psoriasiform acanthosis, thin supra-papillary plates, neutrophils in the stratum corneum, and a superficial perivascular lymphocytic infiltrate, confirming the diagnosis of psoriasis (b). H&E: hematoxylin and eosin.

On the other hand, a urinalysis and CMP were ordered to evaluate renal function and rule out tubulointerstitial nephritis and uveitis (TINU) syndrome. Patients with TINU can present at a young age with bilateral anterior uveitis [27, 28]. However, uveitis in TINU has been mainly characterized as nongranulomatous and associated with an acute presentation of eye redness, pain, and photophobia [27, 28].

Salek et al. also noted that children with early-onset JPsA can develop a severe form of uveitis that may require management with multiple immunosuppressive medications [9]. In their study, they found that all the patients required the addition of a biologic agent, even after having received treatment with methotrexate and some form of corticosteroid [9]. Similarly, Moretti et al. described a case of early-onset JPsA associated with refractory uveitis [14]. In this case, the child failed to respond to nonsteroidal anti-inflammatory drugs, methotrexate, and etanercept, ultimately requiring the use of adalimumab to achieve sustained clinical remission [14]. These findings are in concordance with those of the SYCAMORE trial on JIA-related uveitis, in which management with adalimumab plus methotrexate was associated with a lower rate of treatment failure compared to management with methotrexate alone [29]. Hence, biological therapies may serve as valuable alternatives when there is an insufficient response to conventional treatment [30]. In conclusion, bilateral granulomatous iridocyclitis may be a rare presentation of ocular involvement in patients with early-onset JPsA. However, young patients with bilateral uveitis should be evaluated for other possible systemic associations, such as sarcoidosis and TINU syndrome. As highlighted in our case, a cutaneous biopsy may help establish a tissue diagnosis for patients with uveitis, particularly those with skin manifestations [31, 32].

## Consent

Written consent to publish the case report was obtained. This report does not contain any personal information that could lead to the identification of the patient.

## Authors' Contributions

All the authors attest that they meet the current ICMJE criteria for authorship.

## References

[1] S. T. Angeles-Han, S. Ringold, T. Beukelman et al., "American College of Rheumatology/Arthritis Foundation guideline for the screening, monitoring, and treatment of juvenile idiopathic arthritis–associated uveitis," *Arthritis & Rheumatology*, vol. 71, no. 6, pp. 703–716, 2019.

[2] K. Kotaniemi, A. Savolainen, A. Karma, and K. Aho, "Recent advances in uveitis of juvenile idiopathic arthritis," *Survey of Ophthalmology*, vol. 48, no. 5, pp. 489–502, 2003.

[3] K. Baquet-Walscheid, K. Rothaus, M. Niewerth, J. Klotsche, K. Minden, and A. Heiligenhaus, "Occurrence and risk factors of uveitis in juvenile psoriatic arthritis: data from a population-based nationwide study in Germany," *The Journal of Rheumatology*, vol. 49, no. 7, pp. 719–724, 2022.

[4] A. Abbouda, I. Abicca, C. Fabiani et al., "Psoriasis and psoriatic arthritis-related uveitis: different ophthalmological manifestations and ocular inflammation features," *Seminars in Ophthalmology*, vol. 32, no. 6, pp. 715–720, 2017.

[5] A. Heiligenhaus, M. Niewerth, G. Ganser, C. Heinz, K. Minden, and German Uveitis in Childhood Study Group, "Prevalence and complications of uveitis in juvenile idiopathic arthritis in a population-based nation-wide study in Germany: suggested modification of the current screening guidelines," *Rheumatology*, vol. 46, no. 6, pp. 1015–1019, 2007.

[6] M. L. Stoll, D. Zurakowski, L. E. Nigrovic, D. P. Nichols, R. P. Sundel, and P. A. Nigrovic, "Patients with juvenile psoriatic arthritis comprise two distinct populations," *Arthritis and Rheumatism*, vol. 54, no. 11, pp. 3564–3572, 2006.

[7] D. A. Cabral, R. E. Petty, P. N. Malleson, S. Ensworth, A. Q. McCormick, and M. L. Shroeder, "Visual prognosis in children with chronic anterior uveitis and arthritis," *The Journal of Rheumatology*, vol. 21, no. 12, pp. 2370–2375, 1994.

[8] Y. A. Butbul, P. N. Tyrrell, R. Schneider et al., "Comparison of patients with juvenile psoriatic arthritis and nonpsoriatic juvenile idiopathic arthritis: how different are they?," *The Journal of Rheumatology*, vol. 36, no. 9, pp. 2033–2041, 2009.

[9] S. S. Salek, A. Pradeep, C. Guly, A. V. Ramanan, and J. T. Rosenbaum, "Uveitis and juvenile psoriatic arthritis or psoriasis," *American Journal of Ophthalmology*, vol. 185, pp. 68–74, 2018.

[10] D. Zisman, D. D. Gladman, M. L. Stoll et al., "The juvenile psoriatic arthritis cohort in the CARRA registry: clinical characteristics, classification, and outcomes," *The Journal of Rheumatology*, vol. 44, no. 3, pp. 342–351, 2017.

[11] L. Bravo Ljubetic, J. Peralta Calvo, and F. P. Larrañaga, "Complicated uveitis in late onset juvenile idiopathic psoriatic arthritis," *Archivos de la Sociedad Española de Oftalmología*, vol. 91, no. 4, pp. 195–197, 2016.

[12] J. J. Kanski and G. A. Shun-Shin, "Systemic uveitis syndromes in childhood: an analysis of 340 cases," *Ophthalmology*, vol. 91, no. 10, pp. 1247–1252, 1984.

[13] T. R. Southwood, R. E. Petty, P. N. Malleson et al., "Psoriatic arthritis in children," *Arthritis and Rheumatism*, vol. 32, no. 8, pp. 1007–1013, 1989.

[14] D. Moretti, I. Cianchi, G. Vannucci, R. Cimaz, and G. Simonini, "Psoriatic juvenile idiopathic arthritis associated with uveitis: a case report," *Case Reports in Rheumatology*, vol. 2013, Article ID 595890, 4 pages, 2013.

[15] B. M. Ansell, "Juvenile psoriatic arthritis," *Baillière's Clinical Rheumatology*, vol. 8, no. 2, pp. 317–332, 1994.

[16] Y. Butbul Aviel, P. Tyrrell, R. Schneider et al., "Juvenile psoriatic arthritis (JPsA): juvenile arthritis with psoriasis?," *Pediatric Rheumatology*, vol. 11, no. 1, p. 11, 2013.

[17] F. Brunello, F. Tirelli, L. Pegoraro et al., "New insights on juvenile psoriatic arthritis," *Frontiers in Pediatrics*, vol. 10, 2022.

[18] A. Ogdie and P. Weiss, "The epidemiology of psoriatic arthritis," *Rheumatic Disease Clinics of North America*, vol. 41, no. 4, pp. 545–568, 2015.

[19] J. D. Keenan, H. H. Tessler, and D. A. Goldstein, "Granulomatous inflammation in juvenile idiopathic arthritis-associated uveitis," *Journal of American Association for Pediatric Ophthalmology and Strabismus*, vol. 12, no. 6, pp. 546–550, 2008.

[20] I. Papasavvas and C. P. Herbort Jr., "Granulomatous features in juvenile idiopathic arthritis-associated uveitis is not a rare

occurrence," *Clinical Ophthalmology*, vol. 15, pp. 1055–1059, 2021.

[21] M. R. Dana, J. Merayo-Lloves, D. A. Schaumberg, and C. S. Foster, "Visual outcomes prognosticators in juvenile rheumatoid arthritis-associated uveitis," *Ophthalmology*, vol. 104, no. 2, pp. 236–244, 1997.

[22] V. Jhanji, C. J. Rapuano, and R. B. Vajpayee, "Corneal calcific band keratopathy," *Current Opinion in Ophthalmology*, vol. 22, no. 4, pp. 283–289, 2011.

[23] A. Morris, M. Rogers, G. Fischer, and K. Williams, "Childhood psoriasis: a clinical review of 1262 cases," *Pediatric Dermatology*, vol. 18, no. 3, pp. 188–198, 2001.

[24] R. L. Niederer, S. P. Ma, M. L. Wilsher et al., "Systemic associations of sarcoid uveitis: correlation with uveitis phenotype and ethnicity," *American Journal of Ophthalmology*, vol. 229, pp. 169–175, 2021.

[25] C. P. Herbort, N. A. Rao, M. Mochizuki, and the members of the Scientific Commi, "International criteria for the diagnosis of ocular sarcoidosis: results of the first international workshop on ocular sarcoidosis (IWOS)," *Ocular Immunology and Inflammation*, vol. 17, no. 3, pp. 160–169, 2009.

[26] D. Valeyre, A. Prasse, H. Nunes, Y. Uzunhan, P. Y. Brillet, and J. Müller-Quernheim, "Sarcoidosis," *The Lancet*, vol. 383, no. 9923, pp. 1155–1167, 2014.

[27] D. Amaro, E. Carreño, L. R. Steeples, F. Oliveira-Ramos, C. Marques-Neves, and I. Leal, "Tubulointerstitial nephritis and uveitis (TINU) syndrome: a review," *British Journal of Ophthalmology*, vol. 104, no. 6, pp. 742–747, 2020.

[28] V. Saarela, M. Nuutinen, M. Ala-Houhala, P. Arikoski, K. Rönnholm, and T. Jahnukainen, "Tubulointerstitial nephritis and uveitis syndrome in children: a prospective multicenter study," *Ophthalmology*, vol. 120, no. 7, pp. 1476–1481, 2013.

[29] A. Ramanan, A. D. Dick, A. P. Jones, A. McKay, and P. R. Williamson, "Adalimumab plus methotrexate for uveitis in juvenile idiopathic arthritis," *The New England Journal of Medicine*, vol. 376, no. 17, pp. 1637–1646, 2017.

[30] S. Pasadhika and J. T. Rosenbaum, "Update on the use of systemic biologic agents in the treatment of noninfectious uveitis," *Biologics*, vol. 8, pp. 67–81, 2014.

[31] T. Ohnishi, S. Sato, Z. Tamaki, Y. Uejima, and E. Suganuma, "Juvenile psoriatic arthritis with rash on the hands and knees: diagnostic dilemma," *Clinical Rheumatology*, vol. 40, no. 7, pp. 3021-3022, 2021.

[32] A. G. Elnahry and G. A. Elnahry, "*Granulomatous uveitis*," StatPearls Publishing, 2022.

# 11

# Necrotizing Fasciitis Following Herpes Zoster Ophthalmicus in an Immunocompromised Patient

**Grazia Maria Cozzupoli** ⓘ**, Daniele Gui, Valerio Cozza, Claudio Lodoli, Mariano Alberto Pennisi, Aldo Caporossi, and Benedetto Falsini**

*Fondazione Policlinico Universitario A. Gemelli, Università Cattolica del S. Cuore, Rome, Italy*

Correspondence should be addressed to Grazia Maria Cozzupoli; mgcozzupoli@gmail.com

Academic Editor: Nicola Rosa

Necrotizing fasciitis (NF) is a rare infection that spreads rapidly along the subcutaneous soft tissue planes. NF rarely involves the periorbital region due to the excellent blood supply of this region. We report a case of periorbital necrotising fasciitis following herpes zoster (HZ) in an immunocompromised 70-year-old patient with a dramatically rapid evolution into septic shock. In our patient, the surprisingly rapid spread of the bacterial superinfection led the periorbital cellulitis to turn into frank NF within 2 hours, with an overwhelming evolution. Despite the prompt start of a systemic antibiotic therapy and the immediate surgical intervention, the patient had a septic shock; she was treated in ITU for 31 days and then discharged to a medical ward and eventually died for a mix of complications of the medical treatment and comorbidities. This case is unique because any documented cases of periorbital NF triggered by HZ had never led to a septic shock and death. Ophthalmologists should be aware that even common skin lesions caused by shingles can determine a dramatic clinical picture, in presence of predisposing factors.

## 1. Introduction

Group A $\beta$-haemolytic streptococcus is one of the most common human pathogens. It may cause life-threatening infections with three overlapping clinical presentations: toxic shock syndrome, necrotizing fasciitis (NF), and bacteraemia with no identifiable focus [1].

NF is a rare infection that spreads rapidly along the subcutaneous soft tissue planes. Initially presenting as cellulitis, the infection becomes widespread by bacterial dissection along superficial and deep fasciae [2]. NF presents with pale red, tense, swollen skin and severe pain. Within 1 to 2 days, the skin becomes cyanotic and blue–grey, with irregular erythematous borders [1, 3]. Frank cutaneous gangrene develops within 4 to 5 days, and the skin sloughs due to underlying suppuration by 8 to 10 days [1, 3]. The overwhelming bacterial load leads to marked systemic symptoms that may include shock and organ failure [2]. Early diagnosis and prompt treatment are crucial for the successful management of NF [2].

NF usually involves the extremities, abdominal wall, and groin and rarely involves the head, neck, and periorbital region [4].

We report a case of periorbital NF following herpes zoster (HZ) in an immunosuppressed adult patient with a dramatically rapid evolution into septic shock.

## 2. Case Presentation

A 70-year-old woman affected by Waldenström's Macroglobulinemia, under immunosuppressive therapy with melphalan, was admitted to the Emergency Department of Policlinico Universitario A. Gemelli for severe infection of the facial skin in the periorbital region of left eye. The patient had a medical history of recurrent episodes of herpetic keratitis in the left eye associated with periocular vesicles and erythema due to HZ. Consequently, the patient underwent a deep anterior lamellar keratoplasty, on February 2014, and a penetrating keratoplasty, on June 2016. Since the first surgery,

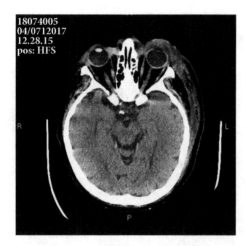

FIGURE 1: Computed tomography showing soft tissue swelling.

the patient had been under prophylactic antiviral therapy with acyclovir. Furthermore, on January 2010, the patient underwent a right dacryocystorhinostomy.

The patient presented to the emergency room having developed periocular blistering, swelling, pain in the same left dermatome of the trigeminal nerve interested in the previous HZ episodes, and also fever in the past 2 days. A diagnosis of shingles was made, and the patient was subsequently prescribed topical and intravenous acyclovir and then discharged.

After 24 hours, the patient represented with worsening of the clinical picture. There were tense periorbital oedema, pain, and erythema spreading to the surrounding areas. The patient was persistently febrile (T≥38.7°C), tachycardic (HR≥105 bpm), and hypotensive (BP≤100/60 mmHg) requiring fluid resuscitation and inotropic support.

A provisional diagnosis of HZ ophthalmicus with secondary bacterial periorbital cellulitis was made. Intravenous piperacillin-tazobactam, clindamycin, linezolid, and acyclovir were initiated.

Non-contrast-enhanced and Iopromide-enhanced cranial computed tomography was urgently performed, showing soft tissue swelling in left periorbital, frontal, temporal, and zygomatic region and at parietal level bilaterally, up to the vertex. The swelling continued caudally to the subcutaneous tissue of the left cheek, reaching the submental and neck region. No evidence of sinus involvement was found (Figure 1).

Despite the adequate fluid administration and the antibiotic and antiviral therapy, in 2 hours the status of the patient evolved into severe hemodynamic instability (HR of 125 bpm, sinus rhythm, BP< 90/40 mmHg) with visible increase in the soft tissue oedema, persistent metabolic acidosis, high blood lactate levels, malaise, and confusion.

The clinical picture of the patient was consistent with the diagnosis of septic shock secondary to periorbital necrotizing fasciitis.

The patient was immediately transferred to the intensive care unit for cardiovascular monitoring. Orotracheal intubation was performed, high-dose adrenaline infusion started,

piperacillin/tazobactam discontinued, and imipenem/cilastatin 1 g intravenously every 6 hours added.

The patient was then referred to the general surgery department and was taken for prompt debridement and fasciotomy for necrotising fasciitis. Two surgical incisions were performed at left frontotemporal and supraclavicular region proceeding with the fasciotomy of temporal and platysma muscle. At the time of the surgery, no purulent discharge was noticed at any levels. All tissue biopsies were reviewed by a consultant pathologist. The patient underwent further surgical debridement after 18 hours. Left upper eyelid showed substantial necrosis of the skin, pretarsal orbicularis muscle, orbital septa, and fat pads. The temporal muscle fascia was also involved by the necrosis and a purulent discharge from the subcutaneous soft tissue at the surgical incisions was observed. Diffuse induration and erythema persisted at left face, neck, and supraclavicular region. Drainage and debridement of the surgical sites were completed and a Negative Pressure Wound Therapy (NPWT) started (Figures 2(a) and 2(b)). The supraclavicular wound was treated with NPWT for 3 days and then substituted by conventional dressings. The frontotemporal wound was treated with NPWT for 10 days (with wound dressing change every 48-72 hrs) and then conventional dressings.

Samples taken from the infected tissues showed group A haemolytic Streptococcus pyogenes infection with histopathological features suggestive of necrotising fasciitis, in keeping with the clinical picture.

On day 7 after surgery, the oedema and erythema of left frontotemporal and supraclavicular region and neck were healed up. Throughout her admission, she received regular ophthalmology review. Ocular bulb integrity and corneal graft remained preserved at all times; an eschar formed on the upper left lid with clear reduction of the periorbital swelling. She was prescribed a tetracycline unguent.

On day 13 after surgery, the patient was diagnosed with postsepsis critical illness myopathy and neuropathy [5], confirmed by electromyography of the deltoid and biceps brachii muscles.

On day 28 after surgery, the limbs resulted in severe hypoperfusion and ischemia, thus into wet gangrene, due to the high-dose adrenaline therapy and, possibly, the underlying Waldenström's Macroglobulinemia, responsible for vasculitis and hyperviscosity syndrome. Contrast-enhanced MRI of the limbs showed a gangrene demarcation line more proximal than clinically expected. Necrosis and ischemic damage extended up to all the limbs muscles, predicting a dismal prognosis in the short term. Given the extent of gangrenous area, the only radical intervention seemed to be the hindquarter and forequarter amputation. However, the team of orthopaedic and general surgeons judged this demolitive procedure disproportioned and contraindicated it. The relatives were informed about the critical conditions of the patient. A bioethics consultant was called in to assess the case. In consideration of the irreversible evolution of the clinical picture, the consultant confirmed the unfavourable risk-benefits ratio of the aforementioned procedure.

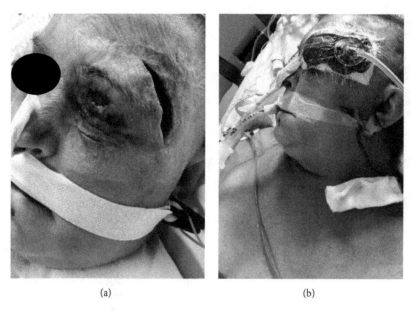

|          |          |
|:--------:|:--------:|
| (a)      | (b)      |

FIGURE 2: (a) The left frontotemporal surgical incision. (b) NPWT dressings positioned at this level.

After 31 days spent in the intensive care unit, the patient was assigned to palliative domiciliary care and died after a total of 61 days from surgery.

## 3. Discussion

A review [6] of 163 patients with NF showed that only 10% involved the head and neck. As described in an observational retrospective case series conducted in 2006 [7], the disease even more rarely involves the eyelids, with only 58 well-documented case reports. In these case reports, the risk factors [8, 9] for developing NF to the eyelids included alcoholism (26%), diabetes mellitus (10%), rheumatologic disease (7%), systemic malignancy (1%), and systemic corticosteroid use (1%). Most patients (52%), however, were healthy, without any predisposing conditions [7].

NF may involve both the eyelids because the subcutaneous tissue over the nose has little resistance to the spread of infection. Of reported cases, 45% had bilateral involvement and 55% had unilateral involvement [7].

NF has a different clinical course in the eyelids than elsewhere in the body due to the very thin eyelid skin with a rich blood supply [2, 4, 7]. The eyelids have little subcutaneous fat, so skin changes and necrosis following infection are visible at an early stage and patients present for medical assistance sooner [10]. Furthermore, the orbicularis muscle acts as a barrier for deep full-thickness spread. Thicker dermis at the eyebrows and malar folds and the dermal adherence at the inferior and lateral margins prevent further extension onto the cheek and forehead [10, 11]. The lid margins are often spared because of the rich blood supply from the marginal arterial arcade [10, 12]. It is because of these anatomic features and early recognition that periorbital NF has a lower mortality rate than truncal or limb NF [4, 10].

Four different case reports [10, 13–15] describe an uncommon association between herpes zoster infection, acting as a trigger, and the development of necrotising fasciitis. In two of the cases mentioned above, the trunk was affected: one patient was a 26-year-old woman without any predisposing conditions [13]; another one was an immunosuppressed 76-year-old woman [14]. In the remaining two cases, the periorbital region was affected: the upper left eyelid of an immunodepressed 53-year-old man [15] (case 1 in Table 1); both eyelids of an immunocompetent 63-year-old woman [10] (case 2 in Table 1).

The vesiculopapular rash arising from herpes zoster may have provided the entry portal for Streptococcal infection in all the cases listed above [10]. Of the two cases involving the periocular region, none resulted in permanent visual impairment or in the development of septic shock.

We compare this patient with two previous cases of periorbital NF following herpes zoster ophthalmic lesions just published (Table 1).

Our patient was immunosuppressed, inasmuch as she was affected by Waldenström's Macroglobulinemia under chronic therapy with melphalan. Notably, the patient had a history of recurrent episodes of HZ ophthalmicus in the same left dermatome of the trigeminal nerve. Interestingly, the incidence of recurrent HZ is increased in patients with malignancy, immunological diseases, human immunodeficiency virus (HIV) infection, diabetes mellitus, and treatment with tumor necrosis factor-$\alpha$ inhibitors [16]. Moreover, Shiraki et al. observed recurrences of HZ in the same dermatome in 16.3% of their patients, and more frequently the recurrences occurred in the left side [16]. The reason for the left-side prevalence is not clear; however, similar observations on right- versus left-side asymmetry have been reported in muscle involvements, such as poliomyelitis of the upper limb, diaphragm paralysis, and neonatal hip instability [16]. Possibly, the patient's status of immunodeficiency and immunosuppression could be involved in allowing for a recurrence of the zoster infection in the same dermatome.

TABLE 1: Comparison between three cases of periorbital NF following cutaneous herpes zoster.

| | Case 1 | Case 2 | Case 3 (present) |
|---|---|---|---|
| Age (yrs)/Gender | 53/M | 63/F | 70/F |
| Immune System | Immunodepressed | Immunocompetent | Immunosuppressed |
| History of ocular diseases | No | No | 2 previous keratoplasties for herpetic keratitis |
| General risk factors | Alcohol abuse | Discoid Lupus Erythematosus | Waldenström's Macroglobulinemia |
| Local risk factors | Periocular shingles lesions, recent eyelid trauma | Periocular shingles lesions | Periocular shingles lesions |
| Periorbital skin lesions localization | Right lower eyelid | Upper eyelids | Left upper eyelid |
| Wound Culture Results | Group A $\beta$-haemolytic streptococcus, staphylococcus aureus | Group A $\beta$-haemolytic streptococcus | Group A $\beta$-haemolytic streptococcus |
| History of Septic Shock | No | No | Yes |
| Time btw. diagnosis of periorbital cellulitis and development of NF | 8 days | 18 hours | 2 hours |
| Systemic Antibiotic Treatment | Co-amoxiclav and acyclovir | Clindamycin, ciprofloxacin and acyclovir | Imipenem/cilastatin, clindamycin, linezolid and acyclovir |
| Surgical Debridement | Debridement, reconstructive full-thickness skin grafting to the lower lid | Debridement, full-thickness skin grafting to the upper lids | Debridement, fasciotomy |
| Outcome | Survived; donor and graft sites healthy. | Survived; donor and graft sites healthy. | Died. |

Also, this condition certainly acted as a predisposing factor for the dramatic evolution of the clinical picture. In our patient, the surprisingly rapid spread of the bacterial superinfection led the periorbital cellulitis to turn into frank NF within 2 hours, with an overwhelming evolution, despite the use of NPWT. Many publications outline the use of NPWT dressings, mainly Vacuum Assisted Closure (V.A.C.®, Acelity and KCI, San Antonio, TX) in the treatment of sternal, sacral, upper and lower extremity, perineal, and abdominal wounds but fewer describe its use in the head and neck region [17]. In 2013, Reiter and Harreus [18] reported on 23 patients treated with VAC therapy in the head and neck, of which six had NF. Byrnside et al. [19] described the use of VAC for necrotizing fasciitis of the face, in which skin was grafted at day 14 to the cheek and temple wounds after sufficient wound bed preparation with the VAC device [17].

This case is unique because any documented cases of periorbital NF triggered by HZ had never resulted in such a massive systemic involvement. Ophthalmologists should be aware that even common lesions caused by shingles can determine a dramatic clinical picture, in presence of predisposing factors.

# References

[1] American Academy of Pediatrics and Committee on Infectious Diseases, "Severe invasive group A streptococcal infections: a subject review," *Pediatrics*, vol. 101, no. 1, pp. 136–140, 1998.

[2] A. L. Bisno and D. L. Stevens, "Streptococcal infections of skin and soft tissues," *The New England Journal of Medicine*, vol. 334, no. 4, pp. 240–245, 1996.

[3] L. Stone, F. Codere, and S. A. Ma, "Streptococcal lid necrosis in previously healthy children," *Canadian Journal of Ophthalmology*, vol. 26, no. 7, pp. 386–390, 1991.

[4] J. W. Kronish and W. M. McLeish, "Eyelid necrosis and periorbital necrotizing fasciitis. Report of a case and review of the literature," *Ophthalmology*, vol. 98, no. 1, pp. 92–98, 1991.

[5] C. L. Kramer, "Intensive Care Unit–Acquired Weakness," *Neurologic Clinics*, vol. 35, no. 4, pp. 723–736, 2017.

[6] B. J. Childers, L. D. Potyondy, R. Nachreiner et al., "Necrotizing fasciitis: a fourteen-year retrospective study of 163 consecutive patients," *The American Surgeon*, vol. 68, no. 2, pp. 109–116, 2002.

[7] V. M. Elner, H. Demirci, J. A. Nerad, and A. S. Hassan, "Periocular necrotizing fasciitis with visual loss: pathogenesis and treatment," *Ophthalmology*, vol. 113, no. 12, pp. 2338–2345, 2006.

[8]  S. H. Factor, O. S. Levine, B. Schwartz et al., "Invasive group a streptococcal disease: Risk factors for adults," *Emerging Infectious Diseases*, vol. 9, no. 8, pp. 970–977, 2003.

[9]  B. Pal, S. Evans, and R. F. Walters, "Necrotising fasciitis of the periorbital region," *Eye*, vol. 15, no. 5, pp. 676-677, 2001.

[10]  V. Fung, Y. Rajapakse, and P. Longhi, "Periorbital necrotising fasciitis following cutaneous herpes zoster," *Journal of Plastic, Reconstructive & Aesthetic Surgery*, vol. 65, no. 1, pp. 106–109, 2012.

[11]  J. A. Luksich, J. B. Holds, and M. E. Hartstein, "Conservative management of necrotizing fasciitis of the eyelids," *Ophthalmology*, vol. 109, no. 11, pp. 2118–2122, 2002.

[12]  D. Lazzeri, S. Lazzeri, M. Figus et al., "Periorbital necrotising fasciitis," *British Journal of Ophthalmology*, vol. 94, no. 12, pp. 1577–1585, 2010.

[13]  G. S. Sewell, V. P. Hsu, and S. R. Jones, "Zoster gangrenosum: Necrotizing fasciitis as a complication of herpes zoster," *American Journal of Medicine*, vol. 108, no. 6, pp. 520-521, 2000.

[14]  P. Jarrett, T. Ha, and F. Oliver, "Necrotizing fasciitis complicating disseminated cutaneous herpes zoster," *Clinical and Experimental Dermatology*, vol. 23, no. 2, pp. 87-88, 1998.

[15]  K. S. Balaggan and S. I. Goolamali, "Periorbital necrotising fasciitis after minor trauma," *Graefe's Archive for Clinical and Experimental Ophthalmology*, vol. 244, no. 2, pp. 268–270, 2006.

[16]  K. Shiraki, N. Toyama, T. Daikoku, and M. Yajima, "Herpes Zoster and Recurrent Herpes Zoster," *Open Forum Infectious Diseases*, vol. 4, no. 1, Article ID ofx007, 2017.

[17]  G. Linkov, J. Cracchiolo, A. F. Fielding, and J. C. Liu, "Facial nerve function preservation with vacuum-assisted closure," *The Journal of Craniofacial Surgery*, vol. 25, no. 4, pp. 1560-1561, 2014.

[18]  M. Reiter and U. Harréus, "Vacuum assisted closure in the management of wound healing disorders in the head and neck: A retrospective analysis of 23 cases," *American Journal of Otolaryngology - Head and Neck Medicine and Surgery*, vol. 34, no. 5, pp. 411–415, 2013.

[19]  V. Byrnside, M. Glasgow, and R. Gurunluoglu, "The Vacuum-Assisted Closure in Treating Craniofacial Wounds," *Journal of Oral and Maxillofacial Surgery*, vol. 68, no. 4, pp. 935–942, 2010.

# 12

# Bilateral Trichotillomania of Eyelashes Triggered by Anxiety due to Nocturnal Enuresis: A Case Report

**Shoko Ubukata, Tatsuya Mimura ⓘ, Emiko Watanabe, Koichi Matsumoto, Makoto Kawashima, Kazuma Kitsu, Mai Nishio, and Atsushi Mizota ⓘ**

*Department of Ophthalmology, Teikyo University School of Medicine, Tokyo 173-8605, Japan*

Correspondence should be addressed to Tatsuya Mimura; mimurat-tky@umin.ac.jp

Academic Editor: Maurizio Battaglia Parodi

*Purpose.* Trichotillomania is a behavioral and mental disorder and is characterized by a recurring habit of pulling out one's hair. The differential diagnosis between trichotillomania and other hair loss conditions such as alopecia areata is difficult for ophthalmologists. We report a rare case of bilateral trichotillomania of the eyelashes that was triggered by anxiety about nocturnal enuresis. *Case Report.* A healthy 9-year-old Japanese boy presented with a bilateral loss of his eyelashes. His parents had believed that his loss of eyelashes was due to alopecia, an autoimmune disorder that results in hair loss, of the eyelashes. Our initial examination revealed that he had suffered from nightly nocturnal enuresis from childhood and was scheduled to go on a school trip the following month. He feared that his school mates might find out about his enuresis, and he said that the anxiety was the cause of the eyelash trichotillomania. The trichotillomania was resolved by discussion among the student, his family, teacher, and school counselor. *Conclusion.* To the best of our knowledge, this is the first report of eyelash trichotillomania caused by anxiety about nocturnal enuresis. Ophthalmologists should be aware that a patient without eyelashes may not be due to alopecia but some anxiety-producing events. In addition, discussion of the anxiety-producing factor among the parents, teacher, and school counselors can resolve the trichotillomania.

## 1. Introduction

Trichotillomania is a hair-pulling mental disorder and is characterized by recurrent, irresistible urges to pull hair out of the body [1, 2]. Patients are fearful to tell their family and doctor, and children with trichotillomania often do not tell their parents. Thus, trichotillomania is frequently misdiagnosed as alopecia areata or other hair loss conditions on initial presentation. The most common site of hair pulling is the scalp, and it occasionally occurs for the eyelashes [3–9]. We report an unusual case of trichotillomania involving the eyelashes caused by anxiety caused by nocturnal enuresis.

## 2. Case Report

The patient was a 9-year-old boy with a history of recurrent episodes of local hair loss which was resolved within 1 to 2 months at the age of 5-6 years. The boy had never scratched his scalp or pulled his hair in front of his parents. Parents thought that the loss of the eyelashes was alopecia, and the boy was followed without receiving any treatment. No abnormalities had been detected in his hair or eyelashes at the age of 7-8 years after entering elementary school.

At the age of 9 years, his parents saw that the eyelashes of the boy were getting fewer but did not notice that he pulled out his eyelashes. His parents were concerned about their son's loss of his eyelashes and visited our hospital.

Our examination showed that there was a complete loss of eyelashes of the upper eyelid of both eyes (Figure 1). His best-corrected visual acuity (BCVA) was 20/20 in both eyes, and his corneas were clear and did not stain with fluorescein. The anterior chamber, iris, and lens were normal. Funduscopy was within normal limits. The skin of the eyelids of both eyes were not swollen, scarred, or desquamated. The pull test of the eyelashes was negative along the edges where the eyelashes were absent and had a normal resistive

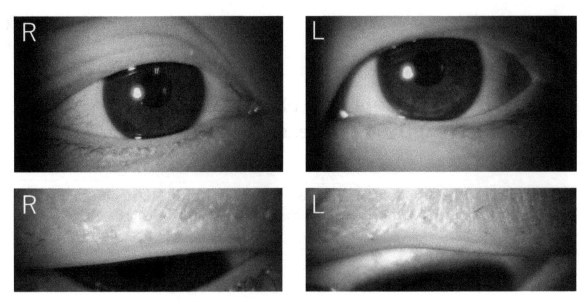

FIGURE 1: Slit-lamp photographs of an 8-year-old boy with trichotillomania of the eyelashes of both eyes. Photograph taken at initial visit.

response. Mycological examination of the eyelid skin was negative. These negative results of alopecia clearly confirmed the diagnosis of trichotillomania.

The mother reported that the boy had suffered from nightly nocturnal enuresis (bedwetting) all of his life, but the frequency was recently reduced to once or twice a month. However, the boy was scheduled to go on a school trip the following month, and the mother noticed that the boy had been depressed and had shown signs of avoiding school.

The boy told us that he had been concerned that his bed wetting might be revealed to his classmates during an overnight school trip. He stated that his stress was reduced by pulling out his eyelashes. We explained to the boy and his mother our diagnosis of trichotillomania and assured them that the condition could be resolved without medications. We suggested that a discussion be held among the parents, his school teacher, and school counselor about his bedwetting especially during the school trip.

One week after the school trip, the boy and mother visited our hospital and reported that no enuresis occurred during the school trip. The boy was followed without any special treatment. The mother reported that the child had not pulled out his eyelashes or hair after the consultation. With the parents' cooperation, the boy also developed control over his bladder during the night and have dry nights by age 10 years.

## 3. Discussion

Eyelash trichotillomania is extremely rare and has never been reported in a Japanese individual. A summary of the case reports on eyelash trichotillomania is presented in Table 1. In our case, the patient had a temporary stress-induced trichotillomania for 1-2 months while in kindergarten. The important causal factors for trichotillomania are stressful social or familial events such as abuse, family conflicts, or death [1, 2]. However, there were no significant stressful life

events in this patient. Thus, this patient is a rare case of recurrent trichotillomania over a three-year period whose latest episode was triggered by an upcoming overnight school trip. He had great anxiety that his nocturnal enuresis will be found out by his classmates.

Trichotillomania is a mental disorder that involves irresistible urges to pull out ones hair [1, 2]. Trichotillomania can develop at all ages, and the age of the first episode of trichotillomania ranges from 9 to 13 years [10]. Our patient developed trichotillomania at the age of 5 years, and this age of onset was quite young compared to cases in general. Our patient was a young boy but there appears to be a female predominance among preadolescents to young adults and 70 to 93% of the patients are girls [11–13].

Trichotillomania can be triggered by different types of neurological disorders and mental disorders such as anxiety, depression, and obsessive–compulsive disorders [14, 15]. Young children with autism spectrum disorder (ASD) may also engage in self-stimulatory trichotillomania [16]. Our patient did not have ASD or any neurological disorders. Most of the symptoms can be resolved after reducing the anxiety, and then trichotillomania generally follows a benign course.

Most young patients with trichotillomania are managed conservatively. Scolding can be counterproductive. Thus, parents and family need to simply ignore the behavior of trichotillomania without pointing out or cautioning the child's behavior. In more severe cases, patients need to be referred to a psychologists or psychiatrists for treatment which may include medications.

In our case, the nocturnal enuresis was associated with the recurrence of trichotillomania. Nocturnal enuresis itself can be frustrating for children because parents may punish their kids for wetting the bed. However, our patient had never been scolded for his nocturnal enuresis by his parents. Thus, it appeared that the patient did not feel nocturnal enuresis itself was stressful. However, the patient was extremely vulnerable

TABLE 1: Summary of case reports of eyelash trichotillomania.

| No | Age/sex (Onset age) | Country | Ocular involvement | Anxiety/ Stress | Therapy | Ocular disease | Other disease | Journal | Year | Author |
|---|---|---|---|---|---|---|---|---|---|---|
| 1 | 33F | Australia | Both | Y | Behavioral therapy | None | Depression | Aust N Z J Ophthalmol | 1995 | Smith |
| 2 | 12M | United Kingdom | Both | N | Psychiatric treatment | None | None | Br J Ophthalmol | 2001 | Patil |
| 3 | 19F | Canada | Right | Y | Treatment of hyperthyroidism | None | hyperthyroidism | Semin Plast Surg | 2007 | Jordan |
| 4 | 6F | Spain | Both | N | antipsychotics or mood stabilizers | None | ADHD, BD | J Can Acad Child Adolesc Psychiatry | 2012 | Olza-Fernández |
| 5 | 55F (12) | United State of America | Both | N | Bimatoprost. | None | None | Optom Vis Sci. | 2013 | Peabody |
| 6 | 12F | Morocco | Left | N | Cognitive - behavioral therapy | None | None | Pan African Medical Journal | 2017 | Touzani |
| 7 | 9M (5) | Japan | Both | Y | None | None | None | | This Case | Ubukata, Mimura |

Age, years; M, male; F, female; Y, yes; N, no: attention-deficit/hyperactivity disorder, ADHD; pediatric bipolar disorder, BD.

to other people's awareness of his enuresis especially his classmates. The boy was worried that his classmates would become aware of his enuresis on the school trip. Therefore, the classroom teacher, school counselor, and the parents needed to care for the children's distress, such as enuresis, throughout their school life.

In conclusion, as best we know, this is the first case report of recurrent bilateral trichotillomania involving the eyelashes triggered by anxiety of nocturnal enuresis. Punishing the child for the nocturnal enuresis can cause anguish; therefore, it is important not to scold or punish the child. Fortunately, our patient had a good outcome following conservative management. However, the management of trichotillomania with emotional distress in children at school may require strong cooperation among the school teacher, patient, and parents.

## Consent

Consent has been obtained.

## References

[1] M. E. Franklin, K. Zagrabbe, and K. L. Benavides, "Trichotillomania and its treatment: a review and recommendations," *Expert Review of Neurotherapeutics*, vol. 11, no. 8, pp. 1165–1174, 2014.

[2] M. Huynh, A. C. Gavino, and M. Magid, "Trichotillomania," *Seminars in Cutaneous Medicine and Surgery*, vol. 32, no. 2, pp. 88–94, 2013.

[3] J. R. Smith, "Trichotillomania: ophthalmic presentation," *Australian & New Zealand Journal of Ophthalmology*, vol. 23, no. 1, pp. 59–61, 1995.

[4] B. B. Patil and T. C. Dowd, "Trichotillomania," *British Journal of Ophthalmology*, vol. 85, no. 11, p. 1386, 2001.

[5] D. R. Jordan, "Eyelash loss," *Seminars in Plastic Surgery*, vol. 21, no. 1, pp. 32–36, 2007.

[6] I. Olza-Fernández, I. Palanca-Maresca, S. Jiménez-Fernández, and M. R. Cazorla-Calleja, "Trichotillomania, bipolar disorder and white matter hyperintensities in a six-year old girl," *Journal of the Canadian Academy of Child and Adolescent Psychiatry*, vol. 21, no. 3, pp. 213–215, 2012.

[7] T. Peabody, S. Reitz, J. Smith, and B. Teti, "Clinical management of trichotillomania with bimatoprost," *Optometry and Vision Science*, vol. 90, no. 6, pp. e167–e171, 2013.

[8] K. D. Touzani, Z. Lamari, F. Chraibi, M. Abdellaoui, and I. B. Andaloussi, "Trichotillomania involving the eyelashes: about a case," *Pan African Medical Journal*, vol. 28, p. 142, 2017.

[9] M. Sławińska, A. Opalska, D. Mehrholz, M. Sobjanek, R. Nowicki, and W. Barańska-Rybak, "Videodermoscopy supports the diagnosis of eyelash trichotillomania," *Journal of the European Academy of Dermatology and Venereology*, vol. 31, no. 11, pp. e477–e478, 2017.

[10] D. E. Sah, J. Koo, and V. H. Price, "Trichotillomania," *Dermatologic Therapy*, vol. 21, no. 1, pp. 13–21, 2008.

[11] G. A. Christenson, T. B. Mackenzie, and J. E. Mitchell, "Characteristics of 60 adult chronic hair pullers," *The American Journal of Psychiatry*, vol. 148, no. 3, pp. 365–370, 1991.

[12] L. J. Cohen, D. J. Stein, D. Simeon et al., "Clinical profile, comorbidity, and treatment history in 123 hair pullers: a survey study," *Journal of Clinical Psychiatry*, vol. 56, no. 7, pp. 319–326, 1995.

[13] S. A. Muller, "Trichotillomania," *Dermatologic Clinics*, vol. 5, no. 3, pp. 595–601, 1987.

[14] G. A. Cnhristenso and S. J. Crow, "The characterization and treatment of trichotillomania," *The Journal of Clinical Psychiatry*, vol. 57, supplement 8, pp. 42–47, 1996.

[15] S. R. Chamberlain, L. Menzies, B. J. Sahakian, and N. A. Fineberg, "Lifting the veil on trichotillomania," *The American Journal of Psychiatry*, vol. 164, no. 4, pp. 568–574, 2007.

[16] R. Masiran, "Autism and trichotillomania in an adolescent boy," *BMJ Case Reports*, vol. 2018, Article ID bcr-2018-226270, 2018.

# Pachychoroid Spectrum Disorder Findings in Patients with Coronavirus Disease 2019

**Mojtaba Abrishami** (ID),[1] **Ramin Daneshvar** (ID),[1] **Nasser Shoeibi** (ID),[1] **Neda Saeedian** (ID),[2] **Hamid Reza Heidarzadeh** (ID),[1] and **Seyedeh Maryam Hosseini** (ID)[1]

[1]*Eye Research Center, Mashhad University of Medical Sciences, Mashhad, Iran*
[2]*Department of Internal Medicine, Faculty of Medicine, Mashhad University of Medical Sciences, Mashhad, Iran*

Correspondence should be addressed to Seyedeh Maryam Hosseini; smaryam_hosseini@yahoo.com

Academic Editor: Stephen G. Schwartz

*Purpose.* To report the occurrence of acute, bilateral, central serous chorioretinopathy (CSC), and pachychoroid spectrum disorder findings in patients with coronavirus disease 2019 (COVID-19). *Methods.* In recovered cases of COVID-19 with visual disturbances, complete ocular examinations with multimodal retinal and choroidal evaluation, including enhanced depth imaging optical coherence tomography, fluorescein or indocyanine green angiography, and blue autofluorescence, were obtained. *Results.* Four COVID-19 recovered patients presented with bilateral blurred vision. Ocular examination and imaging revealed pachychoroid and pachyvessels associated with choroidal hyperpermeability without any obvious intraocular inflammation. Bilateral localized serous retinal detachment was obvious in three cases compatible with pachychoroid associated with CSC manifestation and pachychoroid pigment epitheliopathy in one patient. CSC was resolved with treatment by steroidal antimineralocorticoid (Eplerenone) in two patients and by photodynamic therapy in one patient. None of the patients reported emotional stress and history of corticosteroid consumption. *Conclusion.* Hyperpermeability of the choroid, pachychoroidopathy, or choroidal vessel congestion can be observed or exacerbated in association with COVID-19.

## 1. Introduction

Coronavirus disease 2019 (COVID-19) affects different parts of the body. The ocular findings in this regard were primarily confined to conjunctivitis [1, 2]. However, recent reports have indicated that the retina could also be involved in COVID-19 with the acute vascular lesions of the inner retina, including flame-shaped hemorrhages and cotton wool spots [2, 3]. Further peripapillary retinal vascular involvement in early post-COVID-19 patients has been recently described [2]. Moreover, viral ribonucleic acid (RNA) of severe acute respiratory syndrome coronavirus-2 (SARS-CoV-2) was found in the retinal autopsy sample of deceased cases of COVID-19 [4]. Presence of angiotensin-converting enzyme type 2 (ACE2), as the main receptor for SARS-CoV-2 in the retina, and the presence of its homology, ACE, in the choroid and different cell types of the retina [5], increase the possibility of chorioretinal involvement in patients with COVID-19.

Pachychoroid spectrum encompasses a group of different diseases which consist of central serous chorioretinopathy (CSC), pachychoroid pigment epitheliopathy (PPE), polypoidal choroidal vasculopathy (PCV), pachychoroid neovasculopathy (PNV), peripapillary pachychoroid syndrome (PPS), and focal choroidal excavation (FCE) [6]. CSC is a type of serous retinal detachment that mainly occurs in young to middle-aged males. CSC is usually accompanied by leakage at the level of the retinal pigment epithelium, which can be observed on fluorescein angiography (FA) and indocyanine green angiography (ICGA). Choroidal vascular congestion, prominent venous dilation, and hypercyanescent patches indicating areas of choroidal hyperpermeability are other features in angiographies in pachychoroid spectrum findings [6]. Enhanced depth imaging (EDI) optical coherence tomography (OCT) demonstrates that the choroid is pathologically thickened, and vascular lumens have significantly larger hyporeflective spaces. Generally, it is believed that choroidal hyperpermeability and choroidal vascular changes are the primary pathogenic steps and result in choroidal thickening [6]. There is evidence of the effect of the renin-angiotensin-aldosterone system (RAAS) on pachychoroid disease spectrum diseases [7–9], and as SARS-CoV-2 primarily affects the RAAS, there might be a relationship between these diseases. In this regard, herein we report acute bilateral CSC and pachychoroidopathy-like disorder in confirmed cases of COVID-19.

## 2. Case Presentation

*2.1. Case 1.* A 21-year-old male patient with a history of hospital admission for COVID-19 experienced a decrease in vision and metamorphopsia. He had a history of fever, cough, dyspnea, myalgia, red eye, and eye discomfort for two weeks. Results of his lab tests indicated lymphopenia, increased erythrocyte sedimentation rate (ESR) (48 mm/first hour), and increased C-reactive protein (CRP) (192.3 mg/L). Moreover, the real-time reverse transcription polymerase chain reaction (rRT-PCR) amplification of SARS-CoV-2 virus RNA from a nasopharyngeal (NP) swab sample was positive. He was admitted to the hospital for further supportive treatment due to tachypnea (22 breaths per min), decreased blood oxygen saturation (91%) on room air, and diffuse bilateral ground glass opacities in chest high-resolution computed tomography (HRCT). However, there was no need for intensive care, and after four days, the patient decided to continue his treatment in self-isolation at home. He was further treated at home with oral enteric-coated Naproxen and Azithromycin for one week and did not use any kind of systemic corticosteroids. On the eighth day after discharge, he experienced blurring of vision and metamorphopsia; however, there was no further red eye and ocular discomfort. In his ocular examination, the best corrected visual acuity (BCVA) was 20/25 in the right eye and 20/40 in the left eye.

Furthermore, the intraocular pressure (IOP) and anterior segment slit-lamp examination were normal. In fundus examination, bilateral submacular fluid was obvious without any sign of intraocular inflammation. The EDI-OCT (Spectralis OCT manufactured in Heidelberg Engineering, Heidelberg, Germany) revealed retinal hyperreflective bands in different layers of the retina, serous retinal detachment at the macula, and increased choroidal thickness (Figure 1).

Besides, the FA showed no significant leakage, specific signs of vasculitis, or ocular inflammation. On ICGA, in both eyes, a single hot spot at the center of the fovea appeared since the early phase and lasted until the late phase with multiple late hypercyanesence dots scattered at the macular area and outside of the arcades especially at the superotemporal quadrant of the fundus. Moreover, the hyperpermeability of large choroidal vessels was remarkable. After 3 months, CSC responded very well to Eplerenone

25 mg every 12 hours a day and SRF was resolved completely (Figure 2).

*2.2. Case 2.* A 34-year-old female patient with a history of outpatient treatment for COVID-19 referred with a complaint of paracentral scotoma in her left eye. She had a history of myalgia, chest pain, fever, red eye, and ocular discomfort for 10 days, and rRT-PCR for SARS-CoV-2 virus on a NP swab sample was positive. Based on laboratory evaluation, there were lymphopenia, increased ESR (32 mm/first h), and increased CRP (18 mg/L). The patient had been treated with Azithromycin and Acetaminophen at home in quarantine for two weeks. She had not used systemic corticosteroids in the last two years.

The patient experienced blurred vision in her left eye 10 days after the initiation of systemic symptoms. Visual acuity was 20/20 in both eyes, and according to the slit-lamp examination, the anterior segment was normal. In funduscopic evaluation, two small foci of serous retinal detachments in the macula and sparing of the fovea were found in both eyes. The EDI-OCT results revealed pachychoroid with dilated choroidal vessels in both eyes. Moreover, there was retinal pigment epithelial changes resembling pachychoroid pigment epitheliopathy and hyperreflective bands in the outer plexiform layer (Figure 3).

Furthermore, two foci of subretinal fluid in the superotemporal and inferonasal area of the left fovea were found. In addition, FA results showed hyperfluorescent dots and leakage in both eyes as well as a hyperfluorescent focus superior to the disc in the right eye which also had increased autofluorescence. Further evaluations and EDI-OCT results confirmed the presence of a shallow serous retinal detachment with outer retinal changes. Bilaterally, ICGA demonstrated dilated choroidal vessels in the early phase followed by hyperpermeability of choroidal vessels in the midphase and multiple small hot spots out of the macula in the late phase. Moreover, there was a hot spot in the left eye which corresponded to the inferotemporal serous retinal detachment (Figure 4).

After 5 months, CSC responded to Eplerenone 25 mg every 12 hours and SRF was resolved (Figure 5). However, pachychoroid pigment epitheliopathy changes were not changed.

*2.3. Case 3.* A 41-year-old male patient with a history of outpatient treatment for COVID-19 came with a complaint of decreased vision in his right eye since one week after initiation of systemic symptoms. He had a history of severe headache, myalgia, fever, and ocular discomfort for two weeks and positive rRT-PCR for SARS-CoV-2 virus on a NP swab sample. The patient became systemic symptom free one week after diminution in vision. Based on laboratory evaluation, there were lymphopenia, increased ESR, and increased CRP. The patient had been treated with Azithromycin and Naproxen at home in quarantine for two weeks. She had not yet used systemic corticosteroids.

Because of home self-quarantine, the patient came to us four weeks after decrease in his right eye vision. He also complained of gradual blurred vision and metamophopsia

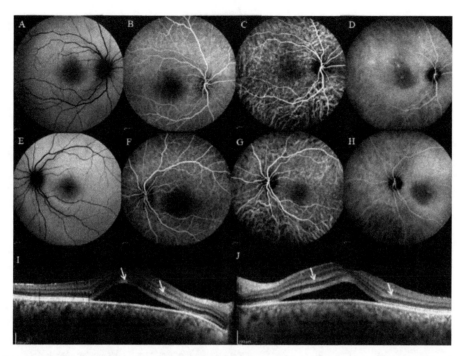

FIGURE 1: (a, e) Fundus autofluorescence (FAF), (b, f) fluorescein angiography (FA), (c, d, g, h) indocyanine green angiography (ICGA), and (i, j) enhanced depth imaging optical coherence tomography (EDI-OCT) of the first case. Retinal hyperreflective bands in different layers of the retina, serous retinal detachment (SRD) at the macula, and increased choroidal thickness on EDI-OCT can be observed. FAF and FA were nearly normal, and the ICGA showed a single hot spot at the center of the fovea. This spot appeared from the early phase and lasted until the late phase with multiple late hypercyanescence dots scattered at the macular area and outside of arcades, especially at superotemporal, and hyperpermeability of large choroidal vessels.

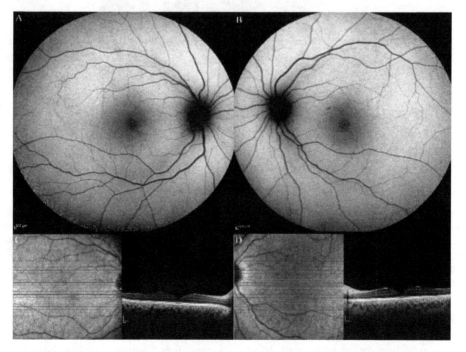

FIGURE 2: (a, b) Fundus autofluorescence and (c, d) enhanced depth imaging optical coherence tomography of the first case following three months of treatment with Eplerenone showing completely resolved SRD. The choroid seems to be still thickened.

in his left eye. In examination, BCVA was 20/32 and 20/20 in the right and left eye, respectively. EDI-OCT revealed pachyvessels in the choroid and SRF in the macula of the right eye and pigment epithelial detachment (PED) in the left eye. ICGA showed bilateral dilatation and hyperpermeability of the choroidal vessels. Moreover, bilateral hypercyanescence as hot spots was obvious bilaterally (Figure 6).

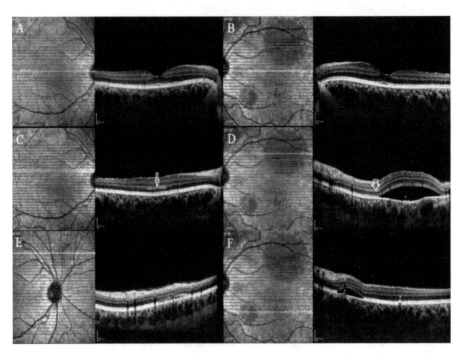

FIGURE 3: Enhanced Depth Imaging Optical Coherence Tomography of the (a, c, e) right and the (b, d, f) left eyes of the second case. Hyperreflective bands of the (c, d, arrows) outer plexiform layer, pachychoroid with dilated choroidal vessels and pachyvessels, and (d, f, asterisks) retinal pigment epithelium changes like pachychoroid pigment epitheliopathy can be seen in both eyes.

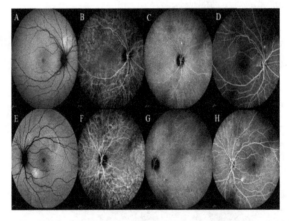

FIGURE 4: (a, e) Fundus autofluorescence, (b, c, f, g) indocyanine green angiography (ICGA), and (d, h) fluorescein angiography (FA) of the (a–d) right and the (e–h) left eye of the second case. The fundus autofluorescence demonstrated hyperautofluorescence foci corresponding to the leakage areas. The FA disclosed hyperfluorescent dots and leakage in both eyes. In the right eye, a hyperfluorescent focus superior to the disc was found on FA and fundus autofluorescence. The ICGA revealed dilation and hyperpermeability of choroidal vessels in the mid- and late phases, multiple small hypercyanescence dots out of the macular area in both eyes, and a hot spot corresponding to an inferotemporal SRD in the left eye.

Photodynamic therapy (PDT) with half-dose of verteporfin was performed for both eyes. Two months later, SRF and PED were completely resolved with small defect in the outer retinal layers and BCVA was improved to 20/20 in the right eye (Figure 7).

*2.4. Case 4.* A 45-year-old female, a staff of eye hospital, with a history of outpatient treatment for COVID-19, was referred with a complaint of ambiguous visual disturbance in both eyes amid her disease period of systemic symptoms.

She had a history of severe headache, myalgia, and fever for two weeks; rRT-PCR for SARS-CoV-2 virus on a NP swab sample was positive. Based on laboratory evaluation, there were lymphopenia, increased ESR, and increased CRP. The patient had been treated with oral Acetaminophen and Hydroxychloroquine at home in quarantine for ten days. She had not yet used systemic corticosteroids.

After return to her job, because of distorted vision, multimodal imaging was performed. Visual acuity was 20/20 in both eyes. She had not consent to take

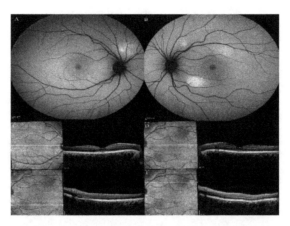

FIGURE 5: (a, b) Fundus autofluorescence and (c–f) enhanced depth imaging optical coherence tomography of the second case after two months of treatment disclosing completely resolved subretinal fluid in different parts of the macula, which were affected before. Choroidal thickening and dilation of choroidal vessels are still visible.

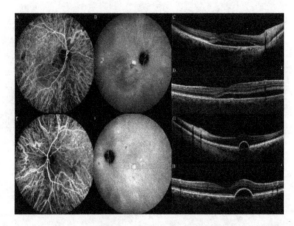

FIGURE 6: The indocyanine green angiography of the third case disclosed dilation and hyperpermeability of choroidal vessels in the early phase associated with multifocal hypercyanescence (hot spots) and diffuse leakage at the posterior pole in the late phase in the (a, b) right and the (e, f) left eyes. Enhanced depth imaging optical coherence tomography revealed (c, d) pachyvessels in the choroid and SRF in the macula of the right eye and (g, h) pigment epithelial detachment (PED) in the left eye.

angiography. She had no history of abnormal vision or any visual abnormalities before COVID disease. In EDI-OCT, bilateral pachychoroid and pachyvessels accompanied by bilateral retinal pigment epithelial (RPE) changes over the pachyvessels and hyperreflectivity of outer retinal layers were obvious. Fundus autofluorescence (FAF) disclosed no abnormality. In infrared reflectance, bilateral hyperreflective dots were visible (Figure 8). The disease course was described for her, and she chose to be followed without any treatment.

## 3. Discussion

This study is a report on acute CSC and pachychoroid spectrum findings in confirmed cases of COVID-19. Despite the fact that conjunctivitis, chemosis, and retinal findings, including inner retinal changes, have been reported in COVID-19 cases [1, 3], however, to the best of our knowledge, there is no report regarding to the subretinal fluid, choroidal hyperpermeability, or choroidopathy similar to the pachychoroid spectrum diseases.

In the first patient with decreased vision, we found bilateral macular subretinal fluid (SRF) and retinal hyperreflective bands in OCT. Regarding to the almost normal FA results without any leakage, we proposed that the underlying cause of these presentations could be choroidal changes. On ICG, hypercyanescence target-shape spots at the fovea were in favor of leakage. Due to the lack of any corresponding leakage in FA, which is a typical finding in patients with CSC, we believe that the mechanisms of SRF a, in this case, might be a choroidopathy, perhaps in the context of viral involvement of the uvea similar to choroidal involvement in Flaviviridae viruses [10].

The second patient was a young female who presented with paracentral scotoma. Pachychoroid, pigment epitheliopathy, CSC, and pachyvessels were found to be associated with retinal fluorescein leakage foci that had correspondent hot spots in ICG angiography. Moreover, multiple tiny peripheral hypercyanescence spots were observed in both patients.

Given the history of COVID-19 in our cases, due to the presence of ACE and ACE2 in the retina and choroid [5], it can be postulated that the choroid may be involved

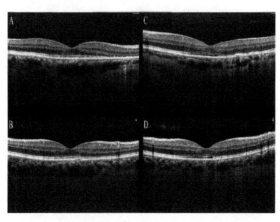

FIGURE 7: Optical coherence tomography of the (a, c) right eye and (b, d) left eye of the third patient one month after photodynamic therapy, even in the (a, b) horizontal or (c, d) vertical, shows complete fluid resorption and also outer retinal atrophy.

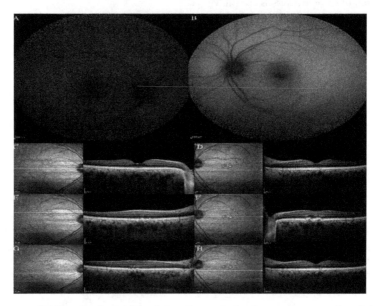

FIGURE 8: Fundus autofluorescence (FAF) and enhanced depth imaging optical coherence tomography of the fourth case. (a, c, e, g) The right eye images. (b, d, f, h) The left eye images. FAF of (a, b) both eyes disclosed no abnormality. In infrared reflectance taken with (c–h) OCT, bilateral hyperreflective dots were visible in both eyes. (c–h) Enhanced depth imaging optical coherence tomography depicted bilateral pachychoroid and pachyvessels accompanied by bilateral small, shallow, and multifocal retinal pigment epithelial (RPE) detachments and changes over the pachyvessels, hyperreflectivity of outer retinal layers, and multiple hyperreflective tiny dots scattered at the inner retinal layers in both eyes.

either in the process of infection with SARS-CoV-2 or the cytokine storm in that setting. Multiple punctate hypercyanescent dots that were scattered at the macular area and beyond as well as the pachyvessels out of the macula were depicted on ICGA indicating a diffuse choroidal disease.

We did not find any sign of chronic CSC in the examination or autofluorescence results of our cases. Moreover, there were no significant pachyvessels on macular EDI-OCT despite the fact that the choroid had been thickened and the sclerochoroidal border was not visible beyond the imaging depth limit. Based on these pieces of evidence, it seems that choroidal hyperpermeability and increased thickness might be caused by an inflammatory process rather than only choroidal vessel dilations in the macular area or exacerbation of old pachychoroidopathy.

In the Flaviviridae family, a group of viruses consists of more than 90 RNA-enveloped viruses similar to the coronaviruses; choroidal involvement has been reported before [10]. It was hypothesized that the virus affects the vessels, and it can pass the blood-retinal barrier. As these viruses modulate retinal innate response, the protective barrier breaches and causes choroidal or retinal pathologies. Bilateral choroidal effusion has been reported from the Dengue virus, a member of this family [11]. Moreover, the multimodal imaging in Dengue fever maculopathy revealed hypocyanescence on the late frames of ICGA without fluorescein leakage accompanied with focal swelling of the outer plexiform and outer nuclear layers and discontinuity in the underlying ellipsoid zone in OCT [12].

Range of reported risk factors for the pathogenesis of CSC is large. Reported etiologies include pregnancy;

endocrine disorders, such as Cushing syndrome; steroid-producing tumors; gastroesophageal disorders; psychologic stress; type A personality; organ transplantation; and multisystem autoimmune diseases, like lupus erythematosus. Medications that were found to be associated with CSC are corticosteroids, antihistamines, phosphodiesterase-5 inhibitors, MEK-inhibitors, sympathomimetic drugs, and antibiotics [6, 13]. In the cases of this study, nonsteroidal anti-inflammatory drugs (NSAIDs) were used since it has been reported that NSAIDs, whether topical [14, 15] or systemic [16, 17], could be effective in the treatment of CSC. Therefore, the use of NSAIDs for the cases of this study might have mitigated the occurrence of CSC. On the other hand, prostaglandin activity was observed in the RPE cells, as well as retinal vasculature [18]; hence, some physicians believe that NSAIDS can delay or prevent spontaneous recovery of CSC in a natural course [19]. However, there is not robust evidence regarding the detrimental effect of systemic NSAIDs on CSC. Therefore, the impact of NSAIDs on the genesis of CSC in these patients is improbable.

Moreover, none of the patients received corticosteroid therapy as these agents were not yet introduced into the COVID-19 treatment protocol at the time. Hence, the pathogenesis of CSC cannot be attributed to systemic corticosteroids. Furthermore, our patients received antibiotics that had been assigned as a risk factor for CSC in a retrospective case-control study [13]. It has been postulated that adaptation to stress, either as psychologic, neuroimmunological, neuroendocrine, or biochemical adaptations, is common in CSC patients. This could explain the higher rate of antibiotic consumption among CSC patients [13]. Furthermore, impaired immunity patients who experienced psychologic stress are more susceptible to infections [20, 21]. Hence, the antibiotic consumption itself may not consider as risk factor, and the confounding effect of stresses may affect more pronouncedly.

There are several plausible theories for SRF accumulation in these cases, including (1) stress caused by the fear of COVID-19 disease, (2) choroidal congestion and hyperpermeability secondary to the viral infection and as a component of systemic, multiorgan involvement in the course of COVID-19 disease [2], and (3) the recurrence of previous CSC. Although neither of our patients was apparently stressed about the disease, however, the first theory could be a possible etiology. Besides, no sign of previous CSC was found in the imaging, examination, or medical history of these cases, and there was also no sufficient evidence to support the third theory. In a recent case series regarding >the spectrum of pulmonary pathology in a cohort of 40 decedents by postmortem autopsy of 40 rRT-PCRs of confirmed COVID-19 cases, vascular congestion and hemangiomatosis-like changes were found in half of them [22]. Moreover, in another postmortem analysis, endotheliitis was found in several organs as a direct consequence of viral involvement, with evidence of the presence of viral inclusion structures, accompanying the host inflammatory response [23]. COVID-19 is associated with widespread microangiopathy; thus, changes of blood flow in the retina and choroid are potential. In recent case-control studies,

alterations of retinal microvasculature are found subsequent to COVID-19 infections compared to healthy control groups [24, 25]. Moreover, in a case-control study in patients stratified to mild, moderate, and severe COVID-19 disease activity and normal controls, patients with moderate and severe disease had decreased macular vascular density (VD) on OCT-angiography (OCT-A) as compared with control subjects or even those who were asymptomatic or paucisymptomatic [26]. These findings raise the possibility of subclinical vascular alterations in individuals who have apparently recovered from COVID-19 infection, and the findings were shown to be associated with the severity of the COVID-19. It is therefore important to monitor these retinal microvasculature changes to ascertain their longitudinal course [27]. Given the presence of ACE and ACE2 receptors in the choroid and retina and with regard to the known role of RAAS in CSC [7, 9], we believe that the second theory is the most probable one. On the other hand, other differential diagnoses including inflammatory uveitic etiologies like Vogt-Koyanagi-Harada disease, age-related macular degeneration, melanoma, or other choroidal masses have been ruled out as these young patients without any other comorbidity, with pachychoroid-like choroidal changes, responded very well to Eplerenone and PDT.

In conclusion, we report four cases of acute CSC in association with COVID-19. It should be noted that in all cases, CSC was simultaneously bilateral. This might have been a simple coincidence or a pathophysiologic correlation between the two entities. Either way, regarding the novelty of COVID-19 and its many unknown faces, every practitioner managing these patients should anticipate various clinical pictures and organ system involvement and treat the variable clinical presentations of COVID-19 as a rule and not an exception. Regarding to accumulative evidences on retinal and choroidal changes due to COVID-19 infection in this report and previous reports [24–28], we could propose the COVID-19 infection as a new etiology for pachychoroid spectrum disorder.

## Abbreviations

| | |
|---|---|
| COVID-19: | Coronavirus disease 2019 |
| OCT: | Optical coherence tomography |
| SARS-CoV-2: | Severe acute respiratory syndrome coronavirus-2 |
| ACE2: | Angiotensin-converting enzyme type 2 |
| ACE: | Angiotensin-converting enzyme |
| CSC: | Central serous chorioretinopathy |
| ICGA: | Indocyanine green angiography |
| EDI-OCT: | Enhanced depth imaging optical coherence tomography |
| rRT-PCR: | Real-time reverse transcription polymerase chain reaction |
| SRF: | Subretinal fluid |
| RAAS: | Renin-angiotensin-aldosterone system |
| PPE: | Pachychoroid pigment epitheliopathy |
| PCV: | Polypoidal choroidal vasculopathy |
| PNV: | Pachychoroid neovasculopathy |

PPS:　　　　Peripapillary pachychoroid syndrome
FCE:　　　　Focal choroidal excavation
ESR:　　　　Erythrocyte sedimentation rate
CRP:　　　　C-reactive protein
NP:　　　　　Nasopharyngeal
HRCT:　　　High-resolution computed tomography
BCVA:　　　Best corrected visual acuity
IOP:　　　　Intraocular pressure
PED:　　　　Pigment epithelial detachment
PDT:　　　　Photodynamic therapy.

## Consent

No written consent has been obtained from the patients as there is no patient identifiable data included in this case series.

## Authors' Contributions

All authors contributed to the conception and design of the study and agreed to be accountable for all the aspects of the report. All authors made critical revisions to the manuscript and declared their final approval.

## Acknowledgments

The authors would like to express their gratitude to Zahra Emamverdian M.Sc., Sepideh Nazari Noghabi M.Sc., Roghaye Kahani B.Sc., and Roya Gholamzadeh B.Sc., the operators of Retinal Imaging Center of Khatam Eye Hospital, Mashhad, Iran. Moreover, the authors appreciate the kind supports of Capt. Alireza Zahmatkesh.

## References

[1] M. Abrishami, F. Tohidinezhad, R. Daneshvar et al., "Ocular manifestations of hospitalized patients with COVID-19 in Northeast of Iran," *Ocular immunology and inflammation*, vol. 28, no. 5, pp. 739–744, 2020.

[2] M. C. Savastano, G. Gambini, A. Savastano et al., "Evidence-based of conjunctival COVID-19 positivity: an Italian experience: Gemelli against COVID group," *European Journal of Ophthalmology*, vol. 23, p. 112067212097654, 2020.

[3] L. A. Pereira, L. C. M. Soares, P. A. Nascimento et al., "Retinal findings in hospitalised patients with severe COVID-19," *British Journal of Ophthalmology*, p. bjophthalmol-2020-317576, 2020.

[4] M. Casagrande, A. Fitzek, K. Püschel et al., "Detection of SARS-CoV-2 in human retinal biopsies of deceased COVID-19 patients," *Ocular Immunology and Inflammation*, vol. 28, no. 5, pp. 721–725, 2020.

[5] R. Choudhary, M. S. Kapoor, A. Singh, and S. H. Bodakhe, "Therapeutic targets of renin-angiotensin system in ocular disorders," *Journal of current ophthalmology*, vol. 29, no. 1, pp. 7–16, 2017.

[6] C. M. G. Cheung, W. K. Lee, H. Koizumi, K. Dansingani, T. Y. Y. Lai, and K. B. Freund, "Pachychoroid disease," *Eye (London, England)*, vol. 33, no. 1, pp. 14–33, 2019.

[7] A. Daruich, A. Matet, A. Moulin et al., "Mechanisms of macular edema: beyond the surface," *Progress in Retinal and Eye Research*, vol. 63, pp. 20–68, 2018.

[8] M. Zhao, I. Célérier, E. Bousquet et al., "Mineralocorticoid receptor is involved in rat and human ocular chorioretinopathy," *The Journal of Clinical Investigation*, vol. 122, no. 7, pp. 2672–2679, 2012.

[9] J. L. Wilkinson-Berka, V. Suphapimol, J. R. Jerome, D. Deliyanti, and M. J. Allingham, "Angiotensin II and aldosterone in retinal vasculopathy and inflammation," *Experimental Eye Research*, vol. 187, p. 107766, 2019.

[10] S. Singh and A. Kumar, "Ocular manifestations of emerging Flaviviruses and the blood-retinal barrier," *Viruses*, vol. 10, no. 10, p. 530, 2018.

[11] V. Cruz-Villegas, A. M. Berrocal, and J. L. Davis, "Bilateral choroidal effusions associated with dengue fever," *Retina*, vol. 23, no. 4, pp. 576–578, 2003.

[12] M. Akanda, S. Gangaputra, S. Kodati, A. Melamud, and H. N. Sen, "Multimodal imaging in dengue-fever-associated maculopathy," *Ocular Immunology and Inflammation*, vol. 26, no. 5, pp. 671–676, 2018.

[13] R. Haimovici, S. Koh, D. R. Gagnon, T. Lehrfeld, S. Wellik, and Central Serous Chorioretinopathy Case-Control Study Group, "Risk factors for central serous chorioretinopathy: a case-control study," *Ophthalmology*, vol. 111, no. 2, pp. 244–249, 2004.

[14] S. H. An and Y. H. Kwon, "Effect of a topical nonsteroidal anti-inflammatory agent (0.1 % pranoprofen) on acute central serous chorioretinopathy," *Graefe's Archive for Clinical and Experimental Ophthalmology*, vol. 254, no. 8, pp. 1489–1496, 2016.

[15] R. Wuarin, V. Kakkassery, A. Consigli et al., "Combined topical anti-inflammatory and oral acetazolamide in the treatment of central serous chorioretinopathy," *Optometry and Vision Science*, vol. 96, no. 7, pp. 500–506, 2019.

[16] A. Caccavale, M. Imparato, F. Romanazzi, A. Negri, A. Porta, and F. Ferentini, "A new strategy of treatment with low-dosage acetyl salicylic acid in patients affected by central serous chorioretinopathy," *Medical Hypotheses*, vol. 73, no. 3, pp. 435–437, 2009.

[17] A. Caccavale, F. Romanazzi, M. Imparato et al., "Low-dose aspirin as treatment for central serous chorioretinopathy," *Clinical Ophthalmology*, vol. 4, pp. 899–903, 2010.

[18] P. Hardy, M. Bhattacharya, D. Abran et al., "Increases in retinovascular prostaglandin receptor functions by cyclooxygenase-1 and -2 inhibition," *Investigative Ophthalmology & Visual Science*, vol. 39, no. 10, pp. 1888–1898, 1998.

[19] P. Venkatesh, "Central serous chorioretinopathy and topical NSAIDs," *Retinal Physician*, vol. 10, no. 8, pp. 24–26, 2013.

[20] M. Freire-Garabal, J. L. Balboa, J. C. Fernandez-Rial, M. J. Núñez, and A. Belmonte, "Effects of alprazolam on influenza virus infection in stressed mice," *Pharmacology, Biochemistry, and Behavior*, vol. 46, no. 1, pp. 167–172, 1993.

[21] S. Cohen, D. A. Tyrrell, and A. P. Smith, "Psychological stress and susceptibility to the common cold," *The New England Journal of Medicine*, vol. 325, no. 9, pp. 606–612, 1991.

[22] S. de Michele, Y. Sun, M. M. Yilmaz et al., "Forty postmortem examinations in COVID-19 patients," *American Journal of Clinical Pathology*, vol. 154, no. 6, pp. 748–760, 2020.

[23] Z. Varga, A. J. Flammer, P. Steiger et al., "Endothelial cell infection and endotheliitis in COVID-19," *Lancet*, vol. 395, no. 10234, pp. 1417-1418, 2020.

[24] M. Abrishami, Z. Emamverdian, N. Shoeibi et al., "Optical coherence tomography angiography analysis of the retina in patients recovered from COVID-19: a case-control study,"

*Canadian Journal of Ophthalmology*, vol. 56, no. 1, pp. 24–30, 2021.

[25] I. C. Turker, C. U. Dogan, D. Guven, O. K. Kutucu, and C. Gul, "Optical coherence tomography angiography findings in patients with COVID-19," *Canadian Journal of Ophthalmology*, vol. 56, no. 2, pp. 83–87, 2021.

[26] M. Á. Zapata, S. Banderas García, A. Sánchez-Moltalvá et al., "Retinal microvascular abnormalities in patients after COVID-19 depending on disease severity," *British Journal of Ophthalmology*, p. bjophthalmol-2020-317953, 2020.

[27] S. S. Sim and C. M. G. Cheung, "Does COVID-19 infection leave a mark on the retinal vasculature?," *Canadian Journal of Ophthalmology*, vol. 56, no. 1, pp. 4-5, 2021.

[28] G. Zamani, S. Ataei Azimi, A. Aminizadeh et al., "Acute macular neuroretinopathy in a patient with acute myeloid leukemia and deceased by COVID-19: a case report," *Journal of Ophthalmic Inflammation and Infection*, vol. 10, no. 1, p. 39, 2020.

# 14

# Fundoscopic Changes in Maroteaux-Lamy Syndrome

**Augusto Magalhães,**[1] **Jorge Meira** ⓘ**,**[1] **Ana Maria Cunha,**[1] **Raul Jorge Moreira,**[1]
**Elisa Leão-Teles,**[2] **Manuel Falcão** ⓘ**,**[1,3] **Jorge Breda,**[1] **and Fernando Falcão-Reis**[1,3]

[1]*Departament of Ophthalmology, Centro Hospitalar Universitário de São João, Porto, Portugal*
[2]*Reference Centre of Inherited Metabolic Diseases, Centro Hospitalar Universitário de São João, Porto, Portugal*
[3]*Department of Surgery and Physiology, Faculty of Medicine of University of Porto, Porto, Portugal*

Correspondence should be addressed to Jorge Meira; jorgesmeira@gmail.com

Academic Editor: Cristiano Giusti

*Purpose.* To describe a clinical case of mucopolysaccharidosis type VI (MPS VI), or Maroteaux-Lamy syndrome, with fundoscopic alterations that may correspond to scleral deposits of glycosaminoglycans. *Materials and Methods.* Clinical case report. *Results.* A 16-year-old girl with MPS VI was examined at the Ophthalmology Department for poor vision due to opacified corneas. Treatment consisted of bilateral penetrating keratoplasty. Retinographies and enhanced depth imaging optical coherence tomography (EDI-OCT) were performed after surgery, suggesting the presence of scleral glycosaminoglycan deposits. The patient evolved with stable corneal and fundoscopic findings. *Conclusions.* To our knowledge, this is the first case of MPS VI described *in vivo* with suspected deposits of glycosaminoglycans in the sclera. Fundoscopic alterations are not usually included in the ocular pathological spectrum of MPS VI. However, with improved control of systemic comorbidities, survival rates of these patients have increased, which in turn has made it possible to observe other changes besides the ones that were classically described. Despite being particularly challenging to manage, efforts should be made to maximizing the visual acuity of these patients, in order to provide them the best possible quality of life.

## 1. Introduction

Mucopolysaccharidoses (MPSs) are a group of disorders caused by inherited defects in lysosomal enzymes resulting in widespread intra and extracellular accumulation of glycosaminoglycans [1].

MPS type VI (MPS VI), or Maroteaux-Lamy syndrome, is a very rare disorder with an incidence ranging from 0.36 to 1.30 per 100,000 [2]. It is an autosomal recessive disorder caused by a deficient activity of the enzyme $N$-acetylgalactosamine 4-sulfatase, which is involved in the degradation of the glycosaminoglycans dermatan sulfate and chondroitin 4-sulfate. Deficient levels of this enzyme lead to the accumulation of partially degraded glycosaminoglycans in tissues and organs, which in turn causes a wide range of clinical manifestations, including abnormal structural development, lung infections, sleep apnoea, cardiac valvular disease, and a characteristic facies, with enlarged tongue, flat nasal bridge, and macrocephaly, that progressively worsens with age. Affected patients are usually said to be intellectually normal [2, 3].

Ocular accumulation of glycosaminoglycans results in progressive corneal opacification and is the main reason for the low visual acuity of these patients as well as the difficulty in observing the retina and optic nerve in detail. Ocular hypertension and glaucoma are also characteristic [4]. Retinal changes are not usually associated with MPS VI [3–5].

## 2. Case Presentation

A 16-year-old caucasian female with biochemical and genetic diagnosis of MPS VI (urinary glycosaminoglycans and decreased arylsulfatase B activity and c.944G> A; pR315Q homozygous mutation in the arylsulfatase B gene) was observed at the Paediatric Ophthalmology clinic with bilateral progressive vision loss in recent years.

The patient had short stature and coarse facial features, typical of MPS disease. Structural abnormalities of the upper respiratory tract had resulted in tracheostomy. Other findings included mild hearing loss, hepatosplenomegaly, cardiac

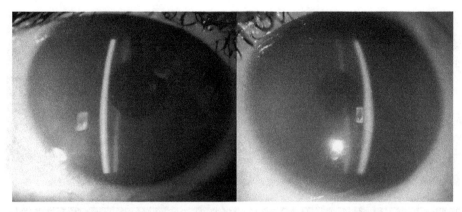

FIGURE 1: Baseline anterior segment photographs. Both corneas are cloudy due to stromal deposits of glycosaminoglycans.

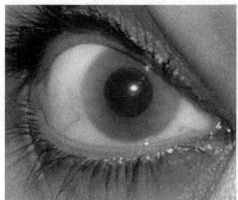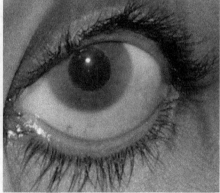

FIGURE 2: Anterior segment photographs after penetrating keratoplasty. There is central transparency of the graft with marked opacity of the peripheral host cornea.

valvular disease, and changes in musculoskeletal development. There was no relevant family history. She was on enzyme replacement therapy with galsufatase 1 mg/kg per week, since the age of ten.

She presented with a best corrected visual acuity (BCVA) of 4/10 (−2.25 × 180) bilaterally. Both corneas were opacified (Figure 1), with increased thickness (central corneal thickness of 741 μm and 779 μm) and intraocular pressure of 34 mmHg and 32 mmHg in the right and left eye, respectively (Goldmann applanation tonometry). She was started on dorzolamide 20 mg/ml + timolol 5 mg/ml. Her corneal opacifications prevented clear ocular fundus evaluation. As corneal opacity progressed, visual acuity decreased to 3/10 in right eye and 1/10 in left eye after two years of follow-up. The patient was submitted to bilateral central penetrating keratoplasty. The trepanation diameter of the donor was 6.50 mm and the trepanation diameter of the recipient cornea was 6.00 mm. (Figure 2). After transplantation, fundoscopic evaluation became possible. Color fundus photography and enhanced depth imaging optical coherence tomography (EDI-OCT) (Figure 3) were performed. Color fundus photography revealed multiple orange patches in the macular area and around the temporal retinal vessels with no specific pattern. However, the retinal periphery was normal. The optic nerves showed a slight symmetrical pallor. EDI-OCT imaging at the location of the orange patches (Figures 3(a) and 3(b)), revealed scleral thickening

associated with choroidal thinning (Figure 3(c)). The retinal pigment epithelium and retina had no apparent changes even in the areas in which the choroidal thinning and scleral thickening were evident. After 8 years of follow-up, the patient's grafts remain transparent with a BCVA of 5/10. IOP has been controlled with a combination of dorzolamide 20 mg/ml and timolol 5 mg/ml (18 mmHg in both eyes).

## 3. Conclusion

The most frequently described ocular manifestations of MPS VI are corneal clouding and ocular hypertension. Retinopathy is not frequently described amongst the usual MPS VI manifestations [1–5]. Poor vision is mainly explained by the corneal changes.

Recently, Lin et al. described retinal pigment epithelium changes in half of the patients with MPS VI [6]. However, the authors do not describe specific fundus characteristics for MPS VI patients, nor do they relate alterations to the OCT changes, that we observed. We hypothesize that scleral thickening and underlying choroidal thinning may result from scleral deposits of glycosaminoglycans. Even though we cannot be sure of the origin of the scleral thinning before a post-mortem analysis, Kenyon et al. in 1972, has described the presence of scleral glycosaminoglycan deposits in post-mortem histology cases [7].

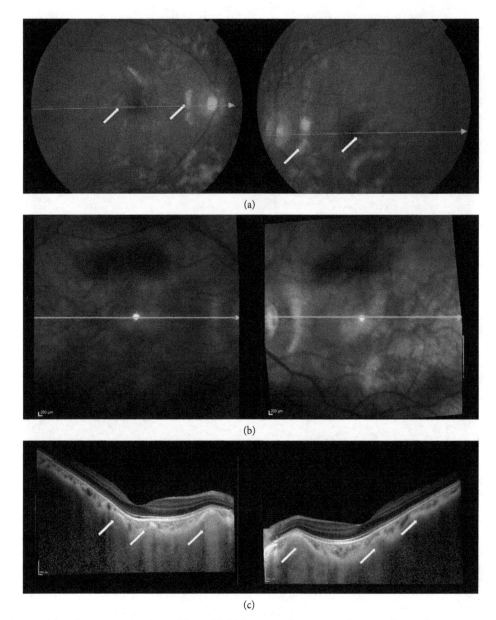

FIGURE 3: (a) Retinographies after penetrating keratoplasty. Multiple areas of orange patches are observed on retinography (arrows). (b) Infrared imaging of the fundus. (c) Enhanced depth imaging optical coherence tomography—the orange patches observed in the retinographies correspond to areas in which deposits of intermediate reflectivity can been seen at the scleral level (white arrows). These lesions are associated with marked choroidal thinning.

The absence of similar case reports in the literature may be due to several reasons. Firstly, these scleral deposits may indeed be uncommon. Secondly, even if present, these deposits are not easily noticed because most patients have severe corneal opacities. Finally, the improved control of systemic comorbidities in the last years increased the life expectancy in these patients, allowing for both the development of new clinical manifestations and a better evaluation of previously unknown characteristics. It is possible that these scleral deposits may be a late manifestation in the course of the disease.

Our patient's retinal and choroid findings have remained stable over the last 2 years; however long-term prognosis of these lesions is still unknown. Due to their external location, they probably will not impair visual function. However, careful follow-up should be advocated in order to detect further changes.

## Disclosure

The study was conducted in the Department of Ophthalmology of São João Hospital, Porto Portugal.

## Authors' Contributions

Augusto Magalhães and Jorge Meira contributed equally to this work and should be considered as equal first authors.

# References

[1] J. L. Ashworth, S. Biswas, E. Wraith, and I. C. Lloyd, "Mucopolysaccharidoses and the eye," *Survey of Ophthalmology*, vol. 51, no. 1, pp. 1–17, 2006.

[2] P. Harmatz, "Mucopolysaccharidosis VI pathophysiology diagnosis and treatment," *Frontiers in Bioscience*, vol. 22, no. 3, pp. 385–406, 2017.

[3] S. Pitz, O. Ogun, L. Arash, E. Miebach, and M. Beck, "Does enzyme replacement therapy influence the ocular changes in type VI mucopolysaccharidosis?" *Graefe's Archive for Clinical and Experimental Ophthalmology*, vol. 247, no. 7, pp. 975–980, 2009.

[4] K. Sornalingam, A. Javed, T. Aslam et al., "Variability in the ocular phenotype in mucopolysaccharidosis," *British Journal of Ophthalmology*, vol. 103, no. 4, pp. 504–510, 2019.

[5] C. Fenzl, K. Teramoto, and M. Moshirfar, "Ocular manifestations and management recommendations of lysosomal storage disorders I: mucopolysaccharidoses," *Clinical Ophthalmology*, pp. 1633–1644, 2015.

[6] H.-Y. Lin, W.-C. Chan, L.-J. Chen et al., "Ophthalmologic manifestations in Taiwanese patients with mucopolysaccharidoses," *Molecular Genetics & Genomic Medicine*, vol. 7, no. 5, p. e00617, 2019.

[7] K. R. Kenyon, T. M. Topping, W. R. Green, and A. E. Maumenee, "Ocular pathology of the Maroteaux-Lamy syndrome (systemic mucopolysaccharidosis type VI). Histologic and ultrastructural report of two cases," *American Journal of Ophthalmology*, vol. 73, no. 5, pp. 718–741, 1972.

# 15

# An Unusual Retinal Vessel Modification in Patients Affected by JIA-Uveitis with a Follow-Up Longer Than 16 Years

Alessandro Abbouda (iD),[1] Irene Abicca,[2] Simone Bruschi (iD),[1] Federico Ricci,[3] Gianluca Aloe (iD),[3] and Maria Pia Paroli (iD)[1]

[1]Department of Ophthalmology, Sapienza University, Umberto I Hospital, Rome, Italy
[2]IRCCS-Fondazione Bietti, Rome, Italy
[3]UOSD Retinal Pathology PTV Foundation Policlinico Tor Vergata University, Rome, Italy

Correspondence should be addressed to Maria Pia Paroli; mpparoli@tiscali.it

Academic Editor: J. Fernando Arevalo

*Purpose.* To report unusual and rare clinical changes of retinal vessel pattern in a series of patients affected by Juvenile Idiopathic Arthritis (JIA) uveitis with a follow-up longer than 16 years. *Methods.* A series of three patients with JIA-uveitis followed at the University of Rome "Sapienza" from 1998 to 2014 were reported. The retinal vessels were analyzed with fluorescein angiography using Heidelberg Retinal Angiogram-2 (HRA-2; Heidelberg Engineering GmBH, Dossenheim, Germany) and the Topcon TRC-50LX retinal camera (Topcon Europe, The Netherlands). A Spectralis Domain OCT (SD-OCT) (Spectralis Family Heidelberg, Germany) was performed to evaluate vessel anatomy. *Results.* Fundus photography showed sheathed vessels localized around the optic disc in every case. Angiography revealed a normal physiology of vessel walls and flow; no sheathing or leakage of dye was observed. SD-OCT demonstrated reflective vessel walls. Vessel lumen appeared patent, and the normal "*hourglass configuration*" was blurred, but identifiable. *Conclusions.* Vessel modifications observed in long-standing JIA-uveitis are not signs of vascular inflammation and are not associated to hypoperfusion. In these cases, ophthalmologists should avoid further invasive investigation and should consider introducing SD-OCT as a routine method to evaluate the vessel changes during the follow-up.

## 1. Introduction

Juvenile Idiopathic Arthritis (JIA) is the most common systemic disease associated with uveitis in childhood. A significant number of patients have already been affected by ocular complications at the time of the diagnosis of uveitis. The ocular complications and visual loss in these patients were investigated in several studies [1–10].

We reported a clinical series of three patients affected by long-term JIA-uveitis with a follow-up of 16 years who developed unusual retinal vessel pattern modifications localized around the optic disc.

## 2. Materials and Method

This study evaluated three patients with diagnosis of JIA-uveitis followed at the University of Rome "Sapienza" from 1998 to 2014. The patients were classified according to the criteria of the International League against Rheumatism (ILAR) [11] and with the International Uveitis Study Group recommendations (IUSG) [12].

Retinal vessels were analyzed with fluorescein angiography using Heidelberg Retinal Angiogram-2 (HRA-2; Heidelberg Engineering GmBH, Dossenheim, Germany) for two patients (cases 1 and 2) and the Topcon TRC-50LX retinal camera (Topcon Europe, The Netherlands) in one patient (case 3). A Spectralis Domain OCT (SD-OCT) (Spectralis Family Acquisition Module, V 5.1.6.0; Heidelberg Engineering, Heidelberg, Germany) was performed to evaluate vessel anatomy [13].

## 3. Case Presentation

Case 1 is a 29-year-old woman with bilateral uveitis onset at 5 years old associated with pauciarticular JIA diagnosed one

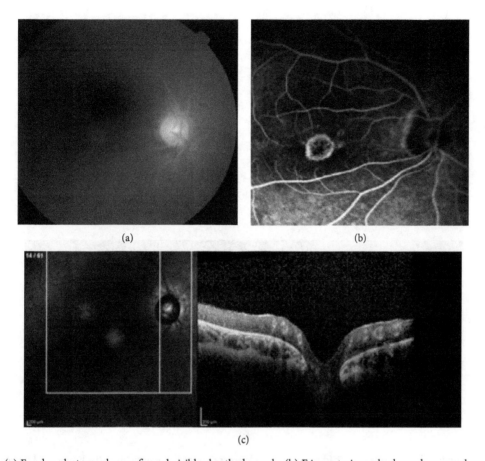

FIGURE 1: Case 1. (a) Fundus photography confirmed visible sheathed vessels. (b) FA; posterior pole showed a normal appearance of vessel walls and flow; no sheathing or leakage of dye was observed at any time. Window effect appears in the foveal area due to atrophy of retinal pigment epithelium subsequent to chronic macular edema. (c) SD-OCT line scan showed very reflective vessel wall. The hyperreflection involves the entire vessel walls, and there is no difference in reflectivity between veins and arteries. Vessel lumen appears patent, and the internal hourglass configuration is blurred, but identifiable.

year before. She referred to our centre at the age of six with bilateral cataract, band keratopathy, and glaucoma. Optic disc edema was detected by ocular B-scan echography. Anti-nuclear antibody (ANA) was positive (1:80) and rheumatoid factor (RF) negative. Haplotype HLA-B27 and DR11 antigens were absent. At the age of ten, phacoemulsification was performed in the right eye. During the follow-up, she developed several episodes of macular edema. To control eye inflammation, topical oral and peribulbar steroids were administered. Glaucoma was managed by topical drops. At 25 years old, right fundus examination underlined a sheathing-like aspect of vessels at the emergence of the optic disc. The left eye was not evaluable due to media opacities. Fundus photography, FA, and SD-OCT were performed (Figure 1).

Case 2 is a 21-year-old woman affected by bilateral JIA- uveitis associated to oligoarthritis since the age of six. She presented at our centre with bilateral cataracts, band keratopathy, and seclusio pupillae. ANA were positive (1:40) and RF negative. The haplotype HLA-B27 and DR11 antigens were positive. At the age of eight, she underwent cataract extraction by pars plana lensectomy with anterior vitrectomy in both eyes. At nine years old, she developed optic disc edema in both eyes with

three months of interval between each one. At the age of eleven, macular edema was diagnosed in the left eye. She was treated with oral, topical, and periocular corticosteroids. When she was 21, fundus evaluation showed sheathed vessels emerging from the optic disc in both eyes (Figure 2).

Case 3 is a 20-year-old woman, diagnosed of bilateral JIA-uveitis since the age of five. Articular involvement occurred when the patient was 11 years old. At the first consultation, she had band keratopathy, seclusio pupillae, cataract, and glaucoma in both eyes. Bilateral optic disc edema was found one month after the onset, and it was confirmed using B-scan echography. HLA-B27 was negative and HLA-DR11 positive. ANA were positive (1:320). Lensectomy with pars plana vitrectomy was performed in both eyes at 7 and 8 years of age. At 10 years old, she underwent trabeculectomy in the left eye. Topical and oral corticosteroids were not enough to control eye inflammation. At 11 years old, oral cyclosporine was started then replaced with methotrexate. It was associated to infliximab two years later. At 16 years old, adalimumab was introduced for articular recrudescence. She was followed up regularly, and when she was 20 years old, sheathed vessels around the optic disc appeared in both eyes (Figure 3).

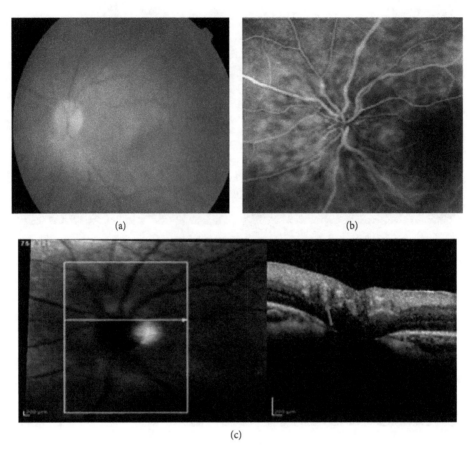

Figure 2: Case 2. (a) Fundus photography described sheathed vessels emerging from the optic disc. (b) FA showed normal vessel walls and flow. (c) The vessel wall reflectivity seemed to be normal or slightly hyperreflective in the SD-OCT linear scan (red arrow).

They all underwent screening tests for systemic vasculitis including antineutrophil cytoplasmic antibodies, anticardiolipin antibody, lupus anticoagulant, anti-DNA antibody, and anti-Ro/SSA and La/SSB antibodies. Screening results were negative in all three cases.

## 4. Discussion

Vasculitic process is not a common feature of this disease, and the differential diagnosis between vasculitis and other vascular modifications is fundamental. FA in active vasculitis includes vascular staining and leakage of dye due to the breakdown of the inner blood-retinal barrier with typical "skip lesions," capillary nonperfusion, retinal neovascularization, and sclerosis of vessels. In our cases, FA evidenced no signs of vascular leakage in both arteries and veins. The process is confined in the area around the optic nerve disc and differs from vasculitis where it is normally located in the middle and peripheral retina. No signs of intraretinal haemorrhages, cotton wool spots, or vascular occlusion were detected.

Normal vessels appear using SD-OCT, with an oval- or round-shaped form and a heterogeneous reflectivity. The top and bottom of the vessel walls, which are vertical to the SD-OCT light source, show the innermost and outermost hyperreflectivity. The interior of vessels shows hourglass-shaped or a double "c" pattern and is due to physiologic blood flow [13, 14]. In our cases, the typical internal hourglass configuration is preserved, indicating that lumen is patent, but consisting diffuse higher reflectivity of the walls was found compared to normal vessels.

Iwasaki et al. [15] described a marked increase and disarrangement of collagen fibrils in the media and adventitia in patients with various vascular diseases. These alterations were associated to the changes on smooth muscle cells and their laminae causing a modification of the transparency of the vessel walls. The lumens of most sheathed vessels were still patent, and the blood cells and endothelial cells appeared to be normal. Regarding our cases, we thought that bilateral optic disc edema during the childhood may induce a progressive collagen fibril disarrangement and confer a sheathed-like aspect to the peripapillary vessels.

Although SD-OCT was a promising additional tool for the assessment of vessel anatomy, it currently can be replaced by swept-source wide-field optical coherence tomography angiography (OCTA). OCTA has the advantage to visualize the blood flow in various layers of the retina without having to inject the dye [16], and recently, capillary nonperfusion in intermediate uveitis has been detected [17]. Unfortunately, when these three patients were followed, OCTA was not available and SD-OCT was the only noninvasive valuable tool for the analysis of sheathed vessels.

SD-OCT optic disc vessel abnormalities in JIA-uveitis patients have not previously been reported in the literature.

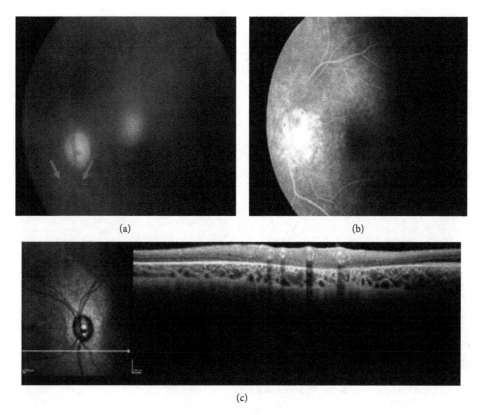

FIGURE 3: Case 3. (a) Sheathed aspect of vessels emerged from the lower bound of the optic nerve head (red arrows), blurred image due to optical opacities. (b) Late stages of the angiogram demonstrate normal fluorescence of the vascular tree. Staining was noted on the inferotemporal border of the optic nerve related to chorioretinal atrophy. (c) SD-OCT scan demonstrated typical internal hourglass configuration and a highly reflective vessel wall in both arterioles and veins.

However, widening of the small peripapillary veins and a significantly larger number of veins without branching were reported in patients with bilateral optic disc edema associated to idiopathic intracranial hypertension and cavernous sinus thrombosis [18].

Overall, based on our cases, we can conclude that SD-OCT could be introduced as a routine study method to evaluate vessel wall reflectivity for the long-term follow-up of JIA- uveitis before performing further investigations.

## References

[1] A. Heiligenhaus, C. Heinz, C. Edelsten, K. Kotaniemi, and K. Minden, "Review for disease of the year: epidemiology of juvenile idiopathic arthritis and its associated uveitis: the probable risk factors," *Ocular Immunology and Inflammation*, vol. 21, no. 3, pp. 180–191, 2013.

[2] A. Heiligenhaus, M. Niewerth, G. Ganser, C. Heinz, K. Minden, and German Uveitis in Childhood Study Group, "Prevalence and complications of uveitis in juvenile idiopathic arthritis in a population-based nation-wide study in Germany: suggested modification of the current screening guidelines," *Rheumatology*, vol. 46, no. 6, pp. 1015–1019, 2007.

[3] Y. Qian and N. R. Acharya, "Juvenile idiopathic arthritis-associated uveitis," *Current Opinion in Ophthalmology*, vol. 21, no. 6, pp. 468–472, 2010.

[4] J. E. Thorne, F. Woreta, S. R. Kedhar, J. P. Dunn, and D. A. Jabs, "Juvenile idiopathic arthritis-associated uveitis: incidence of ocular complications and visual acuity loss," *American Journal of Ophthalmology*, vol. 143, no. 5, pp. 840–846, 2007.

[5] F. Woreta, J. E. Thorne, D. A. Jabs, S. R. Kedhar, and J. P. Dunn, "Risk factors for ocular complications and poor visual acuity at presentation among patients with uveitis associated with juvenile idiopathic arthritis," *American Journal of Ophthalmology*, vol. 143, no. 4, pp. 647–655.e1, 2007.

[6] M. P. Paroli, A. Abbouda, L. Restivo, A. Sapia, I. Abicca, and P. Pivetti Pezzi, "Juvenile idiopathic arthritis-associated uveitis at an Italian tertiary referral center: clinical features and complications," *Ocular Immunology and Inflammation*, vol. 23, no. 1, pp. 74–81, 2015.

[7] B. E. D, E. Cohen, and F. Behar-Cohen, "Uveitis and juvenile idiopathic arthritis: a cohort study," *Clinical Ophthalmology*, vol. 1, no. 4, pp. 513–518, 2007.

[8] A. Skarin, R. Elborgh, E. Edlund, and E. Bengtsson-Stigmar, "Long-term follow-up of patients with uveitis associated with juvenile idiopathic arthritis: a cohort study," *Ocular Immunology and Inflammation*, vol. 17, no. 2, pp. 104–108, 2009.

[9] M. P. Paroli, C. Fabiani, G. Spinucci, I. Abicca, A. Sapia, and L. Spadea, "Severe macular edema in patients with juvenile idiopathic arthritis-related uveitis," *Case Reports in Ophthalmological Medicine*, vol. 2013, Article ID 803989, 5 pages, 2013.

[10] M. Hoeve, V. Kalinina Ayuso, N. E. Schalij-Delfos, L. I. Los, A. Rothova, and J. H. de Boer, "The clinical course of juvenile idiopathic arthritis-associated uveitis in childhood and puberty," *British Journal of Ophthalmology*, vol. 96, no. 6, pp. 852–856, 2012.

[11] L. Berntson, A. Fasth, B. Andersson-Gäre et al., "Construct validity of ILAR and EULAR criteria in juvenile idiopathic arthritis: a population based incidence study from the Nordic countries. International League of Associations for Rheumatology. European League Against Rheumatism," *The Journal of Rheumatology*, vol. 28, no. 12, pp. 2737–2743, 2001.

[12] E. Bloch-Michel and R. B. Nussenblatt, "International Uveitis Study Group recommendations for the evaluation of intraocular inflammatory disease," *American Journal of Ophthalmology*, vol. 103, no. 2, pp. 234-235, 1987.

[13] T. P. Zhu, Y. H. Tong, H. J. Zhan, and J. Ma, "Update on retinal vessel structure measurement with spectral-domain optical coherence tomography," *Microvascular Research*, vol. 95, pp. 7–14, 2014.

[14] Y. Ouyang, Q. Shao, D. Scharf, A. M. Joussen, and F. M. Heussen, "An easy method to differentiate retinal arteries from veins by spectral domain optical coherence tomography: retrospective, observational case series," *BMC Ophthalmology*, vol. 14, no. 1, p. 66, 2014.

[15] M. Iwasaki, T. Ishibashi, H. Inomata, and Y. Taniguchi, "Ultrastructure of sheathed vessels in the retina from patients with various diseases," *Graefe's Archive for Clinical and Experimental Ophthalmology*, vol. 225, no. 3, pp. 177–184, 1987.

[16] R. F. Spaide, J. M. Klancnik Jr., and M. J. Cooney, "Retinal vascular layers imaged by fluorescein angiography and optical coherence Tomography Angiography," *JAMA Ophthalmol*, vol. 133, no. 1, pp. 45–50, 2015.

[17] M. Tian, C. Tappeiner, M. S. Zinkernagel, W. Huf, S. Wolf, and M. R. Munk, "Evaluation of vascular changes in intermediate uveitis and retinal vasculitis using swept-source wide-field optical coherence tomography angiography," *British Journal of Ophthalmology*, vol. 103, no. 9, pp. 1289–1295, 2019.

[18] A. V. Pilat, F. A. Proudlock, R. J. McLean, M. C. Lawden, and I. Gottlob, "Morphology of retinal vessels in patients with optic nerve head drusen and optic disc edema," *Investigative Opthalmology & Visual Science*, vol. 55, no. 6, pp. 3484–3490, 2014.

# 16

# Arnold-Chiari Malformation Type II and CYP1B1 Congenital Glaucoma: A Possible Association

**Shaikha Aldossari**⊙,[1] **Amani Al Bakri**⊙,[1] and **Yumna Kamal**⊙[2]

[1]*King Khaled Eye Specialist Hospital, Riyadh, Saudi Arabia*
[2]*King Abdulaziz University, Jeddah, Saudi Arabia*

Correspondence should be addressed to Yumna Kamal; ykamal0001@stu.kau.edu.sa

Academic Editor: Cristiano Giusti

*Background.* We describe a case of an infant with Arnold-Chiari Malformation Type II (ACM-II) who was born with lumbosacral myelomeningocele, hydrocephalus, and primary congenital glaucoma (PCG) together with dysmorphic features (scaphocephaly, frontal bossing, hypotelorism, entropion, and flat nasal bridge), which according to our knowledge, is a combination that has yet to be described in literature. *Primary diagnosis.* A 2-year-old female who is known to have ACM-II was referred due to abnormal eye examination done in a peripheral hospital that suggested infantile glaucoma in both eyes. *Findings.* During her last physical exam (postop), she was vitally stable, conscious with good feeding. Ophthalmic assessment revealed buphthalmia, superior paracentral scar, deep anterior chambers (AC), and round pupils with positive red reflex, clear lens, and an IOP of 16, 14 mm Hg, respectively. Neurological exam showed paraparesis and moving upper extremities and has axial hypotonia. Genetic testing showed CYP1B1 gene mutation. *Conclusion.* The aim of reporting this case is to share the findings in this infant as it may be a new association. The main learning message here is that ACM-II patients may present with certain ocular symptoms, including glaucoma-related ones that may mimic neurological disorders. This report brings information that could alert general practitioners, neurologists, and neurosurgeons. A deeper understanding of this rare disorder may aid the diagnosis of cases with similar characteristic physical findings by referring them to an ophthalmology clinic for further evaluation. *Case presentation.* A 2-year-old female who is known to have Arnold Chiari Malformation Type II (ACM- II) was referred due to abnormal eye examination done in a peripheral hospital that suggested infantile glaucoma in both eyes. MRI at 3 months of age showed lumbosacral myelomeningocele and hydrocephalus. Genetic testing confirmed a CYP1B1 mutation. These combinations of symptoms were never described in the literature before.

## 1. Introduction

Chiari malformations are a result of multifactorial etiology, mainly genetic and environmental ones. They are classified based on their morphology and severity of anatomic defects. Chiari I malformation is characterized by abnormally shaped cerebellar tonsils that are displaced below the level of the foramen magnum. Type II, also known as Arnold Chiari Malformation (ACM), is when both the cerebellum and brainstem pass through foramen magnum in the presence of spina bifida. This type has been reported to co-occur with known genetic syndromes involving but not limited to trisomy 18 [1]. Primary pediatric glaucomas are subdivided into many subtypes, one of which is primary congenital glaucoma (PCG) which is defined as the presence of isolated abnormal trabecular meshwork (TM) during first three years of life [2]. It is inherited in an autosomal recessive pattern. Due to the high rate of consanguinity in Saudi Arabia, PCG was found to be highly prevalent, especially those caused by CYP1B1 mutations [3]. The two main genes linked to PCG are cytochrome P450 1B1 gene (CYP1B1) within GLC3A locus and LTBP2 within GLC3C locus. The only two ophthalmic findings that were reported in the literature to be associated with Arnold Chiari Malformation Type II are abnormal ocular motility with impairment of smooth pursuit [4, 5].

## 2. Case Report

A 2-year-old female who is known to have Arnold Chiari Malformation Type II was referred due to abnormal eye examination done in a peripheral hospital that suggested infantile glaucoma in both eyes for which she was put on topical Xolamol and Travatan.

She was born to a healthy 18-year-old woman who had an uncomplicated pregnancy course apart from oligohydramnios at 35 weeks' gestation (amniotic fluid index: 7.7 cm, deepest pool 4.3 cm). Mother denied taking folic acid supplementation before or during first trimester. The patient is a product of full-term cesarean section due to breach presentation and large head size. Good APGAR score 6 and 8 at 1 and 5 minutes, respectively, admitted to NICU for myelomeningocele and hydrocephalus. No history of seizures, developmental delays, or neurological disorders in her family. MRI at 3 months of age showed lumbosacral myelomeningocele and hydrocephalus. Ventriculoperitoneal (VP) shunt was inserted at 2 weeks of age and followed by repair of dorsolumbar myelomeningocele at 3 months of age.

During her last physical exam (postop), she was vitally stable, conscious with good feeding. Ophthalmic assessment revealed buphthalmia, superior paracentral scar, deep anterior chambers (AC), and round pupils with positive red reflex and clear lens, and IOP was 16, 14 mm Hg, respectively. Neurological exam showed paraparesis, moving upper extremities, and has axial hypotonia. Skin evaluation revealed large scar of surgery in the posterior dorsolumbar area from repaired meningomyelocele.

The rest of her physical examination was unremarkable. Patient was in good general condition without any distress. She had abnormally shaped head (scaphocephaly). Anterior fontanel was open and flat. VP shunt present. Tympanic membranes and throat were clear. There was no lymphadenopathy. Chest was clear to auscultation, and no rhonchi or crepitations were heard.

On examination, the patiemt had regular heart rate and rhythm without murmurs, a soft and non-tender abdomen, no organomegaly, and normal extremities.

Axial eye length (AEL) is as follows: OD 24.50 mm and OS 25.18 mm. Lab results showed relative neutropenia of 23% (normal: 40–74%). Genetic testing confirmed CYP1B1 mutation.

Deep sclerectomy (DS) was done at 5 months of age (December 2018) for both eyes at different times, one week apart. Micropulse CPC OD was done at the age of 19 months (February 2020). 11 days post-DS, she developed bilateral shallow choroidal detachment with macular involvement from 7.30 to 10.30 extending from disc to almost anterior equator in the right eye and from 1.30 to 4.30 extending from disc to almost anterior equator (except superior temporally to posterior equator only) in the left eye. Plan was to examine her under sedation in two weeks, and she was put on Pred Forte (prednisolone acetate ophthalmic suspension every 4 hours and Atropine twice daily OU.

One-month post-DS, IOP was digitally high and unmeasurable by the Tonopen due to high reading, and pupil was mid-dilated. B-scan showed bilateral optic disc cupping worse in the left eye and resolution of choroidal detachment. This could either indicate that she is a steroid responder or surgery failure due to dilation. Plan was to taper PF, stop atropine, and start antiglaucoma medication.

Despite adequate compliance to full topical antiglaucoma medications, IOP readings remained continuously high upon follow up in the right eye. At age 29 months (December 2020), patient underwent surgery to insert Aurolab aqueous drainage implant (AAIDI Valve) OD.

Post-AAIDI, the patient was doing well. IOP improved but remained high, patient continued Xolamol OD and Travatan.

The rest of her clinical course was unremarkable to date.

## 3. Discussion

Arnold Chiari Malformation Type II (ACM-II) has many etiologies, one of which is of genetic bases as it was linked to certain genetic syndromes 1. Primary congenital glaucoma occurs most commonly in a sporadic fashion, and only about 10-40% were found to be familial and of autosomal dominant inheritance pattern [6].

In our patient, genetic testing confirmed a cytochrome P4501B1 (CYP1B1) gene mutation, which is present on GLC3A loci. This gene was the first gene to be reported as a cause of primary congenital glaucoma [7, 8].

These two entities might have a possible association since both have genetic bases. A study found that 97 out of 126 Arnold Chiari Malformation patients had ocular disturbances [9], mainly nystagmus, since 70% of Arnold Chiari Malformation patients had it in another study [10], specifically, downbeat nystagmus [11].

When it comes to type II, the only ophthalmic finding that was reported in the literature to be associated with Arnold Chiari Malformation Type II was abnormal ocular motility with impairment of smooth pursuit [4, 5].

However, for type I, previous studies reveal a wider range of clinical findings that involved decreased visual acuity in both eyes [12], restricted eye movement [12], rotational nystagmus [12], megalocornea [12], stage II bilateral papilledema [12], synechial angle-closure glaucoma [13], and acquired esotropia [14].

Although a single case reported glaucoma development in a patient with (ACM-I) [15], another one denied the presence of goniodysgenesis or high IOP in a patient with the same type of malformation [12].

To date, the effect of Arnold Chiari Malformation Type II on iridocorneal angle structures was not described in the literature before, whether these two entities are related to each other or it was a coincidence is still in question.

## Additional Points

*Literature Search.* Databases searched were mainly PubMed and Google Scholar, and search terms used were Arnold-Chiari Malformation Type II (ACM-II), primary congenital glaucoma (PCG), dysmorphic features, and syndrome. Years covered were from 1977 to 2020.

## Consent

Informed consent and IRB approval were obtained.

## Acknowledgments

Special thanks are due to Dr. Amani Al Bakri (Chief of Pediatric Ophthalmology Division at King Khaled Eye Specialist Hospital) who kindly provided necessary editing and guidance in writing this report.

## References

[1] R. S. Tubbs, M. Hill, M. Loukas, M. M. Shoja, and W. J. Oakes, "Volumetric analysis of the posterior cranial fossa in a family with four generations of the Chiari malformation type I," *Journal of Neurosurgery. Pediatrics*, vol. 1, no. 1, pp. 21–24, 2008.

[2] O. B. Badeeb, *Congenital Glaucoma in Saudi Arabia*, King Abdulaziz University press, Jeddah, 2011.

[3] O. M. Badeeb, S. Micheal, R. K. Koenekoop, A. I. den Hollander, and M. T. Hedrawi, "CYP1B1 mutations in patients with primary congenital glaucoma from Saudi Arabia," *BMC Medical Genetics*, vol. 15, no. 1, p. 109, 2014.

[4] M. S. Salman, M. Dennis, and J. A. Sharpe, "The cerebellar dysplasia of Chiari II malformation as revealed by eye movements," *The Canadian Journal of Neurological Sciences*, vol. 36, no. 6, pp. 713–724, 2009.

[5] M. S. Salman, J. A. Sharpe, L. Lillakas, M. J. Steinbach, and M. Dennis, "Smooth ocular pursuit in Chiari type II malformation," *Developmental Medicine & Child Neurology*, vol. 49, no. 4, pp. 289–293, 2007.

[6] C. J. Lewis, A. Hedberg-Buenz, A. P. DeLuca, E. M. Stone, W. L. M. Alward, and J. H. Fingert, "Primary congenital and developmental glaucomas," *Human Molecular Genetics*, vol. 26, no. R1, pp. R28–R36, 2017.

[7] R. N. Weinreb, A. L. Grajewski, M. Papadopoulos, J. Grigg, and S. F. Freedman, *Childhood glaucoma: The 9th Consensus Report of the World Glaucoma Association*, Kugler Publications, Netherlands, 2013.

[8] B. A. Bejjani, L. Xu, D. Armstrong, J. R. Lupski, and L. W. Reneker, "Expression Patterns of Cytochrome P4501B1 (Cyp1b1) in FVB/N Mouse Eyes," *Experimental Eye Research*, vol. 75, no. 3, pp. 249–257, 2002.

[9] T. H. Milhorat, M. W. Chou, E. M. Trinidad et al., "Chiari I malformation Redefined: clinical and radiographic findings for 364 symptomatic patients," *Neurosurgery*, vol. 44, no. 5, pp. 1005–1017, 1999.

[10] B. H. Dobkin, "The adult Chiari malformation," *Bulletin of the Los Angeles Neurological Societies*, vol. 42, no. 1, pp. 23–27, 1977.

[11] A. H. Menezes, W. R. K. Smoker, and G. N. Dyste, "Syringomyelia, Chiari malformations, and hydromyelia, chapter 46," in *Neurological Surgery*, J. R. Youmans, Ed., pp. 1421–1459, W B Saunders Co, Philadelphia, 3rd ed. edition, 1990.

[12] M. Imane, M. Asmae, R. Toufik, and S. Rachid, "Œdème papillaire revelant une malformation d'Arnold Chiari type 1: à propos d'un cas," *The Pan African Medical Journal*, vol. 24, p. 293, 2016.

[13] L. R. Dagi and D. S. Walton, "Anterior Axial Lens Subluxation, Progressive Myopia, and Angle-Closure Glaucoma: Recognition and Treatment of Atypical Presentation of Ectopia Lentis," *Journal of American Association for Pediatric Ophthalmology and Strabismus*, vol. 10, no. 4, pp. 345–350, 2006.

[14] A. R. Lewis, L. B. Kline, and J. A. Sharpe, "Acquired esotropia due to Arnold-Chiari I malformation," *Journal of Neuro-Ophthalmology*, vol. 16, no. 1, pp. 49???54–49???54, 1996.

[15] E. Schijman, "History, anatomic forms, and pathogenesis of Chiari I malformations," *Child's Nervous System*, vol. 20, no. 5, pp. 323–328, 2004.

# 17

# Neovascular Glaucoma from Ocular Ischemic Syndrome Treated with Serial Monthly Intravitreal Bevacizumab and Panretinal Photocoagulation: A Case Report

**Hassaan Asif⊙, Zhuangjun Si⊙, Steven Quan, Pathik Amin, David Dao, Lincoln Shaw, Dimitra Skondra, and Mary Qiu⊙**

*Department of Ophthalmology and Visual Science, University of Chicago, Chicago, Illinois, USA*

Correspondence should be addressed to Mary Qiu; mary.qiu@gmail.com

Academic Editor: Kevin J. Blinder

*Purpose.* To describe a case of open-angle neovascular glaucoma (NVG) secondary to ocular ischemic syndrome (OIS) treated with a planned series of 6 monthly anti-VEGF injections with interspersed panretinal photocoagulation (PRP) sessions. We term this treatment protocol the Salvaging Conventional Outflow Pathway in Neovascular Glaucoma (SCOPING) Protocol, and this is our (MQ and DS) standard of care for all NVG patients presenting with partially or completely open angles. *Case.* A 66-year-old man's right eye had a visual acuity of 20/50, intraocular pressure (IOP) of 42 mmHg on 0 IOP-lowering medications, and neovascularization of the iris and angle with no peripheral anterior synechiae. Fundoscopy revealed midperipheral dot-blot hemorrhages without diabetic retinopathy or vein occlusion. Fluorescein angiography revealed peripheral retinal nonperfusion in both eyes. The patient was diagnosed with open-angle NVG secondary to OIS and treated with 6 serial monthly anti-VEGF injections interspersed with 4 PRP sessions, after which his anterior segment neovascularization regressed and IOP normalized on 0 medications. Ten weeks after the last injection, the anterior segment neovascularization and elevated IOP recurred, so he underwent 4 more monthly anti-VEGF injections and 4 PRP sessions, after which his anterior segment neovascularization regressed and his IOP normalized on 0 medications. However, 6 weeks after the last injection, the anterior segment neovascularization and elevated IOP again recurred, so he was resumed on a third course of lifetime monthly anti-VEGF injections, which may be continued in perpetuity. *Conclusion.* The patient's NVG was quiescent while under the protection of serial anti-VEGF injections with interspersed PRP; however, the disease recurred each time injections were stopped. Therefore, in patients with open-angle NVG secondary to OIS, serial monthly anti-VEGF injections may be necessary combined with PRP to suppress underlying neovascular drive and regress anterior segment neovascularization, maintain physiologic IOP, and prevent synechial angle closure.

## 1. Introduction

Neovascular glaucoma (NVG) is characterized by neovascular proliferation in the anterior segment, specifically the angle (NVA) and iris (NVI), that obstructs aqueous outflow through the trabecular meshwork and closes the angle. Intraocular pressure (IOP) can become profoundly elevated and visual outcomes can be devastating [1]. The underlying etiologies for NVG are conditions that cause retinal ischemia, the two most common being proliferative diabetic retinopathy (PDR) and retinal vein occlusion (RVO) [2].

The third most common etiology is ocular ischemic syndrome (OIS), which is often caused by ipsilateral carotid artery stenosis leading to decreased ocular perfusion [3].

For NVG secondary to PDR or RVO, panretinal photocoagulation (PRP) has been the gold standard treatment to reduce angiogenic signals from the peripheral retina and regress anterior segment neovascularization [4]. In recent years, antivascular endothelial growth factor (VEGF) injections have been shown to promptly regress anterior segment neovascularization within days of administration and have been combined with PRP to treat NVG from PDR and

RVO [5–9]. However, there is a paucity of data regarding the therapeutic effects of anti-VEGF and/or PRP in NVG specifically secondary to OIS.

This case report of a patient with NVG secondary to OIS describes the novel strategy of administering a planned series of 6 monthly anti-VEGF injections with multiple sessions of PRP scheduled in between the injections, so the anti-VEGF injections can provide prompt and sustained antineovascular effect for 6 months until full dense PRP can be performed and take effect. We term this treatment protocol the Salvaging Conventional Outflow Pathway in Neovascular Glaucoma (SCOPING) Protocol, and this is our (MQ and DS) standard of care for all NVG patients presenting with partially or completely open angles.

## 2. Case Presentation

A 66-year-old White man with a history of hyperlipidemia, hypertension, and coronary artery disease with angioplasty and stenting presented to the ophthalmology clinic for a routine eye exam. The right eye (OD) had a history of pars plana vitrectomy for epiretinal membrane 3 years prior and subsequent uncomplicated cataract surgery 6 months afterward. He used no ocular medications at baseline. He reported no visual complaints, pain, discomfort, photophobia, redness, or headache. His visual acuity (VA) was 20/50 OD and 20/20 OS with -6.5 diopter glasses. The IOP was 47 mmHg OD and 15 mmHg OS. The anterior segment exam OD revealed a clear cornea without microcystic edema, a deep and quiet anterior chamber without hyphema, NVI at the pupil margin in multiple locations, NVA throughout an otherwise open angle with no peripheral anterior synechiae (PAS), and a 1 piece PCIOL in the capsular bag with mild posterior capsule opacity (PCO). The anterior segment exam OS was unremarkable with a clear cornea, deep and quiet anterior chamber, no NVI or NVA, and 2+ nuclear sclerosis. The fundus exam of both eyes revealed tilted myopic nerves with a symmetric cup-to-disc ratio of 0.5 in both eyes and a full neuroretinal rim for 360 degrees in both eyes with no focal rim changes that would suggest glaucomatous optic neuropathy in either eye. There was no macular edema, no exudates, no flame-shaped hemorrhages, attenuated but nontortuous retinal vasculature without visible neovascularization at the disc (NVD) or elsewhere (NVE), and mid-peripheral dot blot hemorrhages (DBH) in both eyes (Figure 1). The fundus exam was not consistent with PDR or RVO, and OIS was suspected.

The glaucoma service was consulted, and the patient received 3 rounds of timolol, dorzolamide, and brimonidine in the right eye and 500 mg oral acetazolamide; the IOP improved to 16 mmHg 2 hours later. The retina service was consulted, and fluorescein angiography demonstrated profound peripheral retinal non-perfusion in both eyes with no NVD or NVE (Figure 2). The patient was diagnosed with open-angle NVG secondary to OIS in the right eye and underwent prompt intravitreal injection with 1.25 mg (0.05 ml) bevacizumab (IVB) that day.

The antineovascular branch of the treatment plan with the retina service (DS) was to administer at least 6 monthly

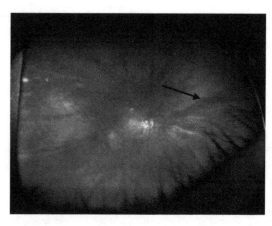

FIGURE 1: Optos fundus photo shows midperipheral retinal hemorrhages in the right eye.

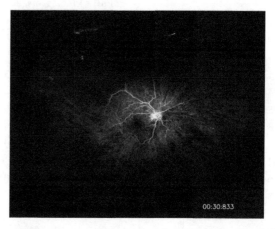

FIGURE 2: Fluorescein angiography at 30 seconds shows peripheral nonperfusion and prolonged filling time.

IVB injections, with multiple sessions of PRP (PASCAL argon laser, Retina 200 lens, parameters described in Table 1) scheduled in between the IVB injections, until the PRP was deemed to be complete. At that point, the IVB injections would be stopped, and the glaucoma service would monitor him for any recurrent anterior segment neovascularization or elevated IOP.

The IOP-control branch of the treatment plan with the glaucoma service (MQ) was to initiate 3 topical IOP-lowering medications (dorzolamide-timolol and brimonidine) and subsequently escalate medical therapy if needed. If the IOP were to become uncontrolled despite maximum tolerated medical therapy and the anterior segment neovascularization was fully regressed at that time, then an angle-based procedure such as gonioscopy-assisted transluminal trabeculotomy would be offered in an attempt to surgically salvage the conventional outflow pathway (consistent with SCOPING Protocol goals) and avoid or delay an aqueous shunt or cyclophotocoagulation, if possible.

A systemic work-up to identify the source of the OIS was performed by the vascular neurology service. A computed tomography angiography demonstrated atherosclerotic calcifications along the bilateral petrous, cavernous, and

TABLE 1: Details of antineovascular and intraocular pressure treatment course of the right eye.

| Weeks after presentation | Treatment | IOP (mmHg) | # Meds | Service(s) |
|---|---|---|---|---|
| First Course | | | | |
| 0 | IVB #1 | 42 | 0 | O->G->R |
| 1 | None | 9 | 3 | G |
| 4 | IVB #2 | 10 | 2 | R |
| 5 | None | 10 | 2 | G |
| 6 | PRP #1 (1118 spots, 225 mW) | 19 | 0 | R |
| 8 | IVB #3 | 19 | 0 | R |
| 10 | PRP #2 (596 spots, 275 mW) | 21 | 0 | R |
| 12 | IVB #4 | 17 | 0 | R |
| 14 | PRP #3 (193 spots, 225 mW) | N/A | 0 | R |
| 16 | IVB #5 | 14 | 0 | R |
| 20 | IVB #6 | 15 | 0 | R |
| 22 | PRP #4 (462 spots, 200 mW) | N/A | 0 | R |
| 24 | None | 19 | 0 | G |
| Second Course | | | | |
| 30 | IVB #1 | 22 | 0 | G->R |
| 31 | PRP #1 (322 spots, 375 mW) | 16 | 0 | R |
| 34 | IVB #2 | 16 | 0 | R |
| 35 | PRP #2 (411 spots, 200 mW) | 13 | 0 | R |
| 38 | IVB #3 | 10 | 0 | R |
| 40 | PRP #3 (560 spots, 200 mW) | N/A | 0 | R |
| 42 | IVB #4 | 18 | 0 | R |
| 46 | PRP #4 (866 spots, 200 mW) | 22 | 0 | R |
| 48 | None | 20 | 0 | G |
| Third Course | | | | |
| 52 | IVB #1 | 27 | 0 | R |
| 54 | None | 14 | 1 | G |
| 56 | IVB #2 | 13 | 0 | R |
| Future | Ongoing serial monthly IVB | | | |

IVB: intravitreal bevacizumab 1.25 mg in 0.05 ml; PRP: panretinal photocoagulation; O: optometry; G: glaucoma; R: retina spot size for PRP was 400 microns in the first course of treatment and 200 microns in the 2nd course of treatment. Duration was 0.5-0.7 seconds.

supraclinoid internal carotid artery (ICA) segments, with multifocal mild and moderate stenoses most pronounced along the bilateral supraclinoid ICA segments. However, the patient was not recommended to pursue neurovascular intervention.

Between Week 0 and Week 22 inclusive, the patient underwent the SCOPING protocol with 6 serial monthly IVB injections interspersed with 4 PRP sessions (Table 1). One day after IVB#1, the visual acuity was still 20/50, the IOP was down from 42 mmHg to 19 mmHg on two IOP-lowering medications, and gonioscopy revealed regressing NVA and no PAS. Throughout the treatment course, the IOP remained physiologic in the teens, even without any IOP-lowering medications after Week 5. He underwent laser capsulotomy at Week 10 for visually significant PCO. At Week 24, two weeks after the SCOPING treatment series, the visual acuity had improved to 20/20, the IOP was 19 mmHg, and gonioscopy revealed fully regressed NVA and no PAS. At this point, his conventional outflow pathway was considered to be "medically salvaged," and no further antineovascular treatment was recommended by the retina

service. He was counseled to continue follow-up with the glaucoma service in 6 weeks.

When the patient presented for follow-up at Week 30, the IOP had risen to 22 mmHg, and gonioscopy revealed recurrent trace NVA in all quadrants and no PAS. He was diagnosed with recurrent anterior segment neovascularization in the setting of stopping serial anti-VEGF injections and underwent a second course of treatment consisting of 4 monthly IVBs and 4 PRP sessions. Only 4 IVBs were planned for this second course rather than 6 because the retina service considered this recurrence to be less severe than the initial presentation. At Week 34, the visual acuity was stable at 20/20, and the IOP was 16 mmHg on no IOP-lowering medications. At Week 38, the IOP was down to 10 mmHg. On Week 48, two weeks after his second course of treatment, the visual acuity was 20/20, the IOP was 20 mmHg, and there was only trace regressing NVA in 2 quadrants on gonioscopy. His conventional outflow pathway was still considered to be "medically salvaged," in line with the goals of the SCOPING protocol.

When the patient followed up four weeks later at Week 52, the IOP was elevated at 27 mmHg with new NVI and NVA. Considering the repeated recurrent anterior segment neovascularization with elevated IOP, despite a total of 10 IVB injections and more than 4000 total spots of PRP over the span of 52 weeks, the retina service recommended a third "course" of treatment, this time with serial monthly IVB injections in perpetuity (Table 1). Two weeks after IVB#1 of this third series, his IOP was 14 mmHg on one IOP-lowering medication, and the NVI and NVA had regressed yet again. The patient's timolol was stopped, and he was recommended to follow-up with retina monthly in perpetuity for serial monthly IVB injections. At the next retina follow-up visit at Week 56, which is his most recent follow-up to date, the VA OD was still 20/20, and the IOP OD was 13 on 0 IOP-lowering medications. The patient underwent the next IVB injection as planned, and his conventional outflow pathway is still considered to be "medically salvaged."

## 3. Discussion

For decades, PRP has been the mainstay treatment for NVG, as it has been shown to reverse anterior segment neovascularization and bring elevated IOP levels back to baseline if the angle is not already completely synechially closed [4]. More recently, anti-VEGF injections, including bevacizumab, have been shown to provide rapid-onset antineovascular effects, including regression of anterior segment neovascularization and reduction of IOP if the angle is not already synechially closed [10–12]. However, there is a paucity of literature regarding the treatment of NVG specifically secondary to OIS using PRP and/or anti-VEGF injections. One paper reports that PRP might be viable for patients with neovascularization secondary to common carotid artery occlusion, and another reports that IVB rapidly reduces NVI in patients with OIS [13, 14].

Furthermore, OIS complicates otherwise well-established treatments for NVG. Only 36% of patients with OIS and open angles have regressed NVI and IOP control after PRP [15]. One study did not find retinal capillary dropout in any eyes with OIS, even in patients with diabetes mellitus. Because FA-proven retinal capillary dropout prompts the usage of PRP in cases of NVG secondary to PDR, this suggests that PRP may not always be indicated in cases of NVG secondary to OIS [16]. However, in OIS eyes with FA-proven retinal non-perfusion, PRP is still the preferred treatment [17].

Recently, there have been many studies in the literature regarding using a combination of PRP and anti-VEGF injections for treating NVG. In a study by Ehlers et al., all 11 patients who received same-day IVB and PRP had regressed neovascularization, whereas only 2 of 12 patients who received PRP-alone had regressed neovascularization at an average follow-up of 118 and 143 days, respectively ($p < 0.001$) [5]. The combination group also had better IOP control at follow-up ($p < 0.005$). Of these patients, 3 in the combination group and 4 in the PRP-alone group had OIS. Another retrospective case series by Vasudev et al.

reports similar results, comparing 14 eyes that received PRP within 1 week of IVB and 15 that received PRP-alone [7]. At 1-month follow-up, the combination group had more regression of NVI than the PRP-alone group ($p < 0.005$), and at 6-month follow-up, the combination group had a significantly lower IOP than the PRP-alone group ($p < 0.05$). In this study, only 1 eye in the combination group had OIS. Other studies utilizing a combination of PRP and anti-VEGF have also reported prompt regression of NVI and IOP control [6, 8, 9]. To date, there are no studies in the literature focused on the combination of PRP and anti-VEGF in treating NVG secondary to OIS, especially not any studies that stratify outcomes by angle status.

In this report, we describe our strategy of treating NVG secondary to OIS with 2 courses of serial monthly IVB adjunced with numerous PRP sessions. The quick regression of this patient's anterior segment neovascularization is likely due to the rapid mechanism-of-action of bevacizumab that has previously been reported. The patient's IOP promptly improved from 42 mmHg on 0 IOP-lowering medications on the day of the acute presentation to 19 mmHg on 0 IOP-lowering medications 1 day after the first injection. Out of an abundance of caution, the patient was kept on 2-3 classes of IOP-lowering medications for the first 5 weeks, but it is likely that his IOP would have remained physiologic in this first month even without any IOP-lowering medications, since the therapeutic effects of each IVB lasts approximately 1 month.

Of note, even after multiple sessions of PRP totaling over 4000 spots, when the IVBs were halted for more than 4 weeks after the first and second course of the SCOPING treatment protocol, there was recurrence of anterior segment neovascularization and elevated IOP. Each time, resumption of IVBs rapidly normalized the IOP and induced rapid regression of the anterior segment neovascularization. Fortunately, no PAS developed, and the angle still remained 100% open during this time frame. This case suggests that full dense PRP in the setting of his OIS was not sufficient to completely and permanently suppress the underlying neovascular drive, and he may require ongoing serial monthly IVBs in perpetuity to keep the disease quiescent. Our observations suggest that in patients with NVG secondary to OIS (in contrast to PDR and RVO), regression of neovascularization and IOP control may largely depend on serial anti-VEGF injections, and full dense PRP may not be adequately effective. This conclusion also depends on the angle being mostly open upon presentation, because if the angle were already mostly synechially closed upon presentation, then anti-neovascular treatments, whether it be PRP or anti-VEGF injections, would not be expected to lower the IOP.

There are numerous limitations to this case report. This patient is scheduled to undergo serial monthly IVB in perpetuity, so follow-up exams including monitoring for anterior segment neovascularization and elevated IOP are needed to determine long-term effectiveness of this treatment strategy. Additionally, future studies are needed with larger treatment groups to confirm our findings, but this can be challenging due to the relatively rare nature of NVG secondary to OIS. Importantly, this patient presented with a 100% open angle, so all findings in this report may only be pertinent to patients with open-angle NVG secondary to OIS. More evidence is needed regarding the best treatment strategy in eyes with NVG secondary to OIS presenting with angles that are already partially or totally synechially closed. This highlights the need for an updated standardized nomenclature for various stages of NVG to help clinicians and researchers better categorize their broad spectrum of "NVG" patients for both research trials and clinical practice [18].

In conclusion, antineovascular treatment plans combining prompt serial monthly anti-VEGF injections with interspersed PRP can rapidly reverse anterior segment neovascularization and may provide long-term IOP control and prevent progressive synechial angle closure in patients with open-angle NVG secondary to OIS. This may prove to be an effective alternative for patients that have previously undergone PRP-alone without sustained success. If there is a planned hiatus of more than 4 weeks between antineovascular treatments with the retina service, close follow-up is recommended with an anterior segment service (glaucoma, comprehensive) to monitor for recurrent anterior segment neovascularization and elevated IOP in the absence of serial monthly IVBs in perpetuity.

## Consent

Written consent to publish this case report was obtained from the patient.

## Acknowledgments

Funding for the publication of this work was provided by the University of Chicago Bucksbaum Institute for Clinical Excellence (JE95793).

## References

[1] S. J. Havens and V. Gulati, "Neovascular glaucoma," *Developments in Ophthalmology*, vol. 55, pp. 196–204, 2016.

[2] S. Senthil, T. Dada, T. Das et al., "Neovascular glaucoma - a review," *Indian Journal of Ophthalmology*, vol. 69, no. 3, pp. 525–534, 2021.

[3] B. Terelak-Borys, K. Skonieczna, and I. Grabska-Liberek, "Ocular ischemic syndrome - a systematic review," *Medical Science Monitor*, vol. 18, no. 8, pp. RA138–RA144, 2012.

[4] L. C. Olmos and R. K. Lee, "Medical and surgical treatment of neovascular glaucoma," *International Ophthalmology Clinics*, vol. 51, no. 3, pp. 27–36, 2011.

[5] J. P. Ehlers, M. J. Spirn, A. Lam, A. Sivalingam, M. A. Samuel, and W. Tasman, "Combination intravitreal bevacizumab/panretinal photocoagulation versus panretinal photocoagulation alone in the treatment of neovascular glaucoma," *Retina*, vol. 28, no. 5, pp. 696–702, 2008.

[6] M. E. Gheith, G. A. Siam, D. S. de Barros, S. J. Garg, and M. R. Moster, "Role of intravitreal bevacizumab in neovascular glaucoma," *Journal of Ocular Pharmacology and Therapeutics*, vol. 23, no. 5, pp. 487–491, 2007.

[7] D. Vasudev, M. P. Blair, J. Galasso, R. Kapur, and T. Vajaranant, "Intravitreal bevacizumab for neovascular glaucoma," *Journal of Ocular Pharmacology and Therapeutics*, vol. 25, no. 5, pp. 453–458, 2009.

[8] S. Ciftci, Y. B. Sakalar, K. Unlu, U. Keklikci, I. Caca, and E. Dogan, "Intravitreal bevacizumab combined with panretinal photocoagulation in the treatment of open angle neovascular glaucoma," *European Journal of Ophthalmology*, vol. 19, no. 6, pp. 1028–1033, 2009.

[9] L. C. Olmos, M. S. Sayed, A. L. Moraczewski et al., "Long-term outcomes of neovascular glaucoma treated with and without intravitreal bevacizumab," *Eye (London, England)*, vol. 30, no. 3, pp. 463–472, 2016.

[10] A. L. Moraczewski, R. K. Lee, P. F. Palmberg, P. J. Rosenfeld, and W. J. Feuer, "Outcomes of treatment of neovascular glaucoma with intravitreal bevacizumab," *British Journal of Ophthalmology*, vol. 93, no. 5, pp. 589–593, 2009.

[11] T. Wakabayashi, Y. Oshima, H. Sakaguchi et al., "Intravitreal bevacizumab to treat iris neovascularization and neovascular glaucoma secondary to ischemic retinal diseases in 41 consecutive cases," *Ophthalmology*, vol. 115, no. 9, pp. 1571–1580.e3, 2008.

[12] S. Duch, O. Buchacra, E. Milla, D. Andreu, and J. Tellez, "Intracameral bevacizumab (Avastin) for neovascular glaucoma," *Journal of Glaucoma*, vol. 18, no. 2, pp. 140–143, 2009.

[13] J. E. Carter, "Panretinal photocoagulation for progressive ocular neovascularization secondary to occlusion of the common carotid artery," *Annals of Ophthalmology*, vol. 16, no. 6, pp. 572–576, 1984.

[14] L. Amselem, J. Montero, M. Diaz-Llopis et al., "Intravitreal bevacizumab (Avastin) injection in ocular ischemic syndrome," *American Journal of Ophthalmology*, vol. 144, no. 1, pp. 122–124, 2007.

[15] G. Sood and A. B. Siddik, *Ocular ischemic syndrome*, StatPearls Publishing, Treasure Island (FL), 2022.

[16] J. B. Mizener, P. Podhajsky, and S. S. Hayreh, "Ocular ischemic syndrome," *Ophthalmology*, vol. 104, no. 5, pp. 859–864, 1997.

[17] R. Malhotra and K. Gregory-Evans, "Management of ocular ischaemic syndrome," *The British Journal of Ophthalmology*, vol. 84, no. 12, pp. 1428–1431, 2000.

[18] M. Qiu, A. G. Shukla, and C. Q. Sun, "Improving outcomes in neovascular glaucoma," *Ophthalmology Glaucoma*, vol. 5, no. 21, pp. 125–127, 2022.

# 18

# Nonarteritic Anterior Ischemic Optic Neuropathy following COVID-19 Vaccination: Consequence or Coincidence

**Rika Tsukii, Yuka Kasuya, and Shinji Makino** ⓘ

*Department of Ophthalmology, Jichi Medical University, Shimotsuke, Tochigi, Japan*

Correspondence should be addressed to Shinji Makino; makichan@jichi.ac.jp

Academic Editor: Kamal Kishore

To report a patient with nonarteritic anterior ischemic optic neuropathy (NA-AION) occurring soon after the COVID-19 vaccination. A 55-year-old woman presented with a 4-day history of inferior visual field disturbance in the right eye 7 days after receiving the first dose of Pfizer-BioNTech COVID-19 vaccine. Examination revealed a best-corrected visual acuity of 20/20 in both eyes. A relative afferent pupillary defect was observed in the right eye. Fundoscopy revealed diffuse optic disc swelling in the right eye, which was prominent above the optic disc. Goldmann visual field testing identified an inferior altitudinal visual field defect with I/2 isopter in the right eye. Although typical complete inferior visual field defect was not detected, a diagnosis of NA-AION was made. The patient was followed without any treatment. During the 2-month follow-up period, the optic disc swelling was gradually improved, and visual acuity was maintained 20/20; however, the optic disc looked diffusely pale in the right eye. Although it is uncertain whether the development of NA-AION after COVID-19 vaccination was consequential or coincidental, we speculate that the close temporal relationship with COVID-19 vaccination suggests the possibility of vasculopathy on the microvascular network of optic nerve head as background of inflammatory or immune-mediated element to the timing of the onset of NA-AION. The aim of this case report is to present this biological plausibility and to elucidate potential ophthalmological complications.

## 1. Introduction

Severe acute respiratory syndrome coronavirus 2 (SARS-CoV-2) infection and the resulting coronavirus disease 2019 (COVID-19) pandemic hit the world by storm, and Japan was no exception. Currently, there has been a tremendous increase in reports of ophthalmic manifestations related with COVID-19 and its vaccination [1–3].

Nonarteritic anterior ischemic optic neuropathy (NA-AION) is an important cause of acute visual loss in middle-aged and elderly populations [4]. Typically, NA-AION is associated with risk factors such as systemic hypertension, diabetes mellitus, and optic disc morphology (small and crowded optic disc) [4].

Here, we report a case of NA-AION occurring soon after the COVID-19 vaccination.

## 2. Case Presentation

A 55-year-old woman presented with a 4-day history of inferior visual field disturbance in the right eye 7 days after receiving the first dose of Pfizer-BioNTech COVID-19 vaccine (BNT162b2 mRNA COVID-19 vaccine). Her personal and family histories as well as physical examination results were unremarkable. She had no other health complaints. Examination revealed a best-corrected visual acuity of 20/20 in both eyes. A relative afferent pupillary defect was observed in the right eye. There was no abnormal ocular motility in either eye. Fundoscopy revealed diffuse optic disc swelling in the right eye, which was prominent above the optic disc (Figure 1(a)). In contrast, no abnormal findings were observed in the left eye (Figure 1(b)). Optical coherence tomography confirmed optic disc swelling in the right eye.

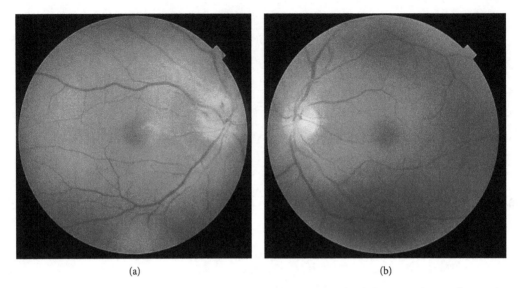

FIGURE 1: Photographs of the right (a) and left (b) fundus on initial examination. Note the diffuse optic disc swelling in the right eye, which was prominent above the optic disc.

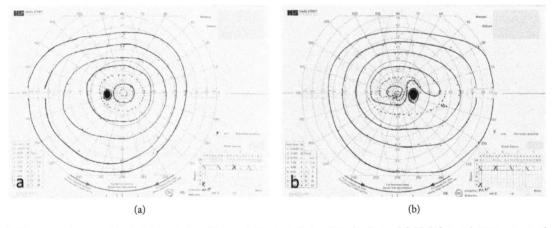

FIGURE 2: Goldmann perimetry of the left (a) and right (b) eyes. Note the inferior altitudinal visual field defect with I/2 isopter in the right eye.

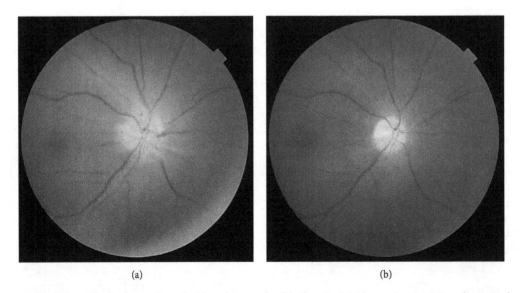

FIGURE 3: Photographs of the right fundus on 2 weeks (a) and 2 months (b) after the initial examination. Note the optic disc swelling was gradually improved; however, the optic disc looked diffusely pale.

However, no abnormal findings were observed in the right macula. Goldmann visual field testing identified an inferior altitudinal visual field defect with I/2 isopter in the right eye (Figure 2). The average critical flicker frequency value was 34 Hz in the right eye and 37 Hz in the left eye. Cranial and orbital MRI showed no abnormal findings. Laboratory examination revealed erythrocyte sedimentation rate was 11 mm/h, and C-reactive protein (CRP) level was 0.02 mg/L (reference range; 0-0.14). Myeloperoxidase-antineutrophil cytoplasmic antibody (MPO-ANCA) was 16.0 U/mL (reference range, <3.5) and proteinase 3- (PR3-) ANCA was 1.0 U/mL (reference range, <3.5). Fluorescein angiography, color vison test, cardiac echography, carotid doppler, and specialized blood coagulation examination were not available in this case.

Although typical complete inferior visual field defect was not detected nor above-mentioned examinations were not conducted, based on patient's history and the aforementioned examinations, a diagnosis of NA-AION was made. The patient was followed without any treatment. During the 2-month follow-up period, the optic disc swelling was gradually improved, and visual acuity was maintained 20/20; however, the optic disc looked diffusely pale in the right eye (Figure 3).

## 3. Discussion

NA-AION is thought to develop due to circulatory insufficiency of the posterior ciliary arteries supplying the optic nerve. Having small, crowded optic disc or other vasculopathies are risk factors for developing NA-AION. Although in the present case, the relatively young patient did not have any vasculopathic risk factors, she developed NA-AION following COVID-19 vaccination.

The occurrence and significance of autoimmune manifestations after the administration of viral vaccines remain controversial. Only two previous cases of NA-AION following influenza vaccination have been reported in the literature [5, 6]. These authors proposed an immune complex-mediated vasculopathy as a likely mechanism.

Previous cases of NA-AION in the setting of COVID-19 infection were reported in the literature [7–9]. SARS-CoV-2 can cause significant inflammation resulting in hypercoagulability manifesting as pulmonary embolism, deep-vein thrombosis, ischemic strokes, or myocardial infarcts [7]. As mentioned, patients with COVID-19 infection can manifest with hypercoagulability and hypoxemia, both of which may contribute to the development of NA-AION.

In contrast, various adverse effects have been reported with COVID-19 vaccine [2, 3], but these events' specific mechanism and frequency have not been investigated thoroughly. A previous case of arteritic anterior ischemic optic neuropathy following COVID-19 vaccination was reported [10]; however, this is the first reported case of NA-AION which was temporally related to the COVID-19 vaccination in Japan.

COVID-19 vaccines result in producing high levels of neutralizing antibodies after injection. These neutralizing antibodies recognize and target the spike proteins in the virus, killing it before the virus is disseminated and cause illness [10]. Neutralizing antibodies against SARS-CoV-2 spike proteins and/or activated T-helper-1 cells after vaccination can crossreact with proteins and antigens in large arteries, outer retinal layers, and retinal pigment epithelial cell [10]. Although it is uncertain whether the development of NA-AION after COVID-19 vaccination was consequential or coincidental, we speculate that the close temporal relationship with COVID-19 vaccination suggests the possibility of vasculopathy on the microvascular network of optic nerve head as background of inflammatory or immune-mediated element to the timing of the onset of NA-AION.

Finally, the aim of this case report is to present this biological plausibility and to elucidate potential ophthalmological complications.

## Consent

We obtained written and informed consent from the patient for the publication of case details and images.

## References

[1] M. Sen, S. G. Honavar, N. Sharma, and M. S. Sachdev, "COVID-19 and eye: a review of ophthalmic manifestations of COVID-19," *Indian Journal of Ophthalmology*, vol. 69, no. 3, pp. 488–509, 2021.

[2] N. G. Kounis, I. Koniari, C. de Gregorio et al., "Allergic reactions to current available COVID-19 vaccinations: pathophysiology, causality, and therapeutic considerations," *Vaccines*, vol. 9, no. 3, p. 221, 2021.

[3] C. Y. C. Chau, L. L. W. Chow, S. Sridhar, and K. C. Shih, "Ophthalmological considerations for COVID-19 vaccination in patients with inflammatory eye diseases and autoimmune disorders," *Ophthalmology and Therapy*, vol. 10, no. 2, pp. 201–209, 2021.

[4] S. S. Hayreh, "Ischemic optic neuropathy," *Progress in Retinal and Eye Research*, vol. 28, no. 1, pp. 34–62, 2009.

[5] A. Kawasaki, V. A. Purvin, and R. Tang, "Bilateral anterior ischemic optic neuropathy following influenza vaccination," *Journal of Neuro-Ophthalmology*, vol. 18, no. 1, pp. 56–59, 1998.

[6] G. Manasseh, D. Donovan, E. H. Shao, and S. R. Taylor, "Bilateral sequential non-arteritic anterior ischaemic optic neuropathy following repeat influenza vaccination," *Case reports in Ophthalmology*, vol. 5, no. 2, pp. 267–269, 2014.

[7] J. Rho, S. C. Dryden, C. D. McGuffey, B. T. Fowler, and J. Fleming, "A case of non-arteritic anterior ischemic optic neuropathy with COVID-19," *Cureus*, vol. 12, article e11950, 2020.

[8] L. Moschetta, G. Fasolino, and R. W. Kuijpers, "Non-arteritic anterior ischaemic optic neuropathy sequential to SARS-CoV-2 virus pneumonia: preventable by endothelial protection?," *BML Case Reports*, vol. 14, no. 7, article e240542, 2021.

[9] K. M. Clarke, V. Riga, A. L. Shirodkar, and J. Meyer, "Proning related bilateral anterior ischaemic optic neuropathy in a patient with COVID-19 related acute respiratory distress syndrome," *BMC Ophthalmology*, vol. 21, no. 1, p. 276, 2021.

[10] A. Maleki, S. Look-Why, A. Manhapra, and C. S. Foster,
     "COVID-19 recombinant mRNA vaccines and serious ocular
     inflammatory side effects: real or coincidence?," *Journal of
     Ophthalmic & Vision Research*, vol. 16, no. 3, pp. 490–501,
     2021.

# 19

# Toxic Anterior Segment Syndrome with Intracameral Moxifloxacin: Case Report and Review of the Literature

**Annahita Amireskandari ⓘ, Andrew Bean, and Thomas Mauger**

*Department of Ophthalmology and Visual Sciences, West Virginia University, Morgantown, WV, USA*

Correspondence should be addressed to Annahita Amireskandari; annahita.amireskandari@wvumedicine.org

Academic Editor: Hiroshi Eguchi

A case of severe anterior segment toxicity secondary to high-volume, undiluted intracameral moxifloxacin for endophthalmitis prophylaxis is reported. We examine the other reported cases of toxicity after intracameral moxifloxacin, as well as iris depigmentation and transillumination syndromes after oral and topical fluoroquinolone exposure. Additionally, we review the literature on safety, efficacy, and appropriate dosing of intracameral antibiotics with a focus on moxifloxacin.

## 1. Introduction

Toxic anterior segment syndrome (TASS), though rare, is one of the most dreaded complications of anterior segment surgery. Resulting in often significant anterior segment inflammation, corneal edema, and damage to the iris and angle structures, it has been reported after cataract surgery, penetrating keratoplasty, and intravitreal antivascular endothelial growth factor (VEGF) injections and vitreoretinal surgery. TASS is thought to be the result of toxicity from residue on surgical instruments, disinfectants, medication, and/or preservatives in medications used during surgery [1]. However, the causative agent remains unknown in many cases.

Moxifloxacin is a fourth-generation fluoroquinolone with broad spectrum activity against Gram-positive and Gram-negative bacteria [2]. Vigamox (Alcon, Fort Worth, Texas) is commonly used in the US as an off-label intracameral injection during cataract surgery, as it is preservative free. We present a case of TASS associated with intracameral preservative-free 0.5% moxifloxacin (Vigamox) during otherwise uncomplicated cataract surgery.

## 2. Case Report

A 74-year-old female presented as a referral from an outside ophthalmologist for persistent corneal edema and mydriatic pupil in the left eye after cataract surgery. According to the referring surgeon, the patient underwent routine phacoemulsification and insertion of a single-piece acrylic intraocular lens implant (IOL) (Acrysof UltraSert ACU0T0, Alcon, Fort Worth, TX). Approximately 0.2 ml intracameral preservative-free 1% lidocaine was instilled in the beginning of the case. Intracameral preservative-free moxifloxacin (Vigamox) was used to replace the anterior chamber at the end of the case (a total volume of approximately approximately 0.6 cc). The surgeon was inadvertently given 0.5% undiluted Vigamox in the syringe instead of the ordered 0.1% concentration for all 7 of his cases that day. This error went unnoticed until the following day when all 7 patients had more than the anticipated amount of intraocular inflammation. Though we do not have details regarding the other 6 cases, this patient was noted to have significant corneal edema, elevated intraocular pressure (IOP), and anterior segment inflammation. These signs persisted at her postoperative week one visit, raising concern for TASS. She was initially treated with topical prednisolone acetate, Vigamox, ketorolac, timolol, netarsudil (Rhopressa 0.02%, Aerie Pharmaceuticals, Irvine, CA), and hypertonic saline (Muro 128 0.5%, Bausch + Lomb, Rochester, NY). The anterior chamber inflammation resolved after several weeks, but the corneal edema and fixed, dilated pupil with transillumination defects persisted at 2 months postoperatively. Per the referring provider, she was the only patient of the 7 that day to have persistent corneal edema and iris damage requiring further surgical intervention. To our knowledge, no cultures or PCR was performed postoperatively. Of note, the patient had cataract surgery in the right eye 2 months prior with the same type of IOL (Alcon Acrysof UltraSert ACU0T0) and 0.6 cc of 0.1% intracameral Vigamox without complication.

The patient presented to our institution approximately two months after cataract surgery in the left eye. The uncorrected vision was 20/25 in the right eye and count fingers at 3 feet in the left eye. The left pupil was dilated and slightly irregular with minimal to no reaction to light. The IOP was 15 mmHg in the right eye and 21 mmHg in the left eye. The anterior and posterior segment exams were normal with a centered posterior chamber IOL on the right. The left eye had mild ptosis with mild conjunctival injection. The cornea was noted to have limbus-to-limbus bullous keratopathy. The anterior chamber was deep without frank inflammation. The iris was fixed, dilated and slightly irregular with a large temporal transillumination defect. It was difficult to assess for endothelial pigment deposition given the diffuse corneal bullae. The posterior chamber IOL appeared to be well centered in the capsular bag (see Figure 1). A hazy view posteriorly revealed no obvious abnormalities of the fundus.

It was evident that there was significant corneal endothelial damage, which led to the chronic bullous keratopathy and toxic injury to the iris, resulting in an atonic iris with an irregular pupil in the left eye. After discussion with the patient, the decision was made to proceed with endothelial keratoplasty and iris repair.

The patient did well postoperatively with a well-adhered graft at her postoperative day one visit and clear cornea at her postoperative week one visit. At week one, the IOP was elevated to 28 mmHg so brimonidine was started twice daily (BID). The pressure fluctuated from 19-26 mmHg over the next 3 months so timolol BID was added as well. Prednisolone acetate was tapered slowly and eventually switched to fluorometholone daily. Visual acuity was 20/40-2 in the left eye at postoperative week one and month one visits. She had 2 nylon sutures in the main wound. Figures 2 and 3 were taken at her one-month postoperative visit. At her most recent follow up 9 months after surgery, she remained on fluorometholone daily, timolol BID, and brimonidine BID. Her best corrected visual acuity was 20/25, and IOP was 18 mmHg in the left eye.

## 3. Discussion

The etiology of toxic anterior segment syndrome in this case is thought to be due to instillation of a high volume (approximately 0.6 cc) of undiluted 0.5% intracameral Vigamox. However, other causes of intraocular inflammation should always be considered, especially infectious etiologies. We are not aware that any cultures or PCR was performed for this patient. Additionally, one must also consider contamination or alteration of the intracameral balanced salt solution, lidocaine, and viscoelastics, as well as, detergents or residue on surgical instruments. Given that all cases that day had

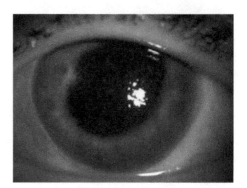

FIGURE 1: Slit lamp photograph of the left eye with diffuse light.

an unexpected amount of postoperative inflammation and the Vigamox concentration was the only known deviation from standard procedure at that particular surgical center, this was thought to be the most likely cause of TASS.

In August 2020, the FDA released a report citing 29 cases of TASS associated with intracameral moxifloxacin use up through December 19, 2019 [3]. Sixteen of these cases involved compounded drugs using moxifloxacin as a bulk substance; 10 involved repackaged Moxeza (Alcon, Fort Worth, Texas) moxifloxacin. There were three cases in which it was unknown whether the moxifloxacin had been repackaged or diluted; two of these were Vigamox, and one was Moxeza. It is important to note that both Vigamox and Moxeza are FDA approved for topical use only [3]. Additionally, Moxeza contains xantham gum which has been associated with TASS [1, 3].

Details of several cases of toxicity with intracameral moxifloxacin have been published this year [4–7]. All 4 of the cases in the series by Sanchez-Sanchez et al. occurred after glaucoma surgery in which patients received Vigamox brand moxifloxacin intracamerally and subconjunctival mitomycin C [4]. Light and Falkenberry presented a case that occurred after pars plana vitrectomy in which the only intraocular medication administered was Vigamox. Regarding the two cases associated with cataract surgery, one involved Vigamox brand moxifloxacin [6]. In the other case by Peñaranda-Henao et al., it was unknown what dose or brand of moxifloxacin was used as the surgery had been performed at an outside institution [7]. It is also unknown whether any other intraocular medications were administered in either of these cases, but 1% preservative-free lidocaine is commonly given intracamerally during cataract surgery. Similar to our patient, all of these cases involved pigment dispersion in the anterior segment. The presence of anterior segment inflammation, pupillary abnormalities, and elevated IOP varied between reports. The individual cases described in these studies are summarized in Table 1.

Multiple reports of uveitis, bilateral acute iris depigmentation (BADI), and/or transillumination (BATI or BAIT) syndromes with *oral* fluoroquinolones use have also been published. These syndromes often include intraocular inflammation, diffuse pigment dispersion onto the corneal endothelium and trabecular meshwork, elevated IOP, pupillary sphincter damage, and iris atony. It is unclear whether the elevated IOP seen in many of these cases is due solely

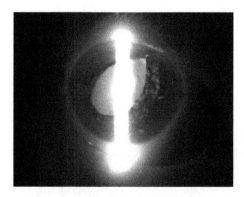

FIGURE 2: Slit lamp photograph with retroillumination of the left eye one month postoperatively.

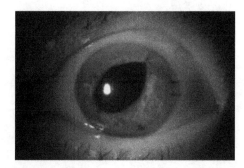

FIGURE 3: Slit lamp photograph of the left eye with diffuse light one month-postoperatively.

to pigment clogging the meshwork or whether there is direct medication toxicity to the trabecular meshwork tissue [8–24]. Of particular interest, a retrospective analysis of 22 cases of acute iris transillumination by Kawali et al. identified 17 cases in which topical ophthalmic fluoroquinolones were used either alone or in conjunction with an oral fluoroquinolone [12].

Opinions regarding the risks and benefits of intracameral moxifloxacin vary greatly. Multiple studies have reported decreased risk of postoperative endophthalmitis with intracameral moxifloxacin use [25–31], though it may be argued that there is more data regarding the use of intracameral cefuroxime [32–35]. While intracameral cefuroxime has been studied more extensively than moxifloxacin and is more cost effective, moxifloxacin may have other benefits. Several authors cite that dose-dependent killing may be an advantage of moxifloxacin over cefuroxime and vancomycin [26, 34]. In addition to their group's clinical experience with moxifloxacin and vancomycin, Arshinoff et al. published an extensive literature review of intracameral vancomycin, cefuroxime, and moxifloxacin during cataract surgery. They concluded that intracameral moxifloxacin is more effective at preventing endophthalmitis compared to vancomycin and cefuroxime, citing that bacterial resistance to moxifloxacin is overcome at a safe level within the anterior chamber [26].

The most effective choice of prophylactic antibiotic remains unclear in the current literature. Bowen et al. performed a meta-analysis of the safety and efficacy of intracameral cefuroxime, moxifloxacin, and vancomycin. The authors note that both cefuroxime and moxifloxacin can be used to

decrease the risk of postoperative endophthalmitis safely [27]. Another in vitro study of bacteria incubated on IOLs showed that all three antibiotics were effective against streptococcus and propionibacteria. They also found that moxifloxacin had broader coverage than cefuroxime and vancomycin, despite being less effective against staphylococcus and pseudomonas at lower doses [36]. Most authors agree that, while retinal toxicity is rare with vancomycin, it should be avoided for routine endophthalmitis prophylaxis during cataract surgery [26, 27, 34].

Regarding volume and concentration of intracameral moxifloxacin, there is some disagreement in the literature about what provides the safest and most efficacious endophthalmitis risk reduction. Several groups have reported favorable safety and efficacy results with undiluted 0.5% moxifloxacin at small doses of 0.03 ml [30] and 0.1 ml [31]. However, Shorstein and Gardner observed that smaller injection volumes of higher concentration moxifloxacin resulted in less precision in the delivered dose. Compared with a 0.5%/0.1 ml intracameral injection, flushing the anterior chamber with 0.15%/0.5 ml provided similar residence times but more consistent anterior chamber concentrations [37]. Matsuura and colleagues examined the safety and efficacy of total replacement of the anterior chamber with 50-500 mcg/ml of moxifloxacin in over 18,000 cataract surgery cases and noted a decreased risk of endophthalmitis. Additionally, there was no significant endothelial cell loss or cases of TASS [38]. They found similar results when flushing that anterior chamber and bag [39]. Arshinoff et al. also found a decreased risk of endophthalmitis with minimal risk of adverse events with 0.3 to 0.4 cc of diluted (3.0 cc Vigamox with 7.0 cc balanced salt solution) moxifloxacin for a final dose equal to 450-699 mcg [25]. Arbisser compared 0.1% moxifloxacin to cataract surgery without intracameral antibiotics and found no significant adverse events with moxifloxacin administration [40].

Both animal and human studies have provided conflicting results regarding moxifloxacin's effects on anterior segment structures. Akal et al. used a rat model to evaluate the effects of intracameral moxifloxacin and noted higher oxidative stress parameters and apoptotic activity in the corneal tissues of rats receiving moxifloxacin compared to controls [41]. Conversely, another study on rabbit eyes found no significant toxicity to endothelial cells with intracameral cefazolin, levofloxacin, or moxifloxacin compared to controls [42].

Haruki et al. used cultured human endothelial cells to examine the effects of different concentrations of moxifloxacin, levofloxacin, and cefuroxime. They found that moxifloxacin doses of more than 500 mcg/ml caused damage to cell membranes and decreased cell viability. Thus, they recommended using an intracameral dose of 500 mcg/ml or less. Another group studied the effects of moxifloxacin on human endothelium, trabecular meshwork, and retinal pigment epithelial cells and found no toxicity to any of these structures with concentrations up to 150 mcg/ml. The authors argued that, given moxifloxacin's minimum inhibitory concentration to inhibit 90% of the most common pathogens causing postoperative endophthalmitis (MIC 90) [43], a concentration of 150 mcg/ml should be safe and effective at preventing

TABLE 1: Case reports of toxicity associated with intracameral moxifloxacin.

| Publication | Subject | Indication for intracameral moxifloxacin | Moxifloxacin brand | Moxifloxacin dose | Other intra-op medications | Adverse effects (AEs) | Time to onset of AEs | Postoperative medications started prior to onset of AEs |
|---|---|---|---|---|---|---|---|---|
| Light and Falkenberry 2019 | 1 of 1 | Endophthalmitis prophylaxis for PPV for symptomatic floaters | Vigamox | 0.1 ml of 5 mg/ml | None | Decreased VA, AC flare, pigment dispersion in AC and angle, iris TID, iris depigmentation, iris TID, elevated IOP | Post-op week 3 | Unspecified topical steroid, NSAID, fluoroquinolone |
| Peñaranda-Henao et al. 2020 | 1 of 1 | Endophthalmitis prophylaxis for cataract surgery | Unknown | Unknown | Unknown | Ocular pain, headache, elevated IOP, AC inflammation with keratic precipitates, pigment dispersion in the AC and angle, pupil deformation with poor reactivity, iris atrophy and TID, pigmented cells in the anterior vitreous, mild decrease in foveal brightness | Post-op week 2.5 | Oral acyclovir, intramuscular betamethasone, topical prednisolone acetate, topical timolol. Later, acyclovir was switched to valacyclovir |
| Sanchez-Sanchez et al. 2020 | 1 of 4 | Endophthalmitis prophylaxis for express shunt implantation for POAG | Vigamox | 0.1 ml of 5 mg/ml | Subconjunctival mitomycin C 0.2 mg/ml | Pigment dispersion in the AC, filtering bleb, and angle around the express shunt, mild mydriasis with sluggish light reaction | Post-op week 4 | Topical moxifloxacin, diclofenac sodium, prednoslone acetate |
| Sanchez-Sanchez et al. 2020 | 2 of 4 | Endophthalmitis prophylaxis for express shunt implantation for POAG | Vigamox | 0.1 ml of 5 mg/ml | Subconjunctival mitomycin C 0.2 mg/ml | Pigment dispersion in the AC and filtering bleb, fixed middilated pupil | Post-op week 2 | Topical moxifloxacin, diclofenac sodium, prednoslone acetate |
| Sanchez-Sanchez et al. 2020 | 3 of 4 | Endophthalmitis prophylaxis for deep non-penetrating sclerotomies with supraciliary hema implant for glaucoma | Vigamox | 0.1 ml of 5 mg/ml | Subconjunctival mitomycin C 0.2 mg/ml | Pigment dispersion in AC and on endothelium, mydriasis with poor light reaction, iris TID, elevated IOP at post op month 3 secondary to pigment obstruction of the trabeculo-Descemet membrane | Post-op week 4 | Topical moxifloxacin, diclofenac sodium, prednoslone acetate |
| Sanchez-Sanchez et al. 2020 | 4 of 4 | Endophthalmitis prophylaxis for deep non-penetrating sclerotomies with supraciliary hema implant for POAG | Vigamox | 0.1 ml of 5 mg/ml | Subconjunctival mitomycin C 0.2 mg/ml | Pigment dispersion under bleb, TID, irregular pupil | Post-op week 6 | Topical moxifloxacin, diclofenac sodium, prednoslone acetate |
| Zubicoa et al. 2020 | 1 of 1 | Endophthalmitis prophylaxis for cataract surgery | Vigamox | 0.1 ml of 5 mg/ml | Unknown | Eye pain, circumciliary congestion, pigment deposition on the IOL and in the angle, flare, mydriasis, iris TID | Post-op week 3.5 | Unspecified topical steroid |

AC: anterior chamber; AEs: adverse effects; IOP: intraocular pressure; NSAID: nonsteroidal anti-inflammatory; PPV: pars plana vitrectomy; POAG: primary open angle glaucoma; TID: transillumination defect; VA: visual acuity.

endophthalmitis [44]. A very recent in vivo study compared intracameral moxifloxacin doses of 250 mcg/0.1 ml and 500 mcg/0.1 ml during cataract surgery and found no significant difference in endothelial cell count postoperatively. The authors state that a higher concentration should be considered to decrease the risk of endophthalmitis, as both concentrations appeared safe [45]. These results should be interpreted with caution, however, as toxicity from fluoroquinolones may depend on exposure time [46].

The use of intracameral antibiotics still varies greatly among surgeons. As reviewed here, there is conflicting data on the risks and benefits of intracameral moxifloxacin. Regardless of antibiotic choice, it is critical that the specific drug and concentration are checked at each step of preparation. Depending on the surgical center or hospital's protocol for preparing antibiotics, this may involve a hospital or facility pharmacy, operating room nurses, scrub technicians, and/or physicians. By verifying the antibiotic name, whether or not it is preservative free, its concentration, and the planned injection amount at each step of preparation, critical errors are less likely to occur. The surgeon is ultimately the last check in this process and should also verify each of these parameters prior to instilling any medication in the eye. If an error does occur and results in significant anterior segment toxicity as seen with the case presented, initial aggressive control of inflammation and IOP is indicated. Even with a severe inflammatory response, it is often possible to have relatively good outcomes with proper management.

## Consent

The patient provided consent for publication.

## References

[1] C. Y. Park, J. K. Lee, and R. S. Chuck, "Toxic anterior segment syndrome-an updated review," *BMC Ophthalmology*, vol. 18, no. 1, p. 276, 2018.

[2] T. D. M. Pham, Z. M. Ziora, and M. A. T. Blaskovich, "Quinolone antibiotics," *Medchemcomm*, vol. 10, no. 10, pp. 1719–1739, 2019.

[3] United States Food and Drug Administration, "FDA alerts health care professionals of risks associated with intraocular use of compounded moxifloxacin in drug safety and availability," August 2020, https://www.fda.gov/drugs/drug-safety-and-availability/fda-alerts-health-care-professionals-risks-associated-intraocular-use-compounded-moxifloxacin.

[4] C. Sánchez-Sánchez, B. Puerto, C. López-Caballero, and I. Contreras, "Unilateral acute iris depigmentation and transillumination after glaucoma surgery with mitomycin application and intracameral moxifloxacin," *American Journal of Ophthalmology Case Reports*, vol. 18, article 100639, 2020.

[5] J. G. Light and S. M. Falkenberry, "Unilateral bilateral acute iris transillumination-like syndrome after intracameral moxifloxacin injection for intraoperative endophthalmitis prophylaxis," *JCRS Online Case Reports*, vol. 7, no. 1, pp. 3–5, 2019.

[6] A. Zubicoa, M. Echeverria-Palacios, M. Mozo Cuadrado, and E. Compains Silva, "Unilateral acute iris transillumination-like syndrome following intracameral moxifloxacin injection," *Ocular Immunology and Inflammation*, vol. 25, pp. 1-2, 2020.

[7] M. M. D. Peñaranda-Henao, J. M. S. Reyes-Guanes, J. M. D. Muñoz-Ortiz, Á. M. M. D. Gutiérrez, and A. de-la-Torre PhD, "Anterior uveitis due to intracameral moxifloxacin: a case report," *Ocular Immunology and Inflammation*, vol. 29, pp. 1–4, 2020.

[8] C. Altan, B. Basarir, and C. Kesim, "An unexpected complication in bilateral acute iris transillumination: cystoid macular edema," *Indian Journal of Ophthalmology*, vol. 66, no. 6, pp. 869–871, 2018.

[9] B. Eadie, M. Etminan, and F. S. Mikelberg, "Risk for uveitis with oral moxifloxacin: a comparative safety study," *JAMA Ophthalmology*, vol. 133, no. 1, pp. 81–84, 2015.

[10] H. Eser-Ozturk and Y. Sullu, "Over-dose oral moxifloxacin related bilateral acute iris transillumination in a short period," *Glokom-Katarakt/Journal of Glaucoma-Cataract*, vol. 15, p. 51, 2020.

[11] D. M. Hinkle, M. S. Dacey, E. Mandelcorn et al., "Bilateral uveitis associated with fluoroquinolone therapy," *Cutaneous and Ocular Toxicology*, vol. 31, no. 2, pp. 111–116, 2012.

[12] A. Kawali, P. Mahendradas, and R. Shetty, "Acute depigmentation of the iris: a retrospective analysis of 22 cases," *Canadian Journal of Ophthalmology*, vol. 54, no. 1, pp. 33–39, 2019.

[13] R. M. Knape, F. E. Sayyad, and J. L. Davis, "Moxifloxacin and bilateral acute iris transillumination," *Journal of Ophthalmic Inflammation and Infection*, vol. 3, no. 1, p. 10, 2013.

[14] E. O. Kreps, K. Hondeghem, A. Augustinus et al., "Is oral moxifloxacin associated with bilateral acute iris transillumination?," *Acta Ophthalmologica*, vol. 96, no. 4, pp. e547–e548, 2018.

[15] S. Mahanty, A. A. Kawali, S. S. Dakappa et al., "Aqueous humor tyrosinase activity is indicative of iris melanocyte toxicity," *Experimental Eye Research*, vol. 162, pp. 79–85, 2017.

[16] R. Morshedi, D. Bettis, M. Moshirfar, and A. T. Vitale, "Bilateral acute iris transillumination following systemic moxifloxacin for respiratory illness: report of two cases and review of the literature," *Ocular Immunology and Inflammation*, vol. 20, no. 4, pp. 266–272, 2012.

[17] P. Plaza-Ramos, H. Heras-Mulero, P. Fanlo, and A. Zubicoa, "Bilateral acute iris transillumination syndrome. A case report," *Archivos de la Sociedad Española de Oftalmología (English Edition)*, vol. 93, 2018.

[18] A. Perin, V. Lyzogubov, and N. Bora, "In vitro assessment of moxifloxacin toxicity to human iris pigment epithelium," *Investigative Ophthalmology & Visual Science*, vol. 56, article 5729, 2015.

[19] J. M. Perone, D. Chaussard, and G. Hayek, "Bilateral acute iris transillumination (BAIT) syndrome: literature review," *Clinical Ophthalmology*, vol. 13, pp. 935–943, 2019.

[20] H. S. Sandhu, A. J. Brucker, L. Ma, and B. L. VanderBeek, "Oral fluoroquinolones and the risk of uveitis," *JAMA Ophthalmology*, vol. 134, no. 1, pp. 38–43, 2016.

[21] I. Tugal-Tutkun and M. Urgancioglu, "Bilateral acute depigmentation of the iris," *Graefe's Archive for Clinical and Experimental Ophthalmology*, vol. 244, no. 6, pp. 742–746, 2006.

[22] I. Tugal-Tutkun, B. Araz, and M. Taskapili, "Bilateral acute depigmentation of the iris: report of 26 new cases and four-year follow-up of two patients," *Ophthalmology*, vol. 116, no. 8, pp. 1552–1557.e1, 2009.

[23] I. Tugal-Tutkun, S. Onal, and A. Garip, "Bilateral acute iris transillumination," *Archives of Ophthalmology*, vol. 129, no. 10, pp. 1312–1319, 2011.

[24] M. Wefers Bettink-Remeijer, K. Brouwers, L. van Langenhove et al., "Uveitis-like syndrome and iris transillumination after the use of oral moxifloxacin," *Eye*, vol. 23, no. 12, pp. 2260–2262, 2009.

[25] S. A. Arshinoff and M. Modabber, "Dose and administration of intracameral moxifloxacin for prophylaxis of postoperative endophthalmitis," *Journal of Cataract and Refractive Surgery*, vol. 42, no. 12, pp. 1730–1741, 2016.

[26] S. A. Arshinoff, T. Felfeli, and M. Modabber, "Aqueous level abatement profiles of intracameral antibiotics: a comparative mathematical model of moxifloxacin, cefuroxime, and vancomycin with determination of relative efficacies," *Journal of Cataract and Refractive Surgery*, vol. 45, no. 11, pp. 1568–1574, 2019.

[27] R. C. Bowen, A. X. Zhou, S. Bondalapati et al., "Comparative analysis of the safety and efficacy of intracameral cefuroxime, moxifloxacin and vancomycin at the end of cataract surgery: a meta-analysis," *The British Journal of Ophthalmology*, vol. 102, no. 9, pp. 1268–1276, 2018.

[28] V. Galvis, A. Tello, M. A. Sánchez, and P. A. Camacho, "Cohort study of intracameral moxifloxacin in postoperative endophthalmitis prophylaxis," *Ophthalmology and Eye Diseases*, vol. 6, pp. 1–4, 2014.

[29] A. Haripriya, D. F. Chang, S. Namburar, A. Smita, and R. D. Ravindran, "Efficacy of intracameral moxifloxacin endophthalmitis prophylaxis at aravind eye hospital," *Ophthalmology*, vol. 123, no. 2, pp. 302–308, 2016.

[30] M. V. Melega, M. Alves, R. P. C. Lira et al., "Safety and efficacy of intracameral moxifloxacin for prevention of post-cataract endophthalmitis: randomized controlled clinical trial," *Journal of Cataract and Refractive Surgery*, vol. 45, no. 3, pp. 343–350, 2019.

[31] A. X. Zhou, W. B. Messenger, S. Sargent, and B. K. Ambati, "Safety of undiluted intracameral moxifloxacin without postoperative topical antibiotics in cataract surgery," *International Ophthalmology*, vol. 36, no. 4, pp. 493–498, 2016.

[32] R. Braga-Mele, D. F. Chang, B. A. Henderson et al., "Intracameral antibiotics: safety, efficacy, and preparation," *Journal of Cataract and Refractive Surgery*, vol. 40, no. 12, pp. 2134–2142, 2014.

[33] Endophthalmitis Study Group, European Society of Cataract & Refractive Surgeons, "Prophylaxis of postoperative endophthalmitis following cataract surgery: results of the ESCRS multicenter study and identification of risk factors," *Journal of Cataract and Refractive Surgery*, vol. 33, no. 6, pp. 978–988, 2007.

[34] E. T. Nguyen and N. H. Shorstein, "Preparation of intracameral antibiotics for injection," *Journal of Cataract and Refractive Surgery*, vol. 39, no. 11, pp. 1778-1779, 2013.

[35] T. P. O'Brien, S. A. Arshinoff, and F. S. Mah, "Perspectives on antibiotics for postoperative endophthalmitis prophylaxis: potential role of moxifloxacin," *Journal of Cataract and Refractive Surgery*, vol. 33, no. 10, pp. 1790–1800, 2007.

[36] P. E. Libre and S. Mathews, "Endophthalmitis prophylaxis by intracameral antibiotics: in vitro model comparing vancomycin, cefuroxime, and moxifloxacin," *Journal of Cataract and Refractive Surgery*, vol. 43, no. 6, pp. 833–838, 2017.

[37] N. H. Shorstein and S. Gardner, "Injection volume and intracameral moxifloxacin dose," *Journal of Cataract and Refractive Surgery*, vol. 45, no. 10, pp. 1498–1502, 2019.

[38] K. Matsuura, T. Miyoshi, C. Suto, J. Akura, and Y. Inoue, "Efficacy and safety of prophylactic intracameral moxifloxacin injection in Japan," *Journal of Cataract and Refractive Surgery*, vol. 39, no. 11, pp. 1702–1706, 2013.

[39] K. Matsuura, C. Suto, Y. Inoue, S. I. Sasaki, S. Odawara, and T. Gotou, "Safety of intracameral injection of moxifloxacin using total replacement technique (bag and chamber flushing)," *Journal of Ocular Pharmacology and Therapeutics*, vol. 30, no. 9, pp. 771–776, 2014.

[40] L. B. Arbisser, "Safety of intracameral moxifloxacin for prophylaxis of endophthalmitis after cataract surgery," *Journal of Cataract and Refractive Surgery*, vol. 34, no. 7, pp. 1114–1120, 2008.

[41] A. Akal, T. Ulas, T. Goncu et al., "Does moxifloxacin alter oxidant status in the cornea? An experimental study," *Cutaneous and Ocular Toxicology*, vol. 34, no. 2, pp. 139–143, 2015.

[42] S. Y. Kim, Y. H. Park, and Y. C. Lee, "Comparison of the effect of intracameral moxifloxacin, levofloxacin and cefazolin on rabbit corneal endothelial cells," *Clinical & Experimental Ophthalmology*, vol. 36, no. 4, pp. 367–370, 2008.

[43] T. Haruki, D. Miyazaki, K. Matsuura et al., "Comparison of toxicities of moxifloxacin, cefuroxime, and levofloxacin to corneal endothelial cells in vitro," *Journal of Cataract and Refractive Surgery*, vol. 40, no. 11, pp. 1872–1878, 2014.

[44] M. Kernt, A. S. Neubauer, R. G. Liegl et al., "Intracameral moxifloxacin: in vitro safety on human ocular cells," *Cornea*, vol. 28, no. 5, pp. 553–561, 2009.

[45] D. F. Chang, N. V. Prajna, L. B. Szczotka-Flynn et al., "Comparative corneal endothelial cell toxicity of differing intracameral moxifloxacin doses after phacoemulsification," *Journal of Cataract and Refractive Surgery*, vol. 46, no. 3, pp. 355–359, 2020.

[46] E. S. FB, L. C. Carrijo-Carvalho, A. Teixeira, D. de Freitas, and F. R. de Souza Carvalho, "Toxicity of intracameral injection of fourth-generation fluoroquinolones on the corneal endothelium," *Cornea*, vol. 35, no. 12, pp. 1631–1637, 2016.

# 20

# *Chryseobacterium indologenes* Keratitis: Successful Treatment of Multidrug-Resistant Strain

**Ivan J. Lee and Thomas Mauger**⊙

*Department of Ophthalmology, West Virginia University School of Medicine, WVU Eye Institute, 1 Medical Center Dr., Morgantown, WV 26506, USA*

Correspondence should be addressed to Thomas Mauger; thomas.mauger@wvumedicine.org

Academic Editor: Hiroshi Eguchi

A 72-year-old male with history of monocular vision with complete vision loss in his right eye from previous retinal detachment presented with 20/200 vision in the left eye with a corneal ulcer. Culture was obtained, and the patient was started on fortified tobramycin, fortified vancomycin, and amphotericin. Despite the antibiotics, the patient did not significantly improve, after which another culture was obtained before the patient was taken to the surgery for cryotherapy and a partial conjunctival flap. The culture identified *Chryseobacterium indologenes*. There have been fewer than a handful of cases reported in the last three decades with different antibiotic susceptibility profiles. Our patient was successfully treated with ciprofloxacin and ceftazidime with the final vision of 20/40.

## 1. Introduction

*Chryseobacterium indologenes* is an aerobic, gram-negative bacillus that is ubiquitous in nature but is rarely present in the human microflora [1]. While *C. indologenes* is a rare pathogen known to cause different types of infections including bacteremia, meningitis, pneumonia, and indwelling device-associated infections [2], only a few cases of keratitis have been reported to date [3–5], each with varying antibiotic susceptibility profile and clinical course. In this case, we present *C. indologenes* keratitis successfully treated with surgical and pharmacological interventions.

## 2. Case

A 72-year-old male with history of chronic adrenal insufficiency, diabetes mellitus, and monocular vision with complete vision loss in his right eye from previous retinal detachment presented with burning eye pain, redness, and decreased vision of his left eye over a 3-week period. On the initial exam, the patient had 20/200 vision with external findings significant for 3 mm dense round infiltrate in the infero-central cornea with overlying epithelial defect extending superotemporally. Anterior chamber reaction or hypopyon was not observed (Figure 1). The patient was admitted to the hospital and was empirically started on hourly fortified tobramycin 15 mg/ml, fortified vancomycin 50 mg/ml, and amphotericin 0.15% after cultures were performed. Despite the initial treatment for five days, the patient did not significantly improve with no growth in the initial cultures. The decision was made to obtain another set of cultures after holding antibiotic drops for one day, and the patient was started on tobramycin, vancomycin, moxifloxacin, and natamycin eye drops. While awaiting on the second set of cultures, the patient was taken to the surgery for cryotherapy and a partial conjunctival flap due to minimal clinical improvement despite the aforementioned medical management. The patient did well postoperatively with improvement in his symptoms. During this time, the cultures identified *Chryseobacterium indologenes* as the causative organism. A chocolate agar plate was used to isolate the species. A matrix-assisted laser desorption/ionization-time-of-flight mass spectrometer (MALDI-TOF) was implemented for the identification of the species with 99.9% match. The

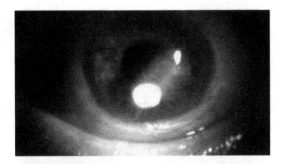

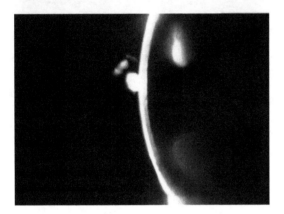

FIGURE 1: Bacterial keratitis at presentation.

TABLE 1: Susceptibility profile for *Chryseobacterium indologenes*.

| Antibiotic | Susceptibility | Disc size for Kirby-Bauer susceptibility* |
|---|---|---|
| Amikacin | Resistant | 13 mm |
| Aztreonam | Resistant | 6 mm |
| Cefepime | Sensitive | 24 mm |
| Ceftazidime | Intermediate | 17 mm |
| Ciprofloxacin | Sensitive | 28 mm |
| Gentamicin | Resistant | 12 mm |
| Meropenem | Sensitive | 26 mm |
| Piperacillin/tazobactam | Sensitive | 31 mm |
| Tobramycin | Resistant | 6 mm |

*Note that the disc size for determination of susceptibility varies for each species.

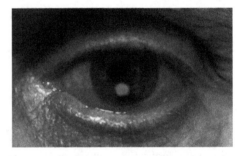

FIGURE 2: Patient at follow-up with 20/40 vision with persisting but improving infiltrate. Partial conjunctival flap is rotated inferiorly.

Kirby-Bauer susceptibility test protocol via a disk diffusion method was applied, in which zone size was measured and interpreted according to the Clinical and Laboratory Standards Institute (CLSI) Performance Standards for Antimicrobial Susceptibility Testing 31st edition (Table 1). The medications were switched to topical ciprofloxacin and ceftazidime accordingly. The flap has rotated fully about 2 weeks after the surgery, exposing 1.7 mm infiltrate with 3 mm epithelial defect overlying the part of the infiltrate. Over the next month, the patient showed slow clinical improvement. An external exam showed gradual clearing of the infiltrate as well as reepithelialization of the surface. At this point, prednisolone acetate 1% was added to his medication regimen. The patient's vision ultimately improved to 20/40, two months after the initial presentation (Figure 2).

## 3. Discussion

*Chryseobacterium indologenes*, formerly known as *Flavobacterium indologenes* or *Flavobacterium aureum*, is an aerobic, nonfermentative, oxidase-positive, and indole-positive gram-negative bacillus that is widely distributed in nature, although rarely present in the human microflora [1]. *C. indologenes* is a rare pathogen known to cause different types of infections including bacteremia, meningitis, pneumonia, and indwelling device-associated infections [2]. Risk factors associated with *C. indologenes* infection includes older age, immunocompromised clinical status including diabetes or systemic steroid treatment, and history of indwelling catheter [6–10], which correlate with our patient with diabetes and chronic steroid treatment for adrenal insufficiency.

The pathogenicity of *Chryseobacterium* species is postulated to involve endotoxin [11, 12] and biofilms [13]. Endotoxins as well as elastase enzymes released by the microorganism cause collagen breakdown, cascading into inflammatory responses of the cornea and eventually corneal perforation if left untreated. The biofilm allows the formation of microbial community that may attach to the solid surface surrounded by extracellular polymeric substances produced by the microorganisms, especially in the setting of indwelling catheter, corroborating the relationship between its mode of virulence and predisposing factor to infection [13]. In addition, *C. indologenes* is intrinsically resistant to carbapenems and cephalosporins by producing molecular class A β-lactamase and class B carbapenem-hydrolyzing β-lactamase (IND1-IND7) [14–17], providing multidrug resistance by nature.

*C. indologenes* have been involved in the development of keratitis. A 47-year-old Asian male suffered corneal perforation despite fortified topical gentamicin and cefazolin for presumed *Pseudomonas aeruginosa* infection. The culture later isolated *C. indologenes* with multiple drug resistance except intermediate response to ceftazidime, which ultimately resolved with hourly ceftazidime eye drops for three weeks [3]. Another 83-year-old female was treated with fortified vancomycin and ceftazidime for bacterial keratitis whose culture ultimately grew *C. indologenes* which was highly resistant to all antibiotics except for trimethoprim-sulfamethoxazole with clinical improvement after one month of the antibiotics [4]. For both cases, susceptibility of strains to antibiotics differed from the strain isolated from our patient, which suggests the standardized treatment for *C. indologenes* to be challenging.

In conclusion, *Chryseobacterium indologenes* is a possibly emerging bacterial cause of keratitis that should be considered for recalcitrant cases in older, immunocompromised groups of patients. Standardization of antimicrobial treatment for *C. indologenes* keratitis remains difficult due to varying susceptibility to antibiotics on a few number of cases reported.

## Consent

Written informed consent was obtained from the patient for publication of this case report and accompanying images. A copy of the written consent is available for review by the editor-in-chief of this journal on request.

## References

[1] P. R. Hsueh, T. R. Hsiue, J. J. Wu et al., "Flavobacterium indologenes bacteremia: clinical and microbiological characteristics," *Clinical Infectious Diseases*, vol. 23, no. 3, pp. 550–555, 1996.

[2] G. B. Christakis, S. P. Perlorentzou, I. Chalkiopoulou, A. Athanasiou, and N. J. Legakis, "Chryseobacterium indologenes non-catheter-related bacteremia in a patient with a solid tumor," *Journal of Clinical Microbiology*, vol. 43, no. 4, pp. 2021–2023, 2005.

[3] P. Chung-Shien Lu and C. J. Cheng-Ho, "*Flavobacterium indologenes* keratitis," *Ophthalmologica*, vol. 211, no. 2, pp. 98–100, 1997.

[4] J. C. Ramos-Esteban, S. Bamba, and B. H. Jeng, "Treatment of multidrug-resistant Flavobacterium indologenes keratitis with trimethoprim-sulfamethoxazole," *Cornea*, vol. 27, no. 9, pp. 1074–1076, 2008.

[5] M. C. Hsieh, S. Y. Yang, Y. L. Liu, and C. P. Lin, "Chryseobacterium indologenes keratitis—a case report," *The Kaohsiung Journal of Medical Sciences*, vol. 36, no. 7, pp. 563-564, 2020.

[6] S. Degandt, F. van Hoecke, J. Colaert, R. D'Souza, I. Pattyn, and M. Boudewijns, "Bacteremia due to *Chryseobacterium indologenes*, a naturally carbapenem- resistant Gram-negative pathogen, in a geriatric patient," *European Geriatric Medicine*, vol. 4, no. 5, pp. 345-346, 2013.

[7] A. M. Asaad, M. S. Z. al-Ayed, and M. A. Qureshi, "Emergence of unusual nonfermenting Gram-negative nosocomial pathogens in a Saudi hospital," *Japanese Journal of Infectious Diseases*, vol. 66, no. 6, pp. 507–511, 2013.

[8] L. A. Cone, A. A. Morrow, M. Benson, B. Younes, and R. Gade-Andavolu, "Chryseobacterium indologenes sepsis due to an infected central catheter in a patient with metastatic breast cancer to the skin," *Infectious Diseases in Clinical Practice*, vol. 15, no. 6, pp. 403–405, 2007.

[9] S. Shah, U. Sarwar, E. A. King, and A. Lat, "Chryseobacterium indologenes subcutaneous port-related bacteremia in a liver transplant patient," *Transplant Infectious Disease*, vol. 14, no. 4, pp. 398–402, 2012.

[10] J. T. Lin, W. S. Wang, C. C. Yen et al., "Chryseobacterium indologenes bacteremia in a bone marrow transplant recipient with chronic graft-versus-host disease," *Scandinavian Journal of Infectious Diseases*, vol. 35, no. 11-12, pp. 882-883, 2003.

[11] T. N. Peters, N. G. Iskander, E. E. Anderson Penno, D. E. Woods, R. A. Moore, and H. V. Gimbel, "Diffuse lamellar keratitis: isolation of endotoxin and demonstration of the inflammatory potential in a rabbit laser in situ keratomileusis model," *Journal of Cataract and Refractive Surgery*, vol. 27, no. 6, pp. 917–923, 2001.

[12] S. Miyazaki, "Biological activities of partially purified elastase produced by Flavobacterium meningosepticum," *Microbiology and Immunology*, vol. 28, no. 10, pp. 1083–1092, 1984.

[13] Y. C. Chang, H. H. Lo, H. Y. Hsieh, and S. M. Chang, "Identification, epidemiological relatedness, and biofilm formation of clinical *Chryseobacterium indologenes* isolates from Central Taiwan," *Journal of Microbiology, Immunology, and Infection*, vol. 48, no. 5, pp. 559–564, 2015.

[14] B. Zeba, F. de Luca, A. Dubus et al., "IND-6, a highly divergent IND-type metallo-$\beta$-lactamase from Chryseobacterium indologenes strain 597 isolated in Burkina Faso," *Antimicrobial Agents and Chemotherapy*, vol. 53, no. 10, pp. 4320–4326, 2009.

[15] M. Perilli, B. Caporale, G. Celenza et al., "Identification and characterization of a new metallo-$\beta$-lactamase, IND-5, from a clinical isolate of Chryseobacterium indologenes," *Antimicrobial Agents and Chemotherapy*, vol. 51, no. 8, pp. 2988–2990, 2007.

[16] T. Matsumoto, M. Nagata, N. Ishimine et al., "Characterization of CIA-1, an ambler class A extended-spectrum $\beta$-lactamase from Chryseobacterium indologenes," *Antimicrobial Agents and Chemotherapy*, vol. 56, no. 1, pp. 588–590, 2012.

[17] Y. Yamaguchi, N. Takashio, J. I. Wachino et al., "Structure of metallo-lactamase IND-7 from a Chryseobacterium indologenes clinical isolate at 1.65-A resolution," *Journal of Biochemistry*, vol. 147, no. 6, pp. 905–915, 2010.

# 21

# Phthisis Bulbi in a Retinitis Pigmentosa Patient after Argus II Implantation

**Logan Vander Woude, Ramak Roohipour⬥, and Gibran Syed Khurshid**

*Department of Ophthalmology, University of Florida, USA*

Correspondence should be addressed to Ramak Roohipour; ramakroohipour@yahoo.com

Academic Editor: J. Fernando Arevalo

*Purpose.* To report a previously unreported complication of phthisis after Argus II prosthesis implantation in a retinitis pigmentosa (RP) patient. *Case.* A 61-year-old male with advanced RP presented to the retina clinic. The patient had a history of vitrectomy in both eyes (OU) in Cuba in 1996. Pre-op visual acuity (VA) was no light perception (NLP) in the right eye and light perception (LP) in the left eye. The patient met the criteria for Argus II implantation and elected to proceed with surgery in his left eye in December 2017. The surgical implantation of the Argus II was successful without any complications. On postoperative day 1, his VA was stable at LP. He was satisfied with his ambulatory vision after the electrodes were turned on. Four months after surgery, the patient was complaining of aching pain; he was found to have preseptal cellulitis and was started on antibiotics. This swelling improved over two weeks, but when the patient returned, he had a two mm hyphema associated with mild ocular inflammation without an inciting event or reason on exam. The hyphema was treated and resolved after two weeks. However, one month after the hyphema resolved, at postoperative month six, the patient's vision in his left eye became NLP and began to demonstrate phthisical changes, including hypotony, Descemet membrane folds, and a vascular posterior capsular membrane. *Discussion.* The theoretical causes of phthisis bulbi after Argus II implantation include fibrous downgrowth, ciliary shut down due to immune reaction, inflammation, or trauma. While the cause of phthisis in this Argus patient is not certain and possibly multifactorial, it is important to note that phthisis is a possible complication of an Argus II implant, as this patient had no other obvious insult or reason for the phthisical change.

## 1. Introduction

Retinitis pigmentosa is an inherited retinal disease characterized by a progressive degeneration of rods, followed by cones and finally RPE. Initially, patients experience nyctalopia and peripheral vision loss, which progresses over time and may lead to complete vision loss. While research for cures is progressing, including gene therapy and stem cell transplantation, currently, there are no preventive or curative treatments on the market [1].

However, with advancing technology, there are ongoing innovations in prosthetic vision. The Argus II is the first FDA-approved device in Europe and the USA for severe or profound vision loss secondary to retinitis pigmentosa. The patient undergoes surgical implantation of a microarray onto the macula, which bypasses the diseased photoreceptors to directly stimulate preserved inner retina layers via epiretinal microelectrodes. Patients wear glasses equipped with a video camera that relays visual input signals to this microarray, which stimulates the inner retinal layers that relay the inputs to the optic nerve and visual pathway. There is a wide range in visual outcomes in patients, but many notice an overall improvement in functional vision [2].

Studies have so far demonstrated robust safety protocols in phase I and II trials with 70% of patients experiencing no major adverse effects. The most common adverse events include conjunctival dehiscence or erosion, hypotony, and presumed endophthalmitis [1, 3]. To the authors' knowledge, there has been no previously reported case of phthisis after implantation of the Argus II.

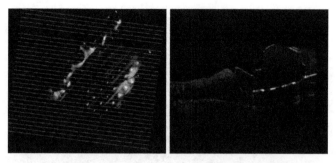

FIGURE 1: OCT image of the patient after Argus implantation.

## 2. Case Presentation

This case presents a 61-year-old male known to the retina clinic with progressive, severe vision loss secondary to RP. The patient has a self-reported history of "experimental vitrectomy" OU in Cuba in 1996, CE/IOL in the right eye (OD) in 2006, and cataract surgery and intraocular lens implant (CE/IOL) in the left eye (OS) in 2010 followed by pars plana vitrectomy (PPV) and removal of retained lens material in 2014, after which the patient was doing well. However, the patient's VA continued to deteriorate to NLP OD and LP OS. Therefore, he elected to have the Argus II implantation, which was done in his better seeing left eye in December 2017.

The following is the procedure details: first, we placed the external electronic case superotemporally and the band was passed under the muscles and secured with Watzke's sleeve in the superonasal quadrant. In order to do so, a 360-degree conjunctival peritomy was performed. The sub-Tenon space was opened in a blunt fashion in all quadrants. The four rectus muscles were identified with the muscle hook and isolated with a 2-0 silk suture. The muscle capsule was cleaned off with Q-tips. Two partial thickness scleral flaps were created inferonasally and superonasally to secure the strip. Electronic case with 2.5 mm silicone strip was passed under the muscles and belts and secured with a silicone sleeve superonasally. The case was tested with a central processing unit under sterile conditions, was secured with two 5-0 mersilene sutures superotemporally and one 5-0 mersilene sutures inferotemporally. Silicone strip was held in inferonasal and superonasal quadrants 12 mm behind the limbus with one 6-0 mersilene. Second, a 23-gauge pars plana vitrectomy with peeling of the posterior hyaloid face was performed. The infusion cannula was inserted at 5 o'clock and confirmed visually to be properly located in vitreous cavity inferotemporally. Two 23-gauge sclerotomies were placed at 10 and 2 o'clock. A 25-gauge chandelier-light source was placed inferiorly with a trocar system. The light pipe and vitrector were inserted in the vitreous cavity. Then after core vitrectomy, the posterior hyaloid face was stained with Kenalog and detached. It was excised successfully up to the periphery. Third, we extended the sclerotomy and passed the electronic array and filament intravitreally by extending the sclerotomy 5 mm superotemporally with a sharp blade 4 mm behind the limbus. The case was tested again with a CPK unit under sterile conditions, and an electronic array with filament was passed through it into the vitreous cavity with silicone

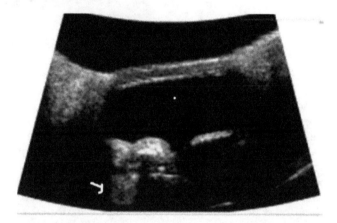

FIGURE 2: UBM image of the patient with hyperreflectivity in the ciliary body adjacent to the supraciliary space with a comet tail artifact (white arrow). It could be due to implant migration anteriorly and fibrous downgrowth.

sleeve-coated forceps. The sclerotomy was then closed with 5-0 mersilene sutures at the edges of the filament. Next, we placed the microelectrode array and perform transretinal and transchoroidal tacking of the array by placing the array on the surface of the macula holding from the manipulating knob with Eckhardt's forceps. It was orientated 45 degrees correctly to the transverse plane of the macula with the left inferior corner at the edge of the optic nerve. At 4 o'clock, 19-gauge sclerotomy was fashioned with an MVR blade. Then, retinal tack was loaded in the tacker, and bimanually, tack was passed through retina and choroid and tacked onto the posterior sclera, while keeping the microarray plate in position. Then, the donor-processed scleral patch was fashioned and secured with 7-0 vicryl. Similar patch was used to cover the coil inferotemporally and secured with 7-0 vicryl. Finally, we closed all sclerotomies and peritomy with 8-0 nylon and 7-0 vicryl, respectively.

The surgical implantation of the Argus II was successful, and the surgery was without complication (Figure 1). On postoperative day one, the patient's VA was LP OS, with elevated intraocular pressure (IOP) of thirty, which returned to normal one week later. At postoperative month one, the vision was stable at LP, with an IOP of seven. The eye was quiet, and the implant was working well; most importantly, the patient was satisfied with his ambulatory vision.

Four months after surgery, the patient presented complaining of aching pain; he was found to have preseptal cellulitis and was started on antibiotics. This cellulitis resolved

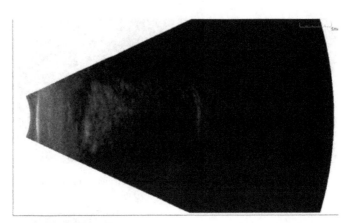

FIGURE 3: Echography of the patient shows intact retina.

over two weeks, but when the patient returned, he had a two mm hyphema associated with mild ocular inflammation without an inciting event or neovascularization on exam. The intraocular lens (IOL) was in the bag, and there was no reason for developing spontaneous hyphema. The hyphema was treated, and two weeks later, it had resolved without apparent incident. However, one month after the hyphema resolved, at postoperative month 6, the patient's VA OS diminished to NLP. In addition, the patient demonstrated phthisical changes, including hypotony (IOP 0 mmHg), Descemet membrane folds, and a vascular sheet posterior to capsular membrane. At no point in the patient's postoperative care, any posterior inflammatory or retinal issues were apparent, including retinal detachment or Argus dehiscence. There was no bleb formation or conjunctival dehiscence. Unfortunately, the phthisical progression affected the Argus II implant, which stopped transmitting the superior field.

The patient was started on steroids, but the eye remained hypotonus, and the patient's phthisical changes continued to progress despite therapy. Exploration of the device was offered to the patient, but the patient refused as it did not have any prognostic value in the setting of advanced retinitis pigmentosa.

## 3. Discussion

While there have been over 100 Argus II implants, there have been no reported cases of phthisis. In the Argus II clinical trial, the documented complications include hypotony, conjunctival erosion or dehiscence, presumed endophthalmitis, retacking, retinal detachment or tear, explants, device failures, uveitis, or corneal decompensation. Of note, most of these complications were clustered in the same patients, while 70% had no complications. It was also realized that the second half of patients had better outcomes likely due to improving surgical techniques [1, 3].

Phthisis is characterized by a shrinkage and disorganization of the globe, typically associated with a squared, opaque, and thickened cornea and sclera, NVI, and retinal detachments. Common causes include trauma, surgery, infection, inflammation, malignancy, retinal detachment, and vascular pathology, which lead to hypotony, inflammatory changes, or violation of the blood-ocular barriers. Pathologically, cells

become disorganized and dysplastic. Early treatment of the cause is the only hope for possible cure, and phthisical eyes quickly become nonfunctional [4].

The etiology of the phthisical changes in this case can have several reasons such as fibrous downgrowth, ciliary shut down due to immune reaction, inflammation, or unreported trauma. It is uncertain why the patient would develop a spontaneous hyphema five months after surgery; it is possible the patient had unreported trauma that caused the hyphema and initiated the phthisical change. It was noted that at the time of the hyphema, the patient had a small inflammatory response, but that resolved within two weeks and was unlikely significant enough to induce enough of an immune response to cause phthisis.

The most probable etiology is that repeated posterior surgeries and the scleral wound for inserting the implant allowed fibrous downgrowth that could have led to phthisis (Figure 2). The patient had an "experimental vitrectomy" in 1996 in Cuba, another PPV for the removal of retained lens material in 2014, and implantation of the Argus II in 2017. It is uncertain what procedure was done in Cuba, but there were no foreign bodies found or issues with his eye before undergoing the third posterior segment surgery for implantation of the Argus II. Perhaps, the 5 mm pars plana sclerotomy used to implant the Argus microarray could have an increased risk of phthisis due to the large wound, and/or insertion of foreign material could stimulate fibrous downgrowth formation. Fibrous downgrowth has been reported by similar mechanisms, including after cases of traumatic corneoscleral wound dehiscence and telescope implantation [5, 6].

The foreign material of the array consists of 60 platinum electrodes embedded in a polyimide, which is theoretically inert. There is also a cable which spans the eye wall to connect the microarray to the Argus II. While this is sutured closed, it is possible the exposed cable, which is composed of a metallized polymer, could lead to phthisis. The composition of the metallized polymer is not reported [1, 3], but it is another possibility that this exposed cable could be reactive or provide the environment for disorganization and phthisical change. The other reason for phthisis after any eye surgery can be due to retinal detachment, but that was ruled out with serial echography and examination (Figure 3).

## 4. Conclusion

While the cause of phthisis in this Argus II patient is not certain and may be multifactorial, it is important to note that phthisis is a possible complication of an Argus II implant, as this patient had no other obvious insult or reason for the phthisical change.

## Additional Points

*Authorship.* All authors attest that they meet the current ICMJE criteria for authorship.

## Consent

Written consent to publish case details was obtained from this patient.

## Acknowledgments

This work was supported in part by an unrestricted grant from Research to Prevent Blindness.

## References

[1] L. da Cruz, J. D. Dorn, M. S. Humayun et al., "Five-year safety and performance results from the Argus II retinal prosthesis system clinical trial," *Ophthalmology*, vol. 123, no. 10, pp. 2248–2254, 2016.

[2] Y. H.-L. Luo and L. da Cruz, "The Argus® II Retinal Prosthesis System," *Progress in Retinal and Eye Research*, vol. 50, pp. 89–107, 2016.

[3] M. S. Humayun, J. D. Dorn, L. da Cruz et al., "Interim results from the international trial of Second Sight's visual prosthesis," *Ophthalmology*, vol. 119, no. 4, pp. 779–788, 2012.

[4] K. Tripathy, R. Chawla, S. Temkar et al., "Phthisis bulbi-a clinicopathological perspective," *Seminars in Ophthalmology*, vol. 33, no. 6, pp. 788–803, 2017.

[5] I. Kremer, J. Zandbank, D. Barash, E. Ben-David, and Y. Yassur, "Extensive fibrous downgrowth after traumatic corneoscleral wound dehiscence," *Annals of Ophthalmology*, vol. 23, no. 12, pp. 465–468, 1991.

[6] M. H. Levy and C. E. Margo, "Fibrous downgrowth complicating implantation of intraocular telescope," *Ophthalmology*, vol. 124, no. 6, p. 895, 2017.

# IgG4-Related Ophthalmic Disease Presenting as Meningitis and Panuveitis

**Maria A. Mavrommatis ⓘ,**[1] **Sarah A. Avila,**[1,2] **and Richard France**[1,2]

[1]*Department of Ophthalmology, Icahn School of Medicine at Mount Sinai, 1 Gustave L. Levy Pl, New York, NY 10029, USA*
[2]*James J Peters VA Medical Center, Department of Ophthalmology, 130 W Kingsbridge Rd, Bronx, NY 10468, USA*

Correspondence should be addressed to Maria A. Mavrommatis; maria.mavrommatis@icahn.mssm.edu

Academic Editor: Claudio Campa

*Purpose.* We report an uncommon case of immunoglobulin gamma 4-related ophthalmic disease (IgG4-ROD) presenting as meningitis and panuveitis. *Observations.* A 35-year-old male with no prior ophthalmic history presented with headaches, altered mental status, and fever of unknown origin. A lumbar puncture (LP) revealed an elevated white count with lymphocytic predominance, confirming a suspected meningitis. After an extensive work-up, he was discharged on oral acyclovir to cover for presumed aseptic meningitis. The patient initially improved, however, bilateral eye pain, redness, and photophobia 2 weeks after discharge prompted his first visit to the ophthalmology clinic. Exam at that time was consistent with bilateral anterior uveitis for which he was given topical prednisolone and cyclopentolate. In addition to the preceding work-up, quantitative immunoglobulin serology including IgG4 levels was added. At follow-up, he was found to have increased ocular inflammation with vitreitis, nerve head edema, and subclinical macular thickening. Visual acuity (VA) had decreased in both eyes. Serology titers for IgG had resulted in a significant elevation in IgG subclass 4 (IgG4). Optical coherence tomography (OCT) and fundus fluorescein angiography (FFA) confirmed posterior retinal involvement. The patient was diagnosed with presumed bilateral panuveitis secondary to IgG4-ROD. *Conclusions and Importance.* IgG4-RD can be a serious condition that requires careful consideration and intuition to diagnose. This report serves to encourage ophthalmologists to consider IgG4-ROD in cases of idiopathic systemic inflammation with ophthalmic involvement.

## 1. Introduction

Immunoglobulin G4-related disease (IgG4-RD) is a recently discovered inflammatory condition characterized by IgG4-mediated fibroinflammation and enlargement of the affected organ [1]. While the notion of IgG4-RD was first recognized in the context of autoimmune pancreatitis [2], the disease has since been connected to inflammatory processes in many other organs, including the orbit and the eye [3]. IgG4-related ophthalmic disease (IgG4-ROD) is the term coined for instances of IgG4-RD resulting in inflammation of the ocular adnexa. IgG4-ROD has multiple clinical presentations, most frequently involving the lacrimal gland, extraocular muscles, orbital bones, and sclera [4]. Few case reports document meningeal involvement and even fewer present with alternative ocular pathology. We report an atypical case of IgG4-ROD presenting as aseptic meningitis and panuveitis.

## 2. Case Report

A 35-year-old male with no prior medical or ophthalmic history presented with headaches, altered mental status, and fever of unknown origin. An extensive work-up for infectious, inflammatory, and neoplastic causes was noncontributory. Labs revealed marked elevations in both erythrocyte sedimentation rate (ESR) and C-reactive protein (CRP), indicating an underlying inflammatory process. Computer tomography (CT) scan of the head showed diffuse inflammation and thickening of the meninges (Figure 1). Lumbar

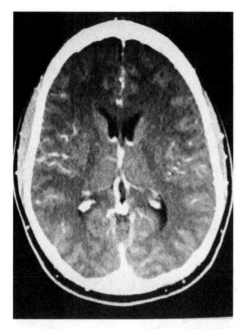

FIGURE 1: CT Scan showing diffuse inflammation and thickening of the meninges.

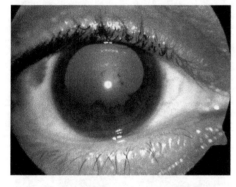

FIGURE 2: External photo of the right eye demonstrating posterior synechiae with pigment on the anterior lens capsule.

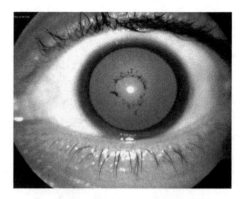

FIGURE 3: External photo of the left eye following synechiolysis with pigmentary right in the anterior lens capsule.

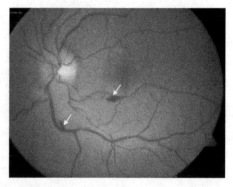

FIGURE 4: Fundus photo of the left eye demonstrating optic nerve head edema with flame hemorrhages along the inferior vascular arcade (white arrows).

puncture (LP) revealed an elevated white count with lymphocytic predominance. He was discharged on a course of oral acyclovir for presumed aseptic meningitis.

The patient initially improved; however, two weeks after discharge, bilateral eye pain, redness, and photophobia prompted his first visit to the ophthalmology clinic. Slit lamp exam was notable for grade 2 anterior chamber cells with flare in both eyes. The right eye showed posterior synechiae with pigment on the anterior lens capsule (Figure 2) while the left eye showed synechiolysis with a residual pigmentary ring on the anterior lens capsule (Figure 3). Dilated fundus exam was within normal limits. He was given topical prednisolone and cyclopentolate for a diagnosis of bilateral anterior uveitis. In addition to his preexisting work-up, quantitative immunoglobulin serology including IgG4 levels was also added given the unexplained systemic inflammation.

At follow-up, his symptoms persisted with a decrease in vision from 20/20 in both eyes to 20/25. He was found to have increased ocular inflammation with persistent anterior chamber cells and subsequent vitreitis and bilateral optic nerve head edema in both eyes (Figures 4 and 5). Optical coherence tomography (OCT) was normal in the right eye but showed subclinical parafoveal thickening in the left eye (Figure 6). Fundus fluorescein angiography (FFA) confirmed posterior retinal involvement with bilateral parafoveal late vascular staining (Figures 7 and 8).

Serology titers for IgG revealed a significant elevation in IgG subclass 4 (IgG4) at 251 mg/dL. A presumed diagnosis of bilateral panuveitis secondary to IgG4-ROD was made. The patient was offered a vitreous biopsy to further confirm the diagnosis, but he declined. He was treated with high dose oral prednisone at 60 mg/day with full resolution in anterior chamber cells, optic nerve head edema (Figures 9 and 10), and OCT macular swelling (Figure 11). The patient's visual acuity returned to 20/20 after treatment.

## 3. Discussion and Conclusion

IgG4-RD is an increasingly recognized immune-mediated condition that can yield destructive inflammation and fibrosis in a number of organs [1]. When the disease manifests in the eye as IgG4-ROD, it typically presents with lacrimal gland, extraocular muscle, and, less commonly, eyelid, orbital

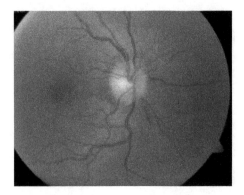

FIGURE 5: Fundus photo of the right eye demonstrating optic nerve head edema.

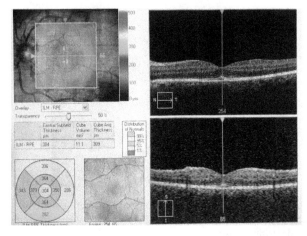

FIGURE 6: OCT Macula of the left eye demonstrating para-foveal macular thickening.

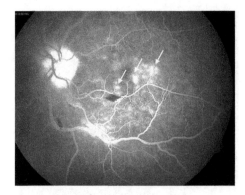

FIGURE 7: Fundus fluorescein angiography of the left eye showing para-foveal late vascular leakage (white arrows) and blockage from flame-hemorrhages.

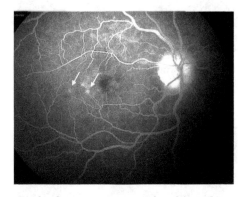

FIGURE 8: Fundus fluorescein angiography of the right eye showing para-foveal late vascular leakage (white arrows).

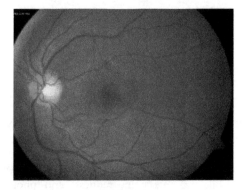

FIGURE 9: Fundus photo of the left eye after treatment showing resolution of the optic nerve head edema.

bone, or scleral involvement [3]. These manifestations can mimic many other conditions, including neoplastic, infectious, and inflammatory diseases. Thus, these require exclusion before a final diagnosis of IgG4-RD can be entertained. Diagnostic criteria put forth by Umehara et al. for IgG4-RD and by Goto et al. for IgG4-ROD can help characterize definitive, probable, and possible IgG4 disease [5, 6]. Furthermore, Yu et al. determined that the optimal cutoff value of IgG4 serum for the diagnosis of IgG4-RD is 248 mg/dL, with a sensitivity and specificity of 77.6% and 92.8%, respectively [7]. They subsequently concluded that 2 or 3 times the upper limit of the normal range of IgG4 level, as was found in the present case, is a useful marker for the diagnosis of IgG4-RD [7]. While serum IgG4 elevated levels significantly aid in the diagnosis, the gold standard for a definitive diagnosis is tissue biopsy. Using serological cut-offs like those put forth by Yu et al. is advantageous in situations when biopsy is difficult or when the patient declines, as in this case.

Here, we describe a rare case of probable IgG4-ROD presenting as meningitis and progressive panuveitis that required an extensive work-up to identify. While IgG4-RD is typically diagnosed by rheumatological specialties, we advise ophthalmologists to consider IgG4-ROD and to add IgG serology to the work-up in cases of idiopathic inflammation.

When the presentation varies beyond the expected, the risk of misdiagnosing the condition heightens, which can be detrimental to the patient's capacity for recovery. A condition like IgG4-ROD can offer an opportunity for elevated collaboration between ophthalmology and rheumatology for a final diagnosis. Despite favorable responses to steroids, long-term management of relapsing IgG4-RD and igG4-ROD patients can be challenging, further supporting the need

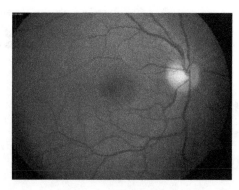

FIGURE 10: Fundus photo of the right eye after treatment showing resolution of the optic nerve head edema.

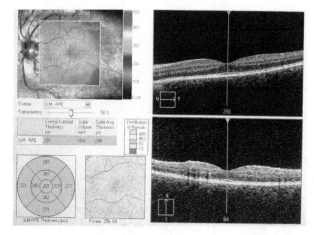

FIGURE 11: OCT Macula of the left eye after treatment demonstrating improved para-foveal macular thickening.

for awareness and multidisciplinary cooperation as it may require immunomodulatory therapy.

## Consent

The patient consented to publication of the case orally.

## Disclosure

All authors attest that they meet the current ICMJE criteria for authorship.

## References

[1] J. H. Stone, Y. Zen, and V. Deshpande, "IgG4-related disease," *The New England Journal of Medicine*, vol. 366, pp. 539–551, 2012.

[2] H. Hamano, S. Kawa, A. Horiuchi et al., "High serum IgG4 concentrations in patients with sclerosing pancreatitis," *The New England Journal of Medicine*, vol. 344, no. 10, pp. 732–738, 2001.

[3] W. Yu, C. Tsai, S. Kao, and C. Liu, "Immunoglobulin G4-related ophthalmic disease," *Taiwan Journal of Ophthalmology*, vol. 8, no. 1, pp. 9–14, 2018.

[4] A. Wu, N. H. Andrew, A. A. McNab, and D. Selva, "IgG4-related ophthalmic disease: pooling of published cases and literature review," *Current Allergy and Asthma Reports*, vol. 15, no. 6, p. 27, 2015.

[5] H. Umehara, K. Okazaki, Y. Masaki et al., "Comprehensive diagnostic criteria for IgG4-related disease (IgG4-RD), 2011," *Modern Rheumatology*, vol. 22, no. 1, pp. 21–30, 2012.

[6] H. Goto, M. Takahira, and A. Azumi, "Diagnostic criteria for IgG4-related ophthalmic disease," *Japanese Journal of Ophthalmology*, vol. 59, no. 1, pp. 1–7, 2015.

[7] K.-H. Yu, T.-M. Chan, P.-H. Tsai, C.-H. Chen, and P.-Y. Chang, "Diagnostic performance of serum IgG4 levels in patients with IgG4-related disease," *Medicine*, vol. 94, no. 41, Article ID e1707, 2015.

# 23

# Varicella Retinal Vasculopathy: Unilateral Cilioretinal Artery Occlusion Despite Acyclovir Therapy Caught using Optical Coherence Tomography-Angiography (OCTA)

**Anadi Khatri ⓘ,[1] Satish Timalsena,[1] Sudhir Gautam,[1] and Muna Kharel[2]**

[1]*Birat Eye Hospital, Biratnagar, Nepal*
[2]*Nepalese Army Institute of Health Sciences, Kathmandu, Nepal*

Correspondence should be addressed to Anadi Khatri; anadikc@gmail.com

Academic Editor: Stephen G. Schwartz

Varicella zoster is known to be associated with vaso-occlusive pathologies, vasculitis, or optic neuritis, leading to profound visual loss. We report a case where a 13-year-old boy who initially presented to us with on and off diminution of vision in his right eye since 3 days and had normal ocular and OCT angiography findings followed up in 5 days with sudden painless diminution of vision in the same eye since one day this time revealing a pale macular region with rest of the retina being normal. Repeated OCT angiography showed loss of the capillary network around the perifoveal region suggesting cilioretinal artery occlusion.

## 1. Introduction

Varicella-zoster virus (VZV) is an exclusively human virus that belongs to the $\alpha$-herpes virus family [1]. VZV is present worldwide and is highly infectious. The primary infection leads to acute varicella or "chickenpox", usually from exposure either through direct contact with a skin lesion or through airborne spread from respiratory droplets [2].

Ocular manifestations of the pathology have been reported in forms of retinal vasculopathy, retinitis, and optic neuritis [3–7]. Cilioretinal artery occlusion in the pediatric population is considered very rare and it is most often associated with hypercoagulable states and embolic phenomena [8]. We present a patient with profound unilateral vision loss due to cilioretinal artery occlusion following varicella zoster infection.

## 2. The Case

A thirteen-year-old boy presented to us with on and off diminution of vision in the right eye (RE) for 3 days. He had recently had varicella zoster (chicken pox) 7 days back for which he had visited pediatrician and dermatologist. He was

on a dose of 400 mg twice daily at the time of presentation but gives history of taking 400 mg for five times initially for 5 days which was appropriate for his body weight of 23 kilograms.

On general evaluation, he had resolving scab marks following varicella zoster dermatitis over the skin of forehead and trunk region. He denies any history of ocular /facial/oral trauma, lightheadedness, or blackouts. The patient party denies observing any abnormal bodily movements or loss of consciousness. The patient does give a history of fever 6 days back which resolved after taking paracetamol. There is no other significant medical or surgical history. Ocular examination revealed a visual acuity of 6/6 in both the eyes (OU). Anterior and posterior segment findings were normal.

Dilated fundus examination revealed normal findings (Figure 1(a)). The patient was advised for OCT angiography (Topcon Medical Systems -Triton™ DRI PLUS SS-OCT) which was normal (Figures 1(b), 1(c), and 1(d)). He was advised for blood examinations including total blood count, peripheral blood smear, CRP, homocysteine levels, lipid profile, and cardiological evaluation. The patient followed up days later with sudden painless diminution of vision in RE. He had a vision of 1/60 RE and 6/6 in the left eye (LE). The anterior segment showed a relative afferent pupillary defect

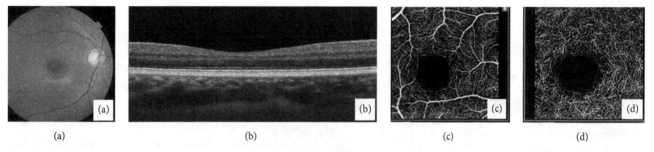

(a)                              (b)                              (c)                              (d)

FIGURE 1: (a)Fundus photo and OCT of macula (b) at initial presentation. Note the well-described perifoveolar capillary plexus in both superficial and deep plexus (c and d).

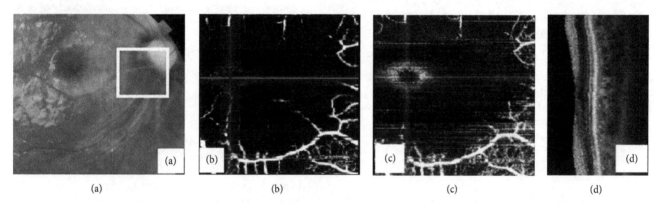

(a)                              (b)                              (c)                              (d)

FIGURE 2: (a) "Ghost-" like cilioretinal vessel(Boxed) impression secondary to occlusion. Note the loss of the perifoveolar capillary plexuses in both superficial and deep plexus (b)and (c) with edema of the perimacular nerve fibre layer(d).

in RE (Grade 3, (Bell's classification)). There was no evidence of vitritis. Dilated fundus examination of RE revealed retinal edema involving the posterior pole with distinctive cherry red-like spot at the foveolar area. The disc was slightly pale. There were arteriolar attenuation and segmentation of blood column within the arterioles (Figure 2(a)). The LE was normal. His blood parameters and cardiovascular and serological reports were normal.

Homocysteine levels and coagulation profile were in the normal range. We planned for FFA but the patient and his party denied going under the procedure and hence we advised for repeating the OCT angiography. OCTA revealed loss of capillary plexus in both superficial and deep retinal layers (Figures 2(b) and 2(c)). Optical coherence tomography revealed massive retinal thickening due to edema with disorganized retinal elements (Figure 2(d)). A diagnosis of right eye cilioretinal artery occlusion was made on the basis of clinical and OCTA findings. Despite treatment with acyclovir and steroids, the vision failed to improve until 4 weeks after which the patient was lost to follow-up.

## 3. Discussion

Retinal artery occlusions (RAO) are most commonly a result of embolic obstruction. Other mechanisms are also known and mainly include exogenous emboli, thrombotic, vasospastic, and vasculitic pathologies [9]. Retinal artery occlusion has been reported as a complication of varicella-zoster infection

in various age groups denoting vaso-occlusive nature of pathology [3–5, 7, 10]. It is also one of the components of the varicella vasculopathy [5].

RAO and branched-RAO have been reported in the pediatric population following chickenpox infection. Jayaram H. et al. have reported bilateral ophthalmic artery occlusion secondary to a probable chicken pox vasculopathy in a child [5]. Similarly, Zamora et al. [3] have reported a case where the patient had multiple recurrent branched retinal artery occlusion secondary to varicella zoster infection. Sebban AI et al. [4] have also reported a similar case with a branch retinal artery following varicella zoster eruptions. Lalit et al. [7] from our region have also reported a case of CRAO with a profound vision loss in a 12-year-old patient who presented within few days after varicella zoster infection with dermatitis causing a profound vision loss.

Our patient presented with unilateral cilioretinal artery occlusion. This was diagnosed with the clinical finding of the fundus and confirmed by OCTA. This is the first case of this pathology to be reported with the use of OCTA. Cilioretinal artery occlusion is considered as the least common variant of RAO [11]. In addition to this rarity, the patient in the first visit had complained about on and off diminution of vision in the same eye for which we performed OCTA which revealed completely normal retinal vasculature architecture. The systemic evaluation had also revealed normal findings. As the patient was already on antiherpetic agents, a continuation of the same medication was advised. Disregard of this, the patient followed up in just a few days with RAO. OCTA showed loss of capillary plexuses in both superficial and deep layer analysis. The presentation of our patient is congruent in many terms with varicella vasculopathy. It has been mentioned that varicella vasculopathy may present as transient ischemic attack with neurological and retinal deficits [10, 12]. A closely related term, postvaricella angiopathy, has been also described in the literature where vaso-occlusive pathologies can occur after several months following chicken pox [10].

Most literatures [2, 3, 7, 10, 13, 14] agree that retinal complications can be treated or prevented with the use of Acyclovir. The patient was already under treatment of this drug and was advised to continue the medication. Yet, the patient presented with cilioretinal artery occlusion in one eye. Studies have suggested that postvaricella vasculopathy is associated with stenosis of the cerebral arteries and also account for nearly 1/3rd of childhood strokes [10, 12, 13]. They have also concluded that in such cases antithrombotic therapy may prevent strokes/transient ischemic attacks (TIA) [13]. The same may hold true for retinal vasculature and a detailed study of retinal vasculatures using fluorescence angiography or OCTA modules may be necessary to confirm this.

## 4. Conclusion

Varicella zoster infections are an established cause for retinal artery occlusions in the pediatric population and can also cause cilioretinal artery occlusion. Use of acyclovir alone may not suffice to prevent vaso-occlusive phenomena and addition of antithrombotic may also be needed. OCTA can be a good noninvasive tool to aid in diagnosis.

## Consent

Consent has been attained and confidentiality of the patient information has been maintained.

## Authors' Contributions

*All authors made an equal contribution in evaluating* and interpreting the OCT findings and critical review of the manuscript. *Dr. Anadi Khatri* was the leader in the drafting of the manuscript.

## Acknowledgments

We would like to thank Mr. Sabin K.C, senior technical staff, for performing the OCT on our patients.

## References

[1] J. Breuer and H. Fifer, "Chickenpox," *BMJ Clinical Evidence*, 2011.

[2] S. A. Pergam, A. P. Limaye, and AST Infectious Diseases Community of Practice, "Varicella zoster virus(VZV) in solid organ transplant recipients," *American Journal of Transplantation*, vol. 9, no. 4, pp. S108–S115, 2009.

[3] R. L. Zamora, L. V. Del Priore, G. A. Storch, L. D. Gelb, and J. Sharp, "Multiple recurrent branch retinal artery occlusions associated with varicella zoster virus," *Retina*, vol. 16, no. 5, pp. 399–404, 1996.

[4] A. I. Sebban, T. J. Sullivan, and M. B. Davison, "Branch retinal artery occlusion in a child," *Australian & New Zealand Journal of Ophthalmology*, vol. 24, no. 3, pp. 283–286, 1996.

[5] H. Jayaram, D. Stanescu-Segal, G. E. Holder, and E. M. Graham, "Bilateral ophthalmic artery occlusions due to probable varicella-zoster virus vasculopathy," *JAMA Ophthalmology*, vol. 130, no. 11, p. 1492, 2012.

[6] R. l. Gurung, "Chicken pox associated bilateral retinal vasculitis in an immunocompetent young male; an unusual case report," *Birat Journal of Health Sciences*, vol. 4, no. 1, pp. 680–682, 2019.

[7] L. Agarwal, N. Agrawal, R. K. Labh, R. Choubey, and B. Agrawal, "Central retinal artery occlusion associated with varicella dermatitis," *Journal of Nepal Paediatric Society*, vol. 36, no. 1, pp. 78–81, 2016.

[8] G. J. Manayath, P. K. Shah, V. Narendran, and R. J. Morris, "Idiopathic pediatric retinal artery occlusion," *Indian Journal of Ophthalmology*, vol. 58, no. 2, pp. 151-152, 2010.

[9] R. G. Julien, "Zona ophthalmique et obliteration de l'artere centrale de la retine," *Bulletin des sociétés d'ophtalmologie de France*, pp. 842-843, 1952.

[10] C. J. Selvakumar, C. Justin, R. Gnanaeswaran, and M. Chandrasekaran, "Post - varicella vasculopathy," *The Journal of the Association of Physicians of India*, vol. 58, pp. 572-573, 2010.

[11] C. M. Greven, M. M. Slusher, and R. G. Weaver, "Retinal arterial occlusion in young adults," *American Journal of Ophthalmology*, vol. 120, pp. 776–783, 1995.

[12] N. Venugopal, "Head injury, varicella vasculopathy: differential diagnosis for pediatric retinal arterial occlusion," *Indian Journal of Ophthalmology*, vol. 65, no. 5, p. 424, 2017.

[13] R. Askalan, S. Laughlin, S. Mayank et al., "Chickenpox and stroke inchildhood: a study of frequency and causation," *Stroke*, vol. 32, no. 6, pp. 1257–1262, 2000.

[14] L. V. Heckler, D. E. Lederer, F. Alwadani, and R. K. Koenekoop, "Idiopathic central retinal artery occlusion in a 6-year-old," *Canadian Journal of Ophthalmology*, vol. 43, no. 3, pp. 375-376, 2008.

# 24

# *Cyphellophora* sp. Isolated from a Corneal Ulcer in the Human Eye

**Satheitra Rajandran** ⓘ,[1,2] **Kursiah Mohd Razali,**[1] **Mushawiahti Mustapha,**[2] **Prem Ananth Palaniappan,**[3] **and Fairuz Amran**[3]

[1]*Department of Ophthalmology, Hospital Raja Permaisuri Bainun, Jalan Raja Ashman Shah, 30450 Ipoh, Perak, Malaysia*
[2]*Department of Ophthalmology, Hospital Canselor Tuanku Muhriz, Jalan Yaacob Latif, Bandar Tun Razak, 56000 Cheras, Kuala Lumpur, Malaysia*
[3]*Institute for Medical Research, Jalan Pahang, 50588 Kuala Lumpur, Wilayah Persekutuan Kuala Lumpur, Malaysia*

Correspondence should be addressed to Satheitra Rajandran; satheitra@gmail.com

Academic Editor: Nicola Rosa

*Cyphellophora* is a black yeast-like fungus with most of the strains being isolated from soil and plants. It tends to cause sooty blotch and flyspeck disease in plants. In humans, it is known to cause superficial skin and nail infections. This report highlights the case of a patient who initially presented with a small corneal abrasion which rapidly progressed into a corneal ulcer after the patient did not respond to the initial conventional treatment. The laboratory results from the corneal scraping found it to be *Cyphellophora* sp.

## 1. Introduction

A corneal ulcer is an inflammatory or infective condition of the cornea resulting in the disruption of the epithelial layer and the corneal stroma [1]. The incidence of corneal ulcers has been estimated to occur 1.5–2 million times per year in developing countries [2]. The etiological agents of the microbial keratitis can be bacteria, fungi, or parasites [1, 2].

Fungal corneal ulcers usually occur in young workers involved in outdoor work, often agricultural work. Often, the fungus that causes a corneal ulcer belongs to the yeast group, e.g., *Candida* sp., or filamentous fungi, e.g., *Fusarium* and *Aspergillus*. A common predisposing factor is trauma to the eye due to organic matter or a soil-contaminated object [3].

*Cyphellophora* belongs to the genus *Cyphellophoraceae* and the order *Chaetothyriales*. It is a black, yeast-like fungus characterised by the production of septated conidia from intercalary or terminal phialides which bear flaring, thin, or conspicuous collarettes. The first generic species *Cyphellophora laciniata* was discovered and isolated from the human skin in 1962 [4, 5].

Plant-associated *Cyphellophora* species such as *C. guyanesis* and *C. vermispora* were commonly found in soil and plants. Most of the strains were known to cause sooty blotch and flyspeck disease which are known to damage certain fruit crops [4].

We describe a rare case of *Cyphellophora* sp. isolated from a patient with a corneal ulcer. This patient initially presented with a corneal abrasion; however, it progressed rapidly into a corneal ulcer. The ulcer did not have the typical presentation of fungal infection and did not respond well to the available topical antifungal eye drops. Here, we highlight the difficulty and the challenges both in the clinical diagnosis and the treatment of this patient.

## 2. Case Report

A 58-year-old male with poorly controlled diabetes mellitus who works as a security guard presented with discomfort and redness in the left eye after a foreign body entered his eye while riding a motorbike. He immediately rinsed out his eye with tap water. On presentation, it was noted that

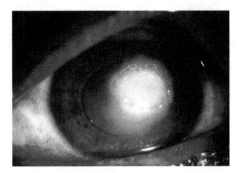

FIGURE 1: Anterior segment picture of the left eye showing a corneal ulcer involving the visual axis.

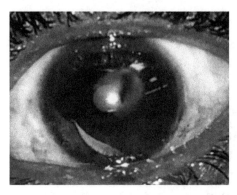

FIGURE 2: Corneal scarring centrally (6 months after the initial presentation).

the left eye vision was 6/36 and the pinhole was 6/18. Examination of the left eye showed a small foreign body (<1 mm) located centrally on the cornea at 12 o'clock at the level of superior pupillary margin. The foreign body was removed, leaving a small epithelial defect. The patient was discharged and prescribed with topical chloramphenicol 0.5% every 4hourly. However, during the subsequent review, it was noted that the epithelial defect persisted.

Ten days later, the patient presented with worsening eye pain and redness. The vision of the left eye was 6/24, and an examination showed a stromal infiltrate measuring 1.7 mm (vertically) and 1.8 mm (horizontally) along with Descemet folds and surrounding corneal haziness. There were no signs of fluffy edges, satellite lesions, or endothelial plaque, which would suggest a fungal infection. Initially, the patient was treated as having infective bacterial keratitis and given hourly topical gentamicin 0.9% and ceftazidime 5%. A corneal scraping was sent for analysis.

Despite intensive hourly topical antibacterial inpatient treatment, the infection progressed into a large corneal ulcer affecting the central visual axis (Figure 1). The visual acuity dropped to 1/60.

The initial lab results of the corneal scraping showed a fungal isolate; however, it had to be sent to the Institute for Medical Research Malaysia (IMR) for identification in view of it being a new strain. The patient was started on hourly topical Amphotericin B 0.15% and hourly Fluconazole 0.2% along with oral Fluconazole 200 mg once daily in addition to the topical treatment. As his diabetic control was very poor, the patient was referred to a medical team and dietitian for optimisation of his diabetes.

Three weeks from the first presentation, the patient was given an intrastromal injection of Amphotericin B (5 μg in 0.1 ml). A week later, he underwent an intracameral administration of 5 μg in 0.1 ml Amphotericin B as he was not responding well to the topical and oral treatments.

Initially, the patient did not show good response to the intrastromal and intracameral injections. However, a week later, the ulcer started responding in addition to the combination of intensive topical antifungal (hourly Fluconazole 0.2% and Amphotericin B 0.15%) and antibacterial (2 hourly gentamicin 0.9% and cefuroxime 5%) eye drops. Four months later, the ulcer had healed completely, leaving a corneal scar (Figure 2). His best corrected visual acuity was 6/24.

The final lab results from IMR suggested an isolate of fungus from *Cyphellophora* sp. The method that was used for microscopic identification of this fungus was culturing on Sabouraud dextrose agar (Figure 3(a)). Lactophenol cotton blue mounting revealed phialides with collarettes bearing septated conidia (Figure 3(b)).

## 3. Discussion

According to the literature, there are only a few reports on *Cyphellophora* causing superficial cutaneous and nail infections in humans. *Cyphellophora laciniata*, *C. pluriseptata*, and *P. ambigua* have been reported to be isolated from superficial lesions in human cutaneous infections [6, 7]. In another instance, the bronchoalveolar lavage fluid from a patient after heart bypass surgery grew *C. fusaroides* [8]. *Cyphellophora suttonii* was also isolated from an ulcerating skin lesion in a patient with sarcoidosis [9].

This was a rare instance of this fungus isolated from an ulcer in the eye. We faced difficulties in the preliminary diagnosis as it did not have typical characteristics of a fungal infection in the eye. It showed a rapid progression of the infection despite being on antibacterial eye drops, which could have also been exacerbated by the patient's poor control of his diabetes. The treatment was challenging as it did not show a good response to any of the initial approaches. Fortunately, the laboratory results aided in the treatment revision. A combination of intensive antifungal and antibacterial eye drops hastened the recovery and healing process, which could suggest a possibility of a mixed infection.

In vitro study analysis of the susceptibility of the fungus *Cyphellophora* sp. showed a good response to caspofungin (minimum inhibitory concentration (MIC) 1.1 μg/ml) and newer types of azoles such as itraconazole and voriconazole (0.1 μg/ml and 0.3 μg/ml, respectively). In the study, it was also noted that the MIC was the highest in susceptibility testing of Fluconazole (27.6 μg/ml) and Amphotericin B (4 μg/ml). This could explain the initial poor response to the treatment in this patient [10]. However, there are no in vivo studies or other similar clinical case reports that could aid in the management.

Cyphellophora sp. Isolated from a Corneal Ulcer in the Human Eye

113

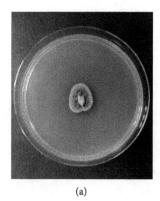 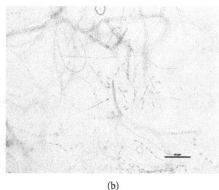

(a) (b)

FIGURE 3: (a) *Cyphellophora* sp. colony growth on Sabouraud dextrose agar. (b) LPCB mount: phialides with collarettes bearing septated conidia (magnification 40x).

## 4. Conclusion

The *Cyphellophora* fungus has now been isolated from a corneal ulcer in a human. The exact nature of the infection and the susceptibility to the antifungal treatment are yet to be learned as this was the first incidence of this fungus in a corneal ulcer in the human eye.

## Consent

Informed consent was obtained from the patient for publication of this case report and all accompanying images.

## References

[1] S. Suwal, D. Bhandari, P. Thapa, M. K. Shrestha, and J. Amatya, "Microbiological profile of corneal ulcer cases diagnosed in a tertiary care ophthalmological institute in Nepal," *BMC Ophthalmology*, vol. 16, no. 1, p. 209, 2016.

[2] H. M. Alkatan and R. S. Al-Essa, "Challenges in the diagnosis of microbial keratitis: a detailed review with update and general guidelines," *Saudi Journal of Ophthalmology*, vol. 33, no. 3, pp. 268–276, 2019.

[3] F. Mohd-Tahir, A. Norhayati, I. Siti-Raihan, and M. Ibrahim, "A 5-year retrospective review of fungal keratitis at Hospital Universiti Sains Malaysia," *Interdisciplinary Perspectives on Infectious Diseases*, vol. 2012, Article ID 851563, 6 pages, 2012.

[4] L. Gao, Y. Ma, W. Zhao et al., "Three new species of *Cyphellophora* (Chaetothyriales) associated with sooty blotch and flyspeck," *PLoS One*, vol. 10, no. 9, article e0136857, 2015.

[5] P. Feng, Q. Lu, M. J. Najafzadeh et al., "Cyphellophora and its relatives in Phialophora: biodiversity and possible role in human infection," *Fungal Diversity*, vol. 65, no. 1, pp. 17–45, 2014.

[6] M. Ameen, "Epidemiology of superficial fungal infections," *Clinics in Dermatology*, vol. 28, no. 2, pp. 197–201, 2010.

[7] A. L. Bittencourt, P. R. Machado, and M. G. Araujo, "Subcutaneous phaeohyphomycosis caused by *Cyphellophora pluriseptata*," *European Journal of Dermatology*, vol. 12, no. 1, pp. 103–106, 2002.

[8] B. C. Sutton, C. K. Campbell, and A. Goldschmied-Reouven, "*Pseudomicrodochium fusarioides* sp. nov., isolated from human bronchial fluid," *Mycopathologia*, vol. 114, no. 3, pp. 159–161, 1991.

[9] L. Ajello, A. A. Padhye, and M. Payne, "Phaeohyphomycosis in a dog caused by *Pseudomicrodochium suttonii* sp. nov," *Mycotaxon*, vol. 12, pp. 131–136, 1980.

[10] P. Feng, M. J. Najafzadeh, J. Sun et al., "In vitro activities of nine antifungal drugs against 81 *Phialophora* and *Cyphellophora* isolates," *Antimicrobial Agents and Chemotherapy*, vol. 56, no. 11, pp. 6044–6047, 2012.

# 25

# Angle Closure Glaucoma in Retinitis Pigmentosa

**Chandni Pradhan,**[1] **Simanta Khadka** ⓘ,[2] **and Purushottam Joshi**[1]

[1]*Mechi Eye Hospital, Birtamod-9, Jhapa, Nepal*
[2]*Bharatpur Eye Hospital, Bharatpur-10, Chitwan, Nepal*

Correspondence should be addressed to Simanta Khadka; simantakhadka@gmail.com

Academic Editor: Cristiano Giusti

*Background.* Angle closure glaucoma (ACG) whether primary or secondary lens induced has rare occurrence in cases with retinitis pigmentosa (RP). *Method.* Five patients with history of diminished vision, ocular pain, and nyctalopia were clinically evaluated. Four patients had unilateral presentations of circumciliary congestion, corneal edema, and high intraocular pressure (IOP), while one had bilateral presentation, respectively. Anterior chambers were shallow; fundoscopy revealed the features of RP and gonioscopy affirmed closed angles in all the cases. The management strategies were individualized based on the specific ocular condition. *Result.* The raised IOP were not well controlled with conventional medical treatment. Neodymium yttrium aluminium garnet laser peripheral iridotomy (LPI) was performed in two patients and in the fellow eye in other two patients as a prophylactic measure. Phacoemulsification surgery with implantation of intraocular lens (IOL) was performed in three patients, whereas phacoemulsification only without IOL and trabeculectomy performed in one patient. Among them, two patients had subluxated lens, where one was managed with capsular tension ring and the other was left aphakic, respectively. However, the vision was not improved significantly in these patients. *Conclusion.* RP may be associated with ACG in rare instances. In these patients, angle closure-related high IOP can have a detrimental effect on the pre-existing visual impairment. However, this can be prevented by thorough clinical examination and timely intervention in those susceptible eyes.

## 1. Introduction

Retinitis pigmentosa (RP) is the term used for a diverse group of progressive hereditary disorders that primarily affect photoreceptors and retinal pigment epithelial (RPE) function. It predominantly affects the rods, followed by subsequent degeneration of cones [1]. The association between RP and glaucoma has been long sought. The first case of RP associated with glaucoma was described by Galezowski in 1862 [2]. Since then there have only been few reports of glaucoma associated with RP. The prevalence of primary open-angle glaucoma with RP ranges from 2 to 12% [3–5]. However, the association of RP and primary angle-closure glaucoma (PACG) has rarely been reported. Badeeb et al. reported the prevalence of 1.03% PACG in RP in patients over 40 years of age [3]. In view of this rarity, the association might be coincidental [4].

Intraocular pressure (IOP) elevation, due to acute angle closure may aggravate the visual impairment in RP patients with pre-existing optic nerve dysfunction [5–7]. Angle closure-related IOP elevation can be prevented by timely intervention in these susceptible eyes. Therefore, understanding the association of angle closure and RP may help preserve visual function in these patients.

Here, we have reported five unusual cases of angle-closure glaucoma (ACG) in RP along with their case-based management. Informed consents of the included patients were obtained, and all the work conducted were in accordance with the Declaration of Helsinki (1964).

## 2. Case Description

*2.1. Case 1.* A 65-year-old female, with a history of nyctalopia presented with a sudden, profound, and painful loss of vision

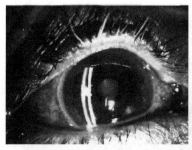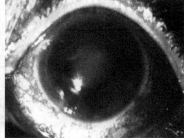

FIGURE 1: Clinical photograph of anterior segment OD and OS of case 1.

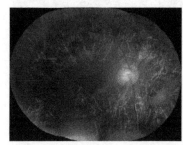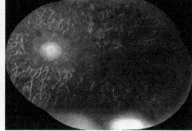

FIGURE 2: Fundus photo OD and OS of case 1.

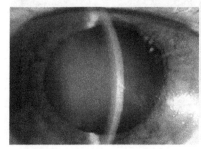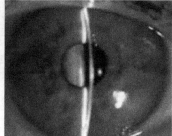

FIGURE 3: Clinical photograph of anterior segment OD and OS of case 2.

OU of three days duration. She recounted a history of poor vision OU since 20 years. On examination, her visual acuity (VA) was hand movement (HM) OU. There was circumciliary congestion (CCC) with corneal edema (Figure 1). The anterior chambers were shallow with Van Herrick (VH) grade two. The pupil was middilated and sluggishly reacting to light OS and presence of posterior subcapsular cataract (PSCC) OU. Goldmann applanation tonometry (GAT) revealed an intraocular pressure (IOP) of 24 mmHg OD and 58 mmHg OS. She was managed with full tolerated antiglaucoma medications (Tab acetazolamide 250 mg, Gtt pilocarpine nitrate 2%, Gtt timolol maleate 0.5%+Gtt brimonidine tartrate 0.1%, and Gtt latanoprost 0.005%) and topical steroids (Gtt prednisolone acetate 1%). The following day, the corneal clarity was enhanced and her IOP was within a normal range of 11 mmHg OD and 12 mmHg OS, respectively. Gonioscopic examination disclosed closed angles in superior, temporal, and nasal quadrants OD, whereas, there was peripheral anterior synechiae (PAS) in all quadrant OS. Fundus examination revealed the cup disc ratio (CDR) 0.5 OD and 0.9 OS. The peripheral vessels were narrow and attenuated OU. There was diffuse RPE atrophy and bony spicules in the posterior pole and midperipheral retina (Figure 2). Neodymium yttrium aluminium garnett (Nd: YAG) laser peripheral iridotomy (LPI) was done OU followed by phacoemulsification with posterior chamber intraocular lens (PCIOL) OD. Her postoperative best corrected visual acuity (BCVA) was 4/60 OD, and IOP was regulated under control OU with topical medications and hence continued.

*2.2. Case 2.* A 55-year-old female with a history of nyctalopia presented with painful loss of vision in RE since two weeks. She had no significant systemic illness or family history of ocular diseases. On examination, VA was HM OD and 6/18 OS. Congestion with corneal edema was evident with shallow AC (VH grade 1), middilated sluggishly reacting pupil, and presence of glaucomflecken with nuclear sclerosis (NS) grade 2 OD. Similarly, AC was also shallow (VH grade 2) and lens opacification of NS grade 2 OS (Figure 3). IOP with applanation was 46 mmHg OD and 17 mmHg OS. The patient was managed with full tolerated antiglaucoma medications. The

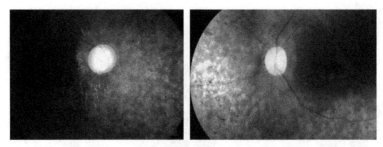

FIGURE 4: Fundus photograph OD and OS of case 2.

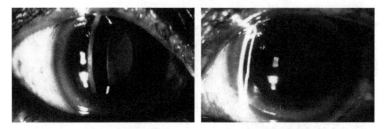

FIGURE 5: Clinical photograph of anterior segment OD and OS of case 3.

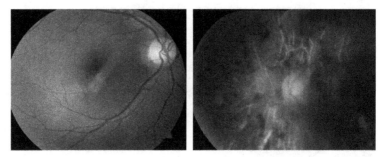

FIGURE 6: Fundus photograph of case 3 with normal looking posterior pole OD and presence of diffuse bony spicules OS.

following day, IOP was persistently high 38 mmHg OD despite medications, but the cornea was relatively clear allowing gonioscopy and fundus examination. On gonioscopy, there was presence of PAS in all quadrants OD. However, the angles were barely visible on indentation OS. On fundus examination, there was waxy pale discs OU, with near total cupping OD and CDR of 0.4 : 1 OS. The vessels were attenuated, and bony spicules diffusely distributed in peripheral retina OU (Figure 4). Prophylactic Nd:YAG LPI was done OS and lens extraction with PCIOL OD. The VA did not improve OD, but IOP declined to 22 mmHg one month past surgery. Antiglaucoma medications were continued OD.

*2.3. Case 3.* A 62-year-old female presented with a history of painless loss of vision OS since 20 years. There was no significant family history. On examination, her BCVA was 6/36 OD and fingers counting close to face (FCCF) OS. Cornea was clear and AC shallow (VH grade 2) OU (Figure 5). Relative afferent pupillary defect (RAPD) was demonstrated during pupillary examination OS. There was nuclear sclerosis (NS) grade 2 OU. Gonioscopy divulged closed angles OD and presence of PAS in superior and temporal quadrants OS with IOP of 12 mmHg OD and 14 mmHg OS. On fundus examination, CDR was 0.3 : 1 OU. Peripheral retina was within

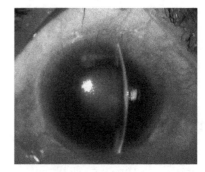

FIGURE 7: Anterior segment OS of case 4.

normal limits OD, but there was presence of diffuse bony spicules OS (Figure 6). The patient mentioned inability to follow up as she was from a very distant area. LPI was done OU, and patient was planned for cataract surgery, but the patient declined.

*2.4. Case 4.* A 44-year-old male had a history of diminished vision OU (OS more marked than OD) since 14 years. He complained of pain and redness OS since one month. On examination, VA was 5/60 OD and HM OS. Anterior

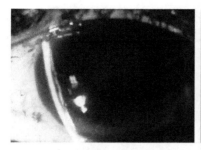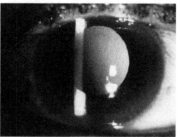

FIGURE 8: Clinical photograph of anterior segment OD and OS of case 5.

segment evaluation revealed shallow AC OD, while there was diffuse corneal edema with shallow AC, middilated pupils OS (Figure 7), and lenticular opacification of NS grade 2 OU. IOP was 16 mmHg OD and 65 mmHg OS, respectively. With commencement of maximum tolerated antiglaucoma medications, the cornea OS cleared allowing gonioscopy which revealed PAS in >270°. On fundus examination, discs were pale OU with CDR of 0.6 : 1 OD and 0.9 : 1 OS, respectively. Other than waxy pallor, the components of classic triad of RP were fulfilled with the presence of attenuated vessels and diffuse bony spicules OU.

Combined cataract surgery and trabeculectomy was planned OS. However, subluxated lens of three-clock hours from 6 to 9 o'clock were noted intraoperatively and implantation of capsular tension ring with PCIOL was possible in the bag at the conclusion of surgery. Prophylactic LPI was done in the fellow eye.

*2.5. Case 5.* A 56-year-old male with complains of nyctalopia and diminished vision since three years. VA was perception of light with inaccurate projection of rays OD; however, there was no perception of light (NPL) OS. There was CCC, corneal edema OD with shallow AC OU. There was grade 3 NS OD, while the fellow eye was aphakic (Figure 8). The pupils were middilated and sluggishly reacting OU. The fundus visibility was very poor OD due to corneal edema and dense NS, and there was posteriorly dislocated lens in vitreous OS. Gonioscopy revealed PAS in three quadrants OS, but hazy media precluded angle evaluation OD. However, the patient denied history of trauma. The IOP was 60 mmHg OD and 35 mmHg OS. The IOP was controlled with maximum tolerated antiglaucoma medications. Combined cataract surgery and trabeculectomy with mitomycin C was performed OD. Intraoperative, subluxation of lens more than 180° from 3 to 10 clock hours was discovered and thorough anterior vitrectomy was performed and the patient was left aphakic. Superior flap with surgical iridectomy was created at superior 12 o'clock position. Postoperative ocular findings were uneventful and revealed no vitreous in AC, but there was no improvement in VA after surgery. The fundus examination post surgery affirmed pale disc with narrow attenuated peripheral vessels and diffuse RPE changes with bony spicules and attenuated arteriole. The presence of sclerosed venules implied probable overlapping sequelae of veno-occlusive disease (Figure 9).

Table 1 represents the ocular biometric parameters of all the subjects included in this series. Table 2 represents

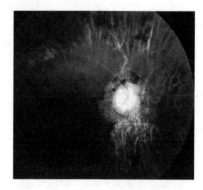

FIGURE 9: Fundus OD of case 5 examined after lens extraction surgery.

summary of the cases with regard to vision, IOP, and management.

## 3. Discussion

We have reviewed five patients of ACG in RP who had visited our hospital at different times between July 2016 and June 2018. Though the literature indicating association between the two conditions are meagre, there are few reports of PACG with RP [3–5]. Among 234 diagnosed cases of RP in our hospital during this period, five cases presented as ACG accounting for prevalence of 2.13% in our series. A prevalence of 1.03% PACG in RP was reported from Canada [3]. Similarly, a five-year study from China showed 2.3% of RP associated with glaucoma, where angle closure was more frequent than open-angle glaucoma [8].

All of our patients were above 40 years, and three were females. It is an established fact that ACG occur more commonly in females. Similar female preponderance was reported to be 54.7% [5] and 56.52% [9] for RP, respectively.

A-scan ocular biometric readings were only included in this series as ultrasonic biomicroscopy (UBM) is not available in our setup. It is also suggested that the simultaneous occurrence of nanophthalmos, angle-closure glaucoma, and pigmentary retinal dystrophy could be a new syndrome [10, 11]. However, none of our patients were nanophthalmic, and the average AL was 21.87 mm OD and 21.38 mm OS, respectively. The role of UBM, where available, can provide reliable information and imaging evidence to evaluate the status of the lens position and determine subluxation for clinical use [12].

TABLE 1: Ocular biometric parameters of the patients.

| S. no. | Age (years) | Gender | Anterior chamber depth (mm) | | Axial length (AL) (mm) | | Lens thickness (mm) | | Central corneal thickness ($\mu$m) | |
|---|---|---|---|---|---|---|---|---|---|---|
| | | | OD | OS | OD | OS | OD | OS | OD | OS |
| 1 | 65 | F | 2.39 | 1.98 | 22.52 | 22.56 | 4.61 | 4.89 | 555 | 536 |
| 2 | 55 | F | 2.34 | 2.12 | 22.9 | 21.86 | 4.98 | 4.82 | 494 | 496 |
| 3 | 63 | F | 2.49 | 2.49 | 20.81 | 20.39 | 4.81 | 5.22 | 535 | 555 |
| 4 | 44 | M | 2.13 | 1.88 | 22.05 | 21.56 | 4.22 | 4.89 | 560 | 590 |
| 5 | 56 | M | 2.15 | 2.8 | 21.08 | 20.54 | 4.83 | — | 552 | 538 |
| Mean | 56.6 ± 8.3 | | 2.3 | 2.25 | 21.87 | 21.38 | 4.69 | 4.95 | 539.2 | 543 |

TABLE 2: Summary of vision, IOP, and management of the cases.

| Case no. | Presenting VA | | Presenting IOP (mm of Hg) | | Management | Final VA | | Final IOP (mm of Hg) | |
|---|---|---|---|---|---|---|---|---|---|
| | OD | OS | OD | OS | | OD | OS | OD | OS |
| 1 | HM | HM | 24 | 58 | OU:LPI, OD:Phaco+PCIOL | 4/60 | HM | 11 | 12 |
| 2 | HM | 6/18 | 46 | 17 | OD:Phaco+PCIOL, OS:LPI | HM | 6/18 | 22 | 17 |
| 3 | 6/36 | FCCF | 12 | 14 | OU:LPI | 6/36 | FCCF | 11 | 12 |
| 4 | 5/60 | HM | 16 | 65 | OD:LPI, OS:Phaco+CTR+PCIOL | 5/60 | HM | 16 | 14 |
| 5 | PL | NPL | 60 | 35 | OD:Phaco+Trab+MMC | PL | NPL | 20 | 18 |

LPI: Nd:YAG laser peripheral iridectomy; Phaco: phacoemulsification; PCIOL: posterior chamber intraocular lens; Trab: trabeculectomy; MMC: mitomycin C.

In this series, two patients had subluxated lens which were identified intraoperatively. There have been reports of lens subluxation in RP, causing anterior luxation of cataractous lens leading to angle closure. It is contemplated that the ultrastructure of the lens in RP is altered, causing lens fibre disorganisation which may contribute to the instability of the lens with anterior displacement and narrowing of angle [13]. Recently, zonular instability is speculated to be the cause behind angle closure in RP patient [14].

Previous theories regarding glaucoma in RP suggest that the migration of pigments is a characteristic feature of retinitis pigmentosa and these pigments in the angle of the anterior chamber has been stressed as a possible etiologic factor in glaucoma [15]. However, not all RP have grave prognosis. Sectoral RP, unilateral RP, and autosomal dominant inherited RPs have very slowly progressive disease course or could even be static [16]. In our series, we encountered only one patient with unilateral presentation.

In patients with RP, the high IOP due to angle closure can cause more visual impairment. Hence, a proper clinical work up, applanation tonometry, gonioscopy and timely intervention in these RP patients could decrease the risk of more damage by the comorbidity of ACG and preserve the ambulatory vision in these susceptible cases.

# References

[1] M. F. Marmor, G. Aguirre, G. Arden et al., "Retinitis pigmentosa, a symposium on terminology and methods of examination," Ophthalmology, vol. 90, no. 2, pp. 126–131, 1983.

[2] C. A. Omphroy, "Sector retinitis pigmentosa and chronic angle-closure glaucoma: a new association," Ophthalmologica, vol. 189, no. 1-2, pp. 12–20, 1984.

[3] O. Badeeb, G. Trope, and M. Musarella, "Primary angle closure glaucoma and retinitis pigmentosa," Acta Ophthalmologica, vol. 71, no. 6, pp. 727–732, 1993.

[4] D. Elder, System of Ophthalmology. Vol XI. Disease of the lens and vitreous, glaucoma and hypotony, CV Mosby Co., St. Louis, 1969.

[5] Y.-C. Ko, C.-J. Liu, D.-K. Hwang, T.-J. Chen, and C. J. Liu, "Increased risk of acute angle closure in retinitis pigmentosa: a population-based case-control study," PLoS One, vol. 9, no. 9, article e107660, 2014.

[6] J. E. Grunwald, A. M. Maguire, and J. Dupont, "Retinal hemodynamics in retinitis pigmentosa," American Journal of Ophthalmology, vol. 122, no. 4, pp. 502–508, 1996.

[7] D. T. L. Quek, V. T. Koh, G. S. Tan, S. A. Perera, T. T. Wong, and T. Aung, "Blindness and long-term progression of visual field defects in Chinese patients with primary angle-closure glaucoma," American Journal of Ophthalmology, vol. 152, no. 3, pp. 463–469, 2011.

[8] D. W. Peng, "Retinitis pigmentosa associated with glaucoma," Chinese Journal of Ophthalmology (Zhonghua yan ke za zhi), vol. 27, no. 5, pp. 262–264, 1992.

[9] J. Xu, Z. Ouyang, Y. Yang et al., "Ocular biometry in primary angle-closure glaucoma associated with retinitis pigmentosa," Journal of Ophthalmology, vol. 2017, Article ID 9164846, 5 pages, 2017.

[10] S. Ghose, M. S. Sachdev, and H. Kumar, "Bilateral nanophthalmos, pigmentary retinal dystrophy and angle closure glaucoma: a new syndrome?," The British Journal of Ophthalmology, vol. 69, no. 8, pp. 624–628, 1985.

[11] A. K. Mandal, T. Das, and V. K. Gothwal, "Angle closure glaucoma in nanophthalmos and pigmentary retinal dystrophy: a rare syndrome," *Indian Journal of Ophthalmology*, vol. 49, p. 271, 2001.

[12] M. Shi, L. Ma, J. Zhang, and Q. Yan, "Role of 25 MHz ultrasound biomicroscopy in the detection of subluxated lenses," *Journal of Ophthalmology*, vol. 2018, Article ID 3760280, 6 pages, 2018.

[13] M. Sira and T. Ho, "Acute angle closure glaucoma secondary to a luxated lens associated with retinitis pigmentosa," *Eye*, vol. 19, no. 4, pp. 472-473, 2005.

[14] L. Devi, J. Mallick, P. Malik, and S. Parija, "Primary angle closure as a presenting feature of retinitis pigmentosa: a rare case report," *Ophthalmology Research: An International Journal*, vol. 7, no. 4, pp. 1–6, 2017.

[15] S. Gartner and A. Schlossman, "Retinitis pigmentosa associated by glaucoma," *American Journal of Ophthalmology*, vol. 32, no. 10, pp. 1337–1350, 1949.

[16] R. A. Pagon, "Retinitis pigmentosa," *Survey of Ophthalmology*, vol. 33, no. 3, pp. 137–177, 1988.

# 26

# Retinal Occlusive Vasculitis in a Patient with Hyperimmunoglobulin E Syndrome

Mohsen Farvardin ⑩,[1] Mohammad Hassan Jalalpour ⑩,[1] Mohammad Reza Khalili ⑩,[1] Golnoush Mahmoudinezhad ⑩,[2] Fereshteh Mosavat ⑩,[3] Soheila Aleyasin ⑩,[3] and Hamidreza Jahanbani-Ardakani ⑩[4,5]

[1]Poostchi Ophthalmology Research Center, Department of Ophthalmology, School of Medicine, Shiraz University of Medical Sciences, Shiraz, Iran
[2]Hamilton Glaucoma Center, Shiley Eye Institute, Viterbi Family Department of Ophthalmology, University of California San Diego, La Jolla, CA, USA
[3]Division of Allergy and Immunology, Department of Pediatrics, School of Medicine, Shiraz University of Medical Sciences, Shiraz, Iran
[4]Department of Ophthalmology, School of Medicine, Shiraz University of Medical Sciences, Shiraz, Iran
[5]Student Research Committee, Shiraz University of Medical Sciences, Shiraz, Iran

Correspondence should be addressed to Hamidreza Jahanbani-Ardakani; hamidreza_jahanbaniardakani@yahoo.com

Academic Editor: Kamal Kishore

*Background.* Hyperimmunoglobulin E syndrome (HIES), or Job's syndrome, is a primary immunodeficiency disorder that is characterized by an elevated level of IgE with values reaching over 2000 IU (normal < 200 IU), eczema, and recurrent staphylococcus infection. Affected individuals are predisposed to infection, autoimmunity, and inflammation. Herein, we report a case of HIES with clinical findings of retinal occlusive vasculitis. *Case Presentation.* A 10-year-old boy with a known case of hyperimmunoglobulin E syndrome had exhibited loss of vision and bilateral dilated fixed pupil. Fundoscopic examination revealed peripheral retinal hemorrhaging, vascular sheathing around the retinal arteries and veins, and vascular occlusion in both eyes. A fluorescein angiography of the right eye showed hyper- and hypofluorescence in the macula and hypofluorescence in the periphery of the retina, peripheral arterial narrowing, and arterial occlusion. A fluorescein angiography of the left eye showed hyper- and hypofluorescence in the supranasal area of the optic disc. Macular optical coherence tomography of the right eye showed inner and outer retinal layer distortion. A genetic study was performed that confirmed mutations of the dedicator of cytokinesis 8 (DOCK 8). HSV polymerase chain reaction testing on aqueous humor and vitreous was negative, and finally, the patient was diagnosed with retinal occlusive vasculitis. *Conclusion.* Occlusive retinal vasculitis should be considered as a differential diagnosis in patients with hyperimmunoglobulin E syndrome presenting with visual loss.

## 1. Introduction

Hyperimmunoglobulin E syndrome (HIES), or Job's syndrome, is a primary immunodeficiency disorder. It was first described in 1966 by Davis and is characterized by an elevated level of IgE with values reaching over 2000 IU (normal < 200 IU), eczema, and recurrent staphylococcus infection. Affected individuals are predisposed to infection, autoimmunity, and inflammation [1, 2]. Herein, we report a case of HIES with clinical findings of retinal occlusive vasculitis.

## 2. Case Presentation

A 10-year-old boy with a known case of HIES was referred to the pediatric ophthalmology clinic at Poostchi Eye Clinic, which is affiliated with Shiraz University of Medical Science

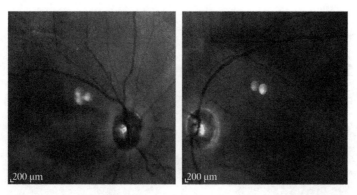

FIGURE 1: Multicolor SLO: (OD) optic nerve pallor, intraretinal hemorrhages, areas of macular whitening, perivascular infiltration, and retinal vein occlusion (thread like); (OS) optic nerve pallor, macular nerve fiber loss, intraretinal hemorrhages, and areas of macular whitening.

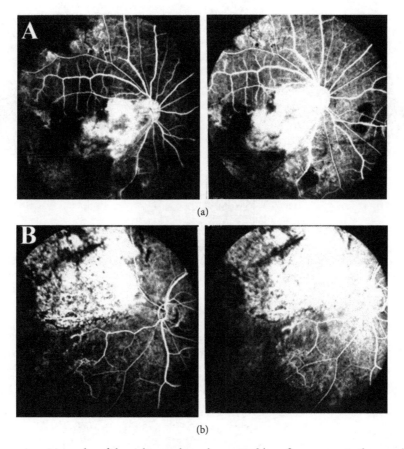

FIGURE 2: (a) Fundus fluorescein angiography of the right eye shows hyper- and hypofluorescence in the macular area in favor of retinal hemorrhage and vascular leakage and peripheral arterial narrowing and occlusion. (b) Fundus fluorescein angiography of the left eye shows hyper- and hypofluorescence that is in favor of vascular leakage, retinal hemorrhage, and ischemia in the supranasal area of the optic disc.

in Shiraz City in Iran. He had exhibited loss of vision and bilateral dilated fix pupils about 1 month before visiting the clinic. His family history revealed that his sister had also been diagnosed with HIES and had succumbed to lymphoma. The patient had been diagnosed with AR-HIES in early childhood. He had presented with eczema, severe dermatitis, recurrent skin abscesses, herpes simplex virus (HSV), gingivostomatitis, and recurrent sinopulmonary infections. He also exhibited a high serum IgE level (600 IU/ml). The NIH hyper IgE score was 40 [3].

An ophthalmic physical examination showed visual acuity of 20/200 in the right eye (OD) and 20/400 in the left eye (OS). Slit lamp examination of both eyes revealed severe meibomian gland dysfunction, blepharitis, and fixed dilated pupils. Funduscopic examination revealed optic nerve pallor, intraretinal hemorrhage, areas of macular

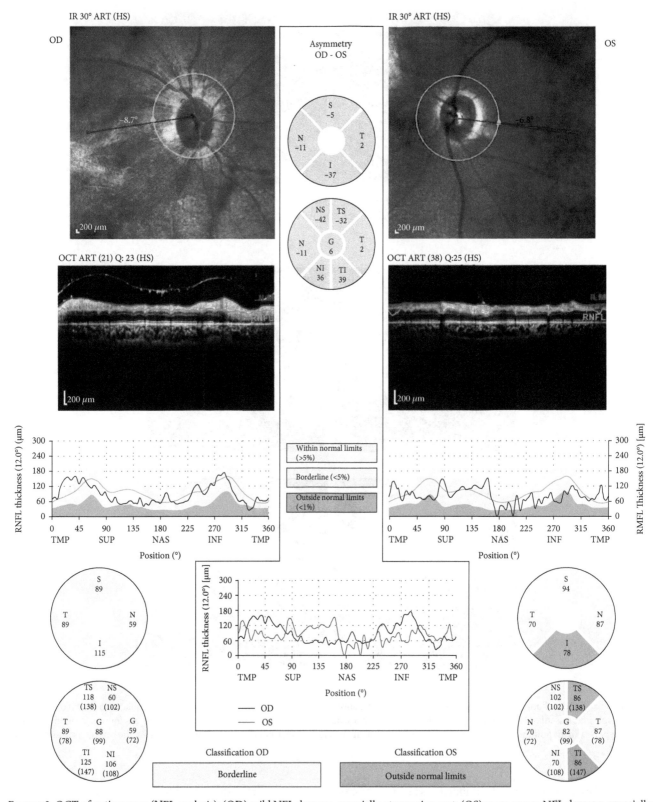

FIGURE 3: OCT of optic nerves (NFL analysis): (OD) mild NFL damage, especially at superior part; (OS) more severe NFL damage, especially at inferior part.

whitening, perivascular infiltration, and retinal vein occlusion. (Figure 1). Fluorescein angiography of the right eye showed hyper- and hypofluorescence that is in favor of vascular leakage and retinal hemorrhage in the macula and

hypofluorescence in the periphery of the retina, peripheral arterial narrowing, and arterial occlusion. Fluorescein angiography of the left eye showed hyper- and hypofluorescence that is in favor of vascular leakage and retinal hemorrhage

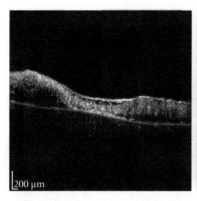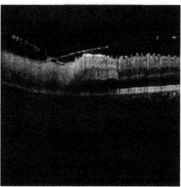

FIGURE 4: OCT of macula: (OD) faint epiretinal membrane, inner and outer retinal layers' distortion with some atrophic areas, and areas of subretinal hyporeflectivity (fluid); (OS) epiretinal membrane, intraretinal hyperreflectivity (hemorrhage), and subretinal hyporeflectivity (fluid).

and ischemia in the supranasal area of the optic disc (Figure 2). Optical coherence tomography (OCT) of optic nerves (NFL analysis) showed retinal nerve fiber damage (NFL) in both eyes (Figure 3). Macular optical coherence tomography of the macula showed epiretinal membrane, inner and outer retinal layers' distortion with some atrophic areas, areas of subretinal hyporeflectivity (fluid), and intraretinal hyperreflectivity (hemorrhage) (Figure 4).

Magnetic resonance imaging of the brain with and without contrast revealed the prominence and dilatation of the cerebral ventricles (lateral and 3rd and 4th ventricles) with possible communicating hydrocephalus, generalized cortical atrophy, and pansinusitis. Magnetic resonance angiography of the brain revealed irregular borders of both posterior cerebral arteries, possible vasculitis, and prominent central and peripheral CSF spaces, suggesting atrophy. A genetic study was performed that confirmed homozygous mutations of the dedicator of cytokinesis 8 (DOCK 8).

To rule out HSV infection, we performed anterior chamber and vitreous tap. The specimen was tested by the microbiological laboratory for HSV PCR and the result was negative. The patient was diagnosed with occlusive retinal vasculitis. Panretinal photocoagulation (PRP) laser treatment was performed to treat the retinal ischemia.

## 3. Discussion and Conclusion

The majority of HIES cases are sporadic; however, autosomal dominant (AD) and autosomal recessive (AR) inherited types have been described in the literature [1]. In 60-70 percent of the AD type, mutation occurs in the STAT3 [4]. In the AR type, which is characterized by persistent viral skin infections and mucocutaneous candidiasis, mutation occurs in the dedicator of cytokinesis 8 (DOCK8) in many cases [4, 5]. DOCK8 mutation-related vasculitis has been previously reported [6].

The prevalence of vascular abnormalities in HIES is unknown. In patients with HIES, vascular abnormalities of the brain, vein, skin, lung, aorta, heart, and foot have been reported [1]. Other ocular manifestations of HIES have been described, including conjunctivitis [7], keratitis, corneal perforation, xanthelasma, undefined eye lid nodules, giant

chalazia, strabismus, and retinal detachment with complicated cataracts and keratoconus [8, 9]. Retinal vasculitis has been described in common variable immunodeficiency [10]. Retinal hemorrhage is also reported as one of the ocular manifestations of hyperimmunoglobulin E syndrome [11]. In addition to vascular abnormality, our patient suffered from MGD, blepharitis, and fixed dilated pupils. The cause in that entity and in our case could be related to autoimmunity or to the occlusion from the high level of IgE as it can induce synthesis of the leukotrienes, chemokines, and cytokines leading to aggregation of the leukocytes and eosinophils with secondary occlusion, and in this setting, the use of omalizumab can potentially control this occlusive process [12].

Our patient was diagnosed with autosomal recessive HIES with DOCK8 mutation. This mutation is associated with a wide spectrum of vascular abnormalities caused by partial T cell deficiency and dysregulation of the immune system, ultimately leading to CNS and systemic vasculitis and lymphoma [13]. Fixed dilated pupils as presented in our patient may have been the result of pupillary sphincter neural damage induced by microangiopathic vasculitis. Central retinal occlusion has previously been reported in autosomal dominant HIES [7]. Our patient was autosomal recessive HIES with sheathing and occlusion of retinal vessels (retinal occlusive vasculitis).

In conclusion, occlusive retinal vasculitis should be considered as a differential diagnosis in patients with hyperimmunoglobulin E syndrome presenting with visual loss. A thorough ophthalmic examination can confirm the diagnosis.

## Consent

Written informed consent was obtained from the patient's parent or guardian for publication of this case report and any accompanying images. A copy of the written consent is available for review by the editor of this journal.

## Authors' Contributions

The authors (M.F., M.R.K, M.H.J., G.S.M.N., F.M., S.A., and H.J.-A.) contributed to the conception, proposal writing, data gathering, manuscript writing, and manuscript revision.

## Acknowledgments

The authors would like to thank Dr. Hassan Saberi (Medical Student, IUMS) for his kind assistance. This study was funded by Shiraz University of Medical Sciences.

## References

[1] H. Yavuz and R. Chee, "A review on the vascular features of the hyperimmunoglobulin E syndrome," *Clinical and Experimental Immunology*, vol. 159, no. 3, pp. 238–244, 2010.

[2] P. F. K. Yong, A. F. Freeman, K. R. Engelhardt, S. Holland, J. M. Puck, and B. Grimbacher, "An update on the hyper-IgE syndromes," *Arthritis Research & Therapy*, vol. 14, no. 6, p. 228, 2012.

[3] A. P. Hsu, J. Davis, J. M. Puck, S. M. Holland, and A. F. Freeman, *STAT3 Hyper IgE Syndrome*, M. P. Adam, H. H. Ardinger, R. A. Pagon, S. E. Wallace, L. J. H. Bean, K. W. Gripp, G. M. Mirzaa, and A. Amemiya, Eds., Seattle (WA): University of Washington, Seattle, 1993-2021.

[4] K. R. Engelhardt, S. McGhee, S. Winkler et al., "Large deletions and point mutations involving the dedicator of cytokinesis 8 (DOCK8) in the autosomal-recessive form of hyper-IgE syndrome," *The Journal of Allergy and Clinical Immunology*, vol. 124, no. 6, pp. 1289–1302.e4, 2009.

[5] H. Hashemi, M. Mohebbi, S. Mehravaran, M. Mazloumi, H. Jahanbani-Ardakani, and S.-H. Abtahi, "Hyperimmunoglobulin E syndrome: genetics, immunopathogenesis, clinical findings, and treatment modalities," *Journal of Research in Medical Sciences*, vol. 22, no. 1, p. 53, 2017.

[6] Q. Zhang, J. C. Davis, I. T. Lamborn, A. F. Freeman, H. Jing, and A. J. Favreau, "Combined immunodeficiency associated with DOCK8 mutations," *The New England Journal of Medicine*, vol. 361, no. 21, pp. 2046–2055, 2009.

[7] B. Grimbacher, S. M. Holland, J. I. Gallin et al., "Hyper-IgE syndrome with recurrent infections–an autosomal dominant multisystem disorder," *The New England Journal of Medicine*, vol. 340, no. 9, pp. 692–702, 1999.

[8] V. Arora, U. R. Kim, H. M. Khazei, and S. Kusagur, "Ophthalmic complications including retinal detachment in hyperimmunoglobulinemia E (Job's) syndrome: case report and review of literature," *Indian Journal of Ophthalmology*, vol. 57, no. 5, pp. 385-386, 2009.

[9] B. Grimbacher, S. M. Holland, and J. M. Puck, "Hyper-IgE syndromes," *Immunological Reviews*, vol. 203, no. 1, pp. 244–250, 2005.

[10] S. Hosseinverdi, H. Hashemi, A. Aghamohammadi, H. D. Ochs, and N. Rezaei, "Ocular involvement in primary immunodeficiency diseases," *Journal of Clinical Immunology*, vol. 34, no. 1, pp. 23–38, 2014.

[11] E. D. Renner, J. M. Puck, S. M. Holland et al., "Autosomal recessive hyperimmunoglobulin E syndrome: a distinct disease entity," *The Journal of Pediatrics*, vol. 144, no. 1, pp. 93–99, 2004.

[12] A. Navinés-Ferrer, E. Serrano-Candelas, G.-J. Molina-Molina, and M. Martín, "IgE-related chronic diseases and anti-IgE-based treatments," *Journal of Immunology Research*, vol. 2016, 12 pages, 2016.

[13] H. C. Su, "Dedicator of cytokinesis 8 (DOCK8) deficiency," *Current Opinion in Allergy and Clinical Immunology*, vol. 10, no. 6, pp. 515–520, 2010.

# 27

# Periorbital Silicone Granulomatosis 30 Years after Acupuncture

Nathan Pirakitikulr⬡,[1] Ann Q. Tran,[1] Armando L. Garcia,[2] Sander R. Dubovy,[2] and Wendy W. Lee[1]

[1]*Division of Oculofacial Plastic and Reconstructive Surgery, Bascom Palmer Eye Institute, University of Miami-Miller School of Medicine, Miami, FL, USA*
[2]*Florida Lions Ocular Pathology Laboratory, Bascom Palmer Eye Institute, University of Miami Miller School of Medicine, Miami, FL, USA*

Correspondence should be addressed to Nathan Pirakitikulr; npiraki@gmail.com

Academic Editor: Nicola Rosa

Silicone-based compounds are commonly used in many medical applications, such as coatings for needles and syringes. Foreign body granulomas are a well-recognized complication of silicone exposure; however, they may be challenging to identify without a clear history. A 61-year-old female patient without prior history of periocular injections, filler, or surgery presented to our oculoplastic clinic with multiple periocular lesions. The patient subsequently underwent excisional biopsy of two prominent lesions, which were identified as granulomas on pathology. Further questioning revealed the cause to be facial acupuncture performed decades prior, and a subsequent targeted exam identified additional lesions at other needling sites. A third lesion was subsequently excised, and there was no recurrence at the last follow-up 3 months postsurgery. Acupuncture is an increasingly common but underrecognized source of silicone exposure and can present up to several decades after exposure as a chronic granulomatous response in a characteristic multifocal pattern.

## 1. Introduction

Silicone-based compounds are commonly used in many medical applications, such as coatings for needles and syringes, as implants and prostheses, and as injectable cosmetic fillers. Foreign body granulomas have been recognized as a complication of silicone exposure since 1964 [1]. They may occur anywhere from months to decades after exposure [2]. Awareness of this risk has led to the decline of free silicone-based injectable fillers in favor of hyaluronic acid- and collagen-based fillers. In this report, we describe a patient without prior filler who presented to our oculoplastic clinic for evaluation of multiple raised periorbital nodules [3]. At the request of the patient, who was concerned the lesions that seemingly arose *de novo* could be malignant, an excisional biopsy was performed. Histopathological evaluation ultimately identified the lesions to be silicone granulomas. Further history revealed an uncommon exposure: facial acupuncture performed three decades prior. To our knowledge, this is the first reported case of multifocal periorbital silicone granulomas arising from prior acupuncture. Patient consent was obtained for publication of the medical photography included in the article. This report adhered to the ethical principles outlined in the Declaration of Helsinki as amended in 2013.

## 2. Case Presentation

A 61-year-old previously healthy Hispanic female presented for oculoplastic evaluation after noting multiple nontender bumps around the left eye associated with intermittent eyelid edema. The patient had no history of trauma and disclosed no prior facial surgeries at the initial visit. Past medical and social history was largely unremarkable. The patient was diagnosed with osteoporosis and was taking calcium supplementation. She reported high stress levels and was taking

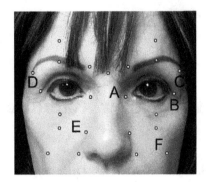

FIGURE 1: Acupuncture trigger points and sites of granuloma formation. Granulomas were found at sites labelled (a)–(f), which correspond to common acupuncture trigger points: (a) jingming, (b) tongziliao, (c, d) taiyang, (e) bitong, and (f) quanliao.

anxiolytics as needed. She had undergone LASIK several years prior for myopia. The patient did not smoke and did not endorse significant sun exposure.

On exam, the patient was found to have multiple nontender, nonpigmented nodules without overlying skin changes at the following locations: below the left medial canthal tendon measuring 1 cm (Figure 1(a)), below the left lateral canthal tendon measuring 0.5 cm (Figure 1(b)), and lateral to the left eyebrow measuring 0.75 cm (Figure 1(c)). The patient subsequently underwent excisional biopsy of both canthal lesions (Figures 1(a) and 1(b)).

Hematoxylin and eosin stain of the two excised specimens revealed fibrovascular tissue containing granulomatous inflammation with foci of clear spaces consistent with silicone oil or other foreign material (Figure 2(a)). No organisms were seen on gram stain, Grocott's methenamine silver stain, or acid-fast staining (Figures 2(b)–2(d)).

At follow-up, the patient disclosed a history of facial acupuncture performed approximately 30 years prior over multiple sessions at a local South Florida spa to relieve stress. The treatment was performed by an acupuncturist licensed by the Florida Board of Acupuncture using single-use disposable acupuncture needles. A comprehensive review of the patient's medical and surgical history revealed a previously undisclosed history of a minifacelift without fat transfer, Botox to the forehead, and permanent eyeliner tattooing. There were no records of other facial cosmetic procedures, and the patient denied any prior periocular lower lid injections or fillers. Given the additional exposure history, the patient was reexamined, and additional nodules along the right brow (Figure 1(d)), right nasolabial groove (Figure 1(e)), and left canine fossa (Figure 1(f)) were found, which corresponded to trigger points commonly used in acupuncture.

The patient underwent additional removal of the right brow lesion (Figure 1(d)), but elected to observe the deeper lesions found in the mid and lower face (Figures 1(e) and 1(f)).

## 3. Discussion

Despite the declining use of silicone-based fillers in cosmetic surgery, silicone granulomas are still frequently encountered

by dermatologists and facial or oculoplastic surgeons. The diagnosis is generally made based on a clear history of exposure, such as through injectable fillers or implants, and characteristic histopathological findings [4]. In the presented case, the prior exposure was not initially disclosed until the histopathological findings prompted a guided review of the patient's history. It is important to ascertain any history of prior acupuncture as patients can be repeatedly exposed to the silicone used to coat needles. In this unique case, the patient presented with multiple periorbital silicone granulomas several decades after facial acupuncture.

Silicone granulomas following acupuncture have been previously described in several parts of the body and in some cases several years after exposure [5, 6], but have not been previously reported in the periocular region despite being a commonly needled site. To our knowledge, this is also the first report of periorbital silicone granulomas occurring decades after exposure. Due to the long span of time between exposure and the patient's clinical presentation, other diagnoses were considered, including cutaneous sarcoidosis. However, a first diagnosis of cutaneous sarcoidosis would have been rare in a 61-year-old patient [7, 8], and the patient had no clinical evidence of scarring at other sites of trauma or surgery. There were no pulmonary or systemic symptoms, and recent routine bloodwork performed by her primary care physician, which included serum calcium, was within normal range. Moreover, the histopathological findings pointed to prior silicone exposure. Notably, the abundance of vacuolated foreign body clear spaces and the absence of asteroid bodies were more consistent with a granulomatous reaction to silicone than sarcoid. In previously published cases of cutaneous sarcoidosis occurring at injection sites, patients were younger, reported a history of scarring at sites of minor trauma, and clinically presented with red-brown papules that on histopathology was predominated by epithelioid granulomas without clear spaces [9–11]. Although serum angiotensin-converting enzyme (ACE) was not checked, it should be noted that an abnormal level would not have been diagnostic of sarcoidosis given the other likely diagnoses.

In addition to prior acupuncture, the patient reported a history of prior eyeliner tattooing, a minifacelift, and Botox. Though these are all potential sources of foreign body granulomas, the identified lesions did not correspond to the involved surgical sites. On histopathology, there was also no evidence of tattoo pigment nor birefringent suture material in any of the specimens as would be expected. Botox-related granulomas are unusual except in the context of sarcoidosis and would have lacked the numerous vacuolated clear spaces seen in our specimen. The patient denied prior facial filler, and the histopathological findings support her history. Commonly encountered fillers display characteristic histopathological findings that are used for identification [4]. Hyaluronic acid filler, for instance, would appear basophilic on hematoxylin-eosin stain. The identification of a clear exposure and material helped assuage concerns for underlying malignant or autoimmune processes and helped preclude further surgical intervention.

Treatment of silicone granulomas varies based on the size and location of the lesions. Small localized lesions are

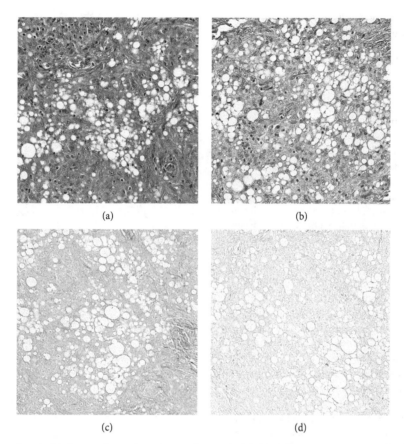

(a)                                  (b)

(c)                                  (d)

FIGURE 2: Histopathology of periorbital granuloma (400x magnification). (a) Hematoxylin and eosin stain demonstrate noncaseating granuloma with multiple foci of clear vacuole-like spaces containing silicone. No organisms were seen on (b) gram, (c) GMS, and (d) acid-fast stains.

commonly excised but may require wide margins due to the risk of progressive scarring if silicone is allowed to migrate through layers of tissue. Disseminated lesions often require medical treatment. These include intralesional steroid injections and oral immunomodulators such as doxycycline, minocycline, celecoxib, allopurinol, and etanercept [12, 13]. Although patients respond well initially, recurrence is common after discontinuation of medical therapy and long-term immunosuppression may be required [14].

Acupuncture use in the United States is rising. According to the 2007 National Health Interview Survey that examined the use of complementary and alternative medicine, approximately 6.3% of the population or 14 million people have undergone a needling procedure [15]. Trigger points on the head, face, and neck are traditionally used to manage headaches, stress, and allergy symptoms [16]. Our patient only received acupuncture to the face. Lesions were found at jingming (Figure 1(a)), tongziliao (Figure 1(b)), taiyang (Figures 1(c) and 1(d)), bitong (Figure 1(e)), and quanliao (Figure 1(f)) which are targeted to alleviate eye strain, headache, stress, allergies, and facial pain, respectively.

Traditional needling practices are also being adapted for cosmetic purposes. Facial cosmetic acupuncture (FCA) has been touted to help with antiaging, skin rejuvenation, and restoration of muscle tone [17]. Although a small clinical trial in Korea has shown positive results based on objective changes on Moire facial topography and patient self-assessment, there is unfortunately an underrecognition of the potential side effects, including disfiguring silicone granulomas [14, 18]. This complication may be prevented with the use of silicone-free acupuncture needles, and early recognition by providers may prevent further disease.

## 4. Conclusions

Silicone granulomas may present decades after exposure and are important to consider on the differential for unexplained multifocal facial masses that follow an unnatural pattern. Diagnosis requires a thorough history, and in particular, providers must be aware of the potential for granuloma formation with the use of silicone-coated acupuncture needles.

## Acknowledgments

The study was financially supported by the Florida Lions Eye Bank, NIH Center Core Grant P30EY014801, and Research to Prevent Blindness Unrestricted Grant.

## References

[1] L. H. Winer, T. H. Sternberg, R. Lehman, and F. L. Ashley, "Tissue reactions to injected silicone liquids," *Archives of Dermatology*, vol. 90, no. 6, pp. 588–593, 1964.

[2] H. C. Hu, H. W. Fang, and Y. H. Chiu, "Delayed-onset edematous foreign body granulomas 40 years after augmentation
rhinoplasty by silicone implant combined with liquid silicone
injection," *Aesthetic Plastic Surgery*, vol. 41, no. 3, pp. 637–
640, 2017.

[3] A. Fallacara, S. Manfredini, E. Durini, and S. Vertuani, "Hyaluronic acid fillers in soft tissue regeneration," *Facial Plastic
Surgery*, vol. 33, no. 1, pp. 087–096, 2017.

[4] L. Requena, C. Requena, L. Christensen, U. S. Zimmermann,
H. Kutzner, and L. Cerroni, "Adverse reactions to injectable
soft tissue fillers," *Journal of the American Academy of Dermatology*, vol. 64, no. 1, pp. 1–34, 2011, quiz 35-6.

[5] M. Yanagihara, T. Fujii, N. Wakamatu, H. Ishizaki,
T. Takehara, and K. Nawate, "Silicone granuloma on the entry
points of acupuncture, venepuncture and surgical needles,"
*Journal of Cutaneous Pathology*, vol. 27, no. 6, pp. 301–305,
2000.

[6] A. J. H. Tschetter, "Silicone granulomas in the setting of acupuncture with silicone-coated needles," *Journal of Clinical
and Investigative Dermatology*, vol. 2, no. 1, 2014.

[7] P. Brito-Zeron, J. Sellares, X. Bosch et al., "Epidemiologic patterns of disease expression in sarcoidosis: age, gender and
ethnicity-related differences," *Clinical and Experimental Rheumatology*, vol. 34, no. 3, pp. 380–388, 2016.

[8] M. H. Noe and M. Rosenbach, "Cutaneous sarcoidosis," *Current Opinion in Pulmonary Medicine*, vol. 23, no. 5, pp. 482–
486, 2017.

[9] H. Zargham and E. O'Brien, "Cutaneous sarcoidosis at insulin
injection sites," *Canadian Medical Association Journal*,
vol. 188, no. 9, p. 674, 2016.

[10] D. Mermin, M. P. Loustalan, and M. S. Doutre, "A case of hyaluronic acid injections triggering cutaneous sarcoidosis at previously treated sites," *Journal of the European Academy of
Dermatology and Venereology*, vol. 31, no. 1, pp. e55–e57,
2017.

[11] V. G. Herbert, N. Blödorn-Schlicht, A. Böer-Auer et al., "Gran-
ulomatöse hautveränderungen an botulinumtoxin-A-injek-
tionsstellen," *Der Hautarzt*, vol. 66, no. 11, pp. 863–866, 2015.

[12] K. Beer, "Delayed onset nodules from liquid injectable silicone:
report of a case, evaluation of associated histopathology and
results of treatment with minocycline and celocoxib," *Journal
of Drugs in Dermatology*, vol. 8, no. 10, pp. 952–954, 2009.

[13] T. A. Chen, C. L. Mercado, K. L. Topping, B. P. Erickson, K. P.
Cockerham, and A. L. Kossler, "Disseminated silicone granu-
lomatosis in the face and orbit," *American Journal of Ophthalmology Case Reports*, vol. 10, pp. 32–34, 2018.

[14] S. Bashey, D. S. Lee, and G. Kim, "Extensive facial sclerosing
lipogranulomatosis as a complication of cosmetic acupuncture," *Dermatologic Surgery*, vol. 41, no. 4, pp. 513–516, 2015.

[15] P. M. Barnes, B. Bloom, and R. L. Nahin, "Complementary and
alternative medicine use among adults and children: United
States, 2007," *National Health Statistics Report*, pp. 1–23, 2008.

[16] A. White, T. M. Cummings, M. Cummings, and J. Filshie, *An
Introduction to Western Medical Acupuncture: Churchill Liv-
ingstone*, 2008.

[17] J. Barrett, "Acupuncture and facial rejuvenation," *Aesthetic
Surgery Journal*, vol. 25, no. 4, pp. 419–424, 2005.

[18] Y. Yun, S. Kim, M. Kim, K. S. Kim, J. S. Park, and I. Choi,
"Effect of facial cosmetic acupuncture on facial elasticity: an
open-label, single-arm pilot study," *Evidence-based Complementary and Alternative Medicine*, vol. 2013, 5 pages, 2013.

# 28

# Oculodentodigital Dysplasia: A Case Report and Major Review of the Eye and Ocular Adnexa Features of 295 Reported Cases

**Virang Kumar ⓘ,[1] Natario L. Couser ⓘ,[2,3,4] and Arti Pandya[5]**

[1]Virginia Commonwealth University School of Medicine, Richmond, VA, USA
[2]Department of Ophthalmology, Virginia Commonwealth University School of Medicine, Richmond, VA, USA
[3]Department of Human and Molecular Genetics, Virginia Commonwealth University School of Medicine, Richmond, VA, USA
[4]Department of Pediatrics, Virginia Commonwealth University School of Medicine, Richmond, VA, USA
[5]Department of Pediatrics, Division of Genetics and Metabolism, School of Medicine, University of North Carolina at Chapel Hill, Chapel Hill, NC, USA

Correspondence should be addressed to Virang Kumar; kumarvk@vcu.edu

Academic Editor: Sandra M. Johnson

Oculodentodigital dysplasia (ODDD) is a rare genetic disorder associated with a characteristic craniofacial profile with variable dental, limb, eye, and ocular adnexa abnormalities. We performed an extensive literature review to highlight key eye features in patients with ODDD and report a new case of a female patient with a heterozygous missense *GJA1* mutation (c.65G>A, p.G22E) and clinical features consistent with the condition. Our patient presented with multiple congenital anomalies including syndactyly, microphthalmia, microcornea, retrognathia, and a small nose with hypoplastic alae and prominent columella; in addition, an omphalocele defect was present, which has not been reported in previous cases. A systematic review of the published cases to date revealed 91 literature reports of 295 individuals with ODDD. There were 73 different *GJA1* mutations associated with these cases, of which the most common were the following missense mutations: c.605G>A (p.R202H) (11%), c.389T>C (p.I130T) (10%), and c.119C>T (p.A40V) (10%). Mutations most commonly affect the extracellular-1 and cytoplasmic-1 domains of connexin-43 (gene product of *GJA1*), predominately manifesting in microphthalmia and microcornea. The syndrome appears with an approximately equal sex ratio. The most common eye features reported among all mutations were microcornea, microphthalmia, short palpebral fissures, and glaucoma.

## 1. Introduction

Oculodentodigital dysplasia (ODDD, OMIM #164200) is a rare disorder mainly characterized by abnormal craniofacial, dental, ocular, and digital development. The autosomal dominant form has been the most frequently reported inheritance pattern, although a few cases of autosomal recessive inheritance have been described [1–3]. Craniofacial abnormalities may include microcephaly, prominent columella, and underdeveloped nasal alae [2–4]. Dental abnormalities, such as hypoplastic enamel, small teeth, and premature loss of teeth, are often present [2–4]. Digit abnormalities may include syndactyly, camptodactyly, and midphalangeal hypoplasia [2–4]. Ophthalmic manifestations are common, such as microcornea and microphthalmia, and may involve a wide spectrum of eye and ocular adnexa structures, although previous analyses of prior cases show that full ocular physical exams were not performed on all patients [3, 5].

The gap junction protein alpha 1 (*GJA1*) gene codes for connexin-43, which is a protein that assists in the transmembrane transport of molecules through gap junctions, and mutations in the GJA1 may cause an alteration of the channel conduction properties [1–3, 6]. We report a case of an 8-month-old female patient with an identified *GJA1* mutation and common clinical features associated with ODDD. This patient had an omphalocele at birth, which has not been reported in previous cases. Her eye features included microphthalmia, microcornea, narrow palpebral fissures, blonde fundus, deep anterior chambers, hyperopia, and epiphora in both eyes secondary to bilateral nasolacrimal

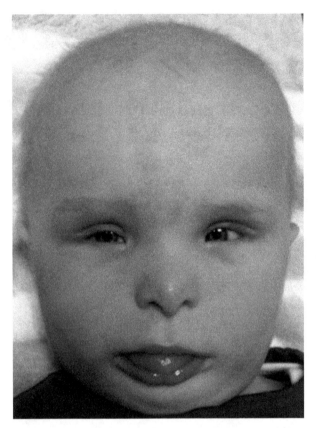

FIGURE 1: Facial photograph of a patient with oculodentodigital dysplasia; note the beaked nose with hypoplastic alae and prominent columella, microphthalmia, microcornea, small palpebral fissures, retrognathia.

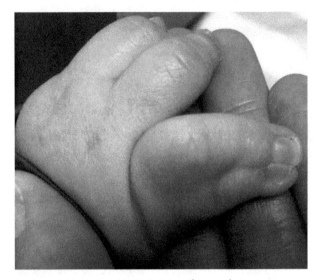

FIGURE 2: Complete syndactyly of the 4$^{th}$ and 5$^{th}$ digits of the right hand.

duct obstructions. We conducted an extensive literature review to summarize the eye features in patients with ODDD reported to date.

## 2. Case Report

The patient, an 8-month-old female, was born to a nonconsanguineous couple from a healthy 37-year-old mother of Native American descent and a healthy 30-year-old father of German and Irish descent. Family history is notable for an older sibling with cleft palate, paternal uncle with autism, paternal second cousin with congenital heart defect, and distant paternal great-great uncle with Down syndrome and webbed/fused 4$^{th}$ and 5$^{th}$ digits of one hand. A normal pregnancy was noted until the second trimester when an omphalocele was detected on ultrasound. A subsequent ultrasound revealed possible syndactyly of the hands. The patient was born at 39 weeks by vaginal delivery with induction. The birth weight was 3.552 kg (75$^{th}$ percentile), birth length was 50 cm (68$^{th}$ percentile), and birth head circumference was 34.5 cm (70$^{th}$ percentile). Apgar scores were 9 at both one minute and five minutes.

Multiple congenital anomalies noted at birth included an omphalocele that measured 4 cm at base and 3.5 cm across with intestines present in the sac, but no liver. The patient had a normocephalic head with sparse wispy hair, a small

nose with hypoplastic alae, a prominent columella, small-appearing palpebral fissures, a small cornea, microphthalmia, a wide anterior fontanelle, and retrognathia (Figure 1). Syndactyly of digits 4 and 5 and webbing of digits 3 and 4 of the right (Figure 2) and left hands were present. Cardiac echocardiogram on the day of birth showed the presence of a mild patent ductus arteriosus, mild patent foramen ovale, and a normal aorta. Feeding difficulties were exacerbated by the presence of the omphalocele; surgical correction was performed on day 2 of life.

An ophthalmologic assessment at 4 months of age was notable for deep anterior chambers, bilateral nasolacrimal duct obstruction, microphthalmia, small 8 mm corneas, a blonde fundus, and moderate hyperopia in both eyes.

At her last examination at 8 months of age, the patient continues to have poor feeding with self-limiting volumes but has improved weight gain. The patient is at the 9$^{th}$ percentile for weight and 12$^{th}$ percentile for length. Cognitive and motor developments are delayed.

Sequencing of the *GJA1* gene (transcript number: NM_000165.3) from patient genomic DNA revealed a heterozygous missense mutation in the *GJA1* gene: c.65G>A (p.G22E). Deletion/duplication analysis of the *GJA1* gene using the aCGH test was negative.

## 3. Methods

We performed a systematic review of the literature to summarize the ocular findings in individuals with ODDD. A PubMed/Medline search of "oculodentodigital syndrome" led us to find a total of 177 articles. No articles were excluded based on the year published. We reviewed the references to identify other articles that did not appear in our original search. 91 articles describing patients with a description consistent with the clinical syndrome, either with or without molecular confirmation of *GJA1* pathogenic variants, were included. Within these selected articles, we identified 295 cases of ODDD with 73 different *GJA1* mutations, including

TABLE 1: *GJA1* variants without clinical information.

| Sources | GJA1 variant | | Cases |
| | Nucleotide | Protein | |
| --- | --- | --- | --- |
| Paznekas et al. [3] | c.7G>A | p.D3N | 1 |
| Paznekas et al. [3] | c.64G>A | p.G22R | 1 |
| Paznekas et al. [3]; Richardson et al. [6] | c.79T>C | p.S27P | 1 |
| Paznekas et al. [3] | c.163A>G | p.N55D | 1 |
| Paznekas et al. [3] | c.174A>C | p.Q58H | 1 |
| Paznekas et al. [3] | c.175C>G | p.P59A | 1 |
| Paznekas et al. [3] | c.221A>T | p.H74L | 1 |
| Paznekas et al. [3] | c.428G>A | p.G143D | 1 |
| Paznekas et al. [3] | c.430A>G | p.K144E | 1 |
| Paznekas et al. [3] | c.434T>G | p.V145G | 1 |
| Paznekas et al. [3] | c.442C>G | p.R148G | 1 |
| Paznekas et al. [3] | c.578C>T | p.P193L | 1 |

TABLE 2: Summary of sex distribution.

| | Males | | Females | | Total |
| --- | --- | --- | --- | --- | --- |
| Individuals with clinical diagnosis of ODDD (with no molecular confirmation) | 14 | 45% | 18 | 56% | 32 |
| Untested individuals with both ODDD phenotype and known relative with molecular confirmation | 52 | 53% | 46 | 47% | 98 |
| Individuals with a molecular confirmed *GJA1* pathogenic variant | 72 | 44% | 93 | 56% | 165 |
| Totals | 138 | 47% | 157 | 53% | 295 |

those that exhibited features of ODDD in the absence of molecular confirmation. Such individuals were either clinically diagnosed or were relatives of individuals with molecularly confirmed *GJA1* pathogenic variants. Twelve reported that *GJA1* gene coding alterations were omitted due to insufficient clinical information and data reported and are listed in Table 1 [3, 6].

## 4. Discussion

Oculodentodigital dysplasia (ODDD) is a rare congenital disorder manifested with developmental anomalies of the eyes, face, dentition, heart, skeletal system, and digits. The syndrome appears to be more common in Caucasian populations with an equal sex ratio [3]. Heterozygous mutation of the *GJA1* gene located at chromosome 6q22.31 has been identified as the most common mutation resulting in ODDD [2, 3]. However, a compound heterozygous individual with missense mutations demonstrated mutations in the *GJA1* gene (p.V41L) and the *GJB2* gene (p.R127H), which encode for connexin-43 and connexin-26, respectively, and has been reported and classified as having overlapping features of Clouston syndrome and ODDD [3, 7].

In addition to the classic phenotypic features of the syndrome, a wide variety of additional physical manifestations

have been observed. Ocular findings of microphthalmia and microcornea have been observed commonly in previous cases [2–4]. Craniofacial anomalies of microcephaly, poor hair growth, hypoplastic nasal alae, and prominent columella have been reported previously [2–4]. Bilateral syndactyly of the 4th and 5th digits is common [2, 3].

A systematic review of the published cases to date (ranging from 1963 to 2019) revealed 91 literature reports of 295 individuals with ODDD [1–91]. Table 2 [1–91] summarizes the sex distribution across all reviewed reports of ODDD. Patients with ODDD present with an approximately equal sex distribution (47% male and 53% female). Of the 295 individuals reported, 32 were clinically diagnosed with ODDD without molecular confirmation, 98 presented with features of ODDD and had a known relative with molecular confirmation of a *GJA1* pathogenic variant, and 165 individuals had a molecularly confirmed *GJA1* pathogenic variant.

There were 73 different *GJA1* mutations identified from the 165 individuals that had a molecularly confirmed *GJA1* pathogenic variant. Table 3 [1–3, 5–71, 92] summarizes the number of patients with each mutation. Patients with confirmed pathogenic variants and their relatives with no molecular confirmation but with features of ODDD were grouped separately. These two groups comprised 263 of the patients included in this study.

The eye features of all 295 patients are summarized in Table 4 [1–91]. The most common ophthalmic manifestations reported were microcornea ($n = 111$), microphthalmia ($n = 110$), short palpebral fissures ($n = 56$), and glaucoma ($n = 51$, 4 closed-angle and 1 open-angle).

Twenty-three patients presented with refractive error, of which isolated myopia was the most frequently noted ($n = 14$), followed by isolated hyperopia ($n = 6$), anisometropia ($n = 2$), and astigmatism ($n = 1$). Forty patients presented with eye movement disorders, with strabismus ($n = 27$, 9 esotropic, 1 exotropic) being the most common, followed by nystagmus ($n = 8$), amblyopia ($n = 3$), Duane syndrome ($n = 2$), and Brown syndrome ($n = 1$). Note that 1 patient had both nystagmus and esotropia [71]. Other common findings included epicanthus ($n = 36$), hypotelorism ($n = 24$), hypertelorism ($n = 22$), madarosis ($n = 19$), cataracts ($n = 17$), persistent pupillary membranes ($n = 13$), shallow anterior chambers ($n = 12$), pale/atrophic irides ($n = 11$), telecanthus ($n = 11$), and uveitis ($n = 10$).

A variety of abnormal findings for the retina and optic disc were noted ($n = 18$), with dysplasia of the retina/fundus ($n = 3$) and pale/atrophic optic discs ($n = 3$) being the most common documented findings.

Of the individuals with molecularly confirmed mutations, the most common mutations present were c.605G>A (p.R202H) (11%; with 1 patient also having a c.717G>A synonymous mutation), c.389T>C (p.I130T) (10%), and c.119C>T (p.A40V) (10%). Table 5 [2, 3, 12, 30, 40, 41, 66, 67, 92] summarizes the eye features present in the patients with these mutations.

Less common features of the phenotype observed in our presented case were also reported in other cases as well. These include nasolacrimal duct abnormalities ($n = 2$), pale/atrophic

Table 3: Reported *GJA1* mutations and sex distribution in ODDD.

| Sources | Multiple mutations? | GJA1 mutation | | | Individuals with a molecular confirmed GJA1 pathogenic variant | | Untested individuals with both ODDD phenotype and known relative with molecular confirmation | | Total individuals with the ODDD phenotype | | | | |
|---|---|---|---|---|---|---|---|---|---|---|---|---|---|
| | | Nucleotide | Protein | Unspecified | Male | Female | Male | Female | Male | | Female | | Total |
| Cavusoglu et al. 2019 | No | c.168_169insT | p.Q57SfsTer6 | N/A | 1 | 0 | 0 | 0 | 1 | 100% | 0 | 0% | 1 |
| Aminabadi et al. 2009 & Aminabadi et al. 2010 | No | N/A | N/A | Missense mutation exon 2 (unspecified) | 1 | 0 | 2 | 1 | 3 | 75% | 1 | 25% | 4 |
| Dwarakanathan et al. 2015 & Furuta et al. 2012 | No | c.75G>T | p.W25C | N/A | 1 | 1 | 0 | 0 | 1 | 50% | 1 | 50% | 2 |
| Quick and Dobersen 2014; National Center for Biotechnology Information 2020 | Yes | c.605G>A c.717G>A | p.R202H p.R239R | N/A | 1 | 0 | 0 | 0 | 1 | 100% | 0 | 0% | 1 |
| Paznekas et al. 2003 & Paznekas et al. 2009 | No | c.605G>A | p.R202H | N/A | 1 | 7 | 4 | 5 | 5 | 29% | 12 | 71% | 17 |
| Jamsheer et al. 2010 | Yes | c.301C>T c.6delT | p.R101X p.G2fsX7 | N/A | 1 | 0 | 0 | 0 | 1 | 100% | 0 | 0% | 1 |
| Jamsheer et al. 2010 | No | c.301C>T | p.R101X | N/A | 0 | 1 | 0 | 0 | 0 | 0% | 1 | 100% | 1 |
| Paznekas et al. 2009; Joss et al. 2008; & Richardson et al. 2006 | No | c.97C>T | p.R33X* | N/A | 0 | 2 | 0 | 0 | 0 | 0% | 2 | 100% | 2 |
| Paznekas et al. 2009; Richardson et al. 2004; Paznekas et al. 2003; & Gladwin et al. 1997 | No | c.93T>C | p.I31M | N/A | 0 | 0 | 4 | 4 | 4 | 50% | 4 | 50% | 8 |
| Wang et al. 2019 | No | c.91A>T | p.I311P | N/A | 1 | 0 | 0 | 0 | 1 | 100% | 0 | 0% | 1 |
| Paznekas et al. 2009 & van Steensel et al. 2005 | No | c.780_781delTG | p.C260fsX306 | N/A | 1 | 2 | 0 | 0 | 1 | 33% | 2 | 67% | 3 |
| Paznekas et al. 2009; Paznekas et al. 2003; & Gorlin et al. 1963 | No | c.68A>C | p.K23T | N/A | 1 | 0 | 0 | 0 | 1 | 100% | 0 | 0% | 1 |
| Dwarakanathan et al. 2015; Paznekas et al. 2009; & Vreeburg et al. 2007 | No | c.689_690delAT | p.Y230fsX236 | N/A | 0 | 3 | 1 | 0 | 1 | 25% | 3 | 75% | 4 |
| This study; Gumus 2018; Paznekas et al. 2009; Paznekas et al. 2003; & Traboulsi and Parks 1990 | No | c.65G>A | p.G22E | N/A | 0 | 3 | 0 | 0 | 0 | 0% | 3 | 100% | 3 |
| Wiest et al. 2006 | No | c.659C>A | p.S220Y | N/A | 0 | 1 | 0 | 0 | 0 | 0% | 1 | 100% | 1 |
| Paznekas et al. 2009; Paznekas et al. 2003; & Norton et al. 1995 | No | c.646G>T | p.V216L | N/A | 1 | 0 | 4 | 1 | 5 | 83% | 1 | 17% | 6 |
| Park et al. 2017; Paznekas et al. 2009; & Paznekas et al. 2003 | No | c.61G>A | p.G21R | N/A | 0 | 2 | 0 | 0 | 0 | 0% | 2 | 100% | 2 |
| Brice et al. 2013 | No | c.617A>G | p.K206R | N/A | 1 | 2 | 1 | 1 | 2 | 40% | 3 | 60% | 5 |

TABLE 3: Continued.

| Sources | Multiple mutations? | GJA1 mutation Nucleotide | Protein | Unspecified | Individuals with a molecular confirmed GJA1 pathogenic variant Male | Female | Untested individuals with both ODDD phenotype and known relative with molecular confirmation Male | Female | Total individuals with the ODDD phenotype Male | Female | Total |
|---|---|---|---|---|---|---|---|---|---|---|---|
| Paznekas et al. 2009 | No | c.602C>T | p.S201F | N/A | 0 | 1 | 0 | 0 | 0% (0) | 100% (1) | 1 |
| Paznekas et al. 2009 & de la Parra et al. 2007 | No | c.5G>T | p.G2V | N/A | 1 | 0 | 0 | 0 | 100% (1) | 0% (0) | 1 |
| Vitiello et al. 2005 & Vingolo et al. 1994 | No | c.581A>C | p.H194P* | N/A | 3 | 5 | 3 | 3 | 43% (6) | 57% (8) | 14 |
| Paznekas et al. 2009; Paznekas et al. 2003; & Judisch et al. 1979 | No | c.52T>C | p.S18P | N/A | 0 | 0 | 1 | 3 | 25% (1) | 75% (3) | 4 |
| Paznekas et al. 2009 & Paznekas et al. 2003 | No | c.50A>C | p.Y17S | N/A | 3 | 4 | 0 | 0 | 43% (3) | 57% (4) | 7 |
| Paznekas et al. 2009 & Debeer et al. 2005 | No | c.504_506delCTT | p.F169del | N/A | 0 | 1 | 0 | 0 | 0% (0) | 100% (1) | 1 |
| Wiest et al. 2006 & Thomsen et al. 1998 | No | c.461C>A | p.T154N | N/A | 0 | 2 | 0 | 1 | 0% (0) | 100% (3) | 3 |
| Paznekas et al. 2009 & van Es et al. 2007 | No | c.460A>G | p.T154A* | N/A | 0 | 2 | 0 | 0 | 0% (0) | 100% (2) | 2 |
| Paznekas et al. 2009; Richardson et al. 2004; Paznekas et al. 2003; Gladwin et al. 1997; & Schrander-Stumpel et al. 1993 | No | c.443G>A | p.R148Q | N/A | 0 | 0 | 2 | 2 | 50% (2) | 50% (2) | 4 |
| Taşdelen et al. 2018 | No | c.442C>T | p.R148Ter | N/A | 1 | 0 | 0 | 0 | 100% (1) | 0% (0) | 1 |
| Paznekas et al. 2009; Debeer et al. 2005; & Spaepen et al. 1991 | No | c.440Y>C | p.M147T | N/A | 0 | 1 | 0 | 0 | 0% (0) | 100% (1) | 1 |
| Paznekas et al. 2009; Richardson et al. 2004; & Brueton et al. 1990 | No | c.427G>A | p.G143S | N/A | 0 | 0 | 8 | 1 | 89% (8) | 11% (1) | 9 |
| Orosz et al. 2018 | No | c.413G>A | p.G138D | N/A | 1 | 0 | 0 | 0 | 100% (1) | 0% (0) | 1 |
| Paznekas et al. 2009; Paznekas et al. 2003; & Shapiro et al. 1997 | No | c.412G>C | p.G138R | N/A | 1 | 2 | 2 | 2 | 43% (3) | 57% (4) | 7 |
| Kogame et al. 2014 | No | c.412G>A | p.G138S | N/A | 1 | 0 | 0 | 0 | 100% (1) | 0% (0) | 1 |
| Paznekas et al. 2009; Richardson et al. 2004; Paznekas et al. 2003; & Gladwin et al. 1997 | No | c.402G>T | p.K134N | N/A | 0 | 0 | 0 | 2 | 0% (0) | 100% (2) | 2 |
| Paznekas et al. 2009 & Paznekas et al. 2003 | No | c.400A>G | p.K134E | N/A | 0 | 1 | 0 | 0 | 0% (0) | 100% (1) | 1 |
| Nishat et al. 2012; Paznekas et al. 2009; Paznekas et al. 2003; & Amador et al. 2008 | No | c.389T>C | p.I130T | N/A | 7 | 4 | 5 | 1 | 71% (12) | 29% (5) | 17 |
| Paznekas et al. 2009; Musa et al. 2008; Wiest et al. 2006; & Loddenkemper et al. 2002 | No | c.338T>C | p.L113P | N/A | 2 | 2 | 1 | 0 | 60% (3) | 40% (2) | 5 |
| Paznekas et al. 2009 & Debeer et al. 2005 | No | c.330G>C | p.E110D | N/A | 2 | 3 | 1 | 2 | 38% (3) | 63% (5) | 8 |
| Paznekas et al. 2009 & Kelly et al. 2006 | No | c.32T>C | p.L11P | N/A | 0 | 1 | 0 | 0 | 0% (0) | 100% (1) | 1 |

TABLE 3: Continued.

| Sources | Multiple mutations? | GJA1 mutation | | | Individuals with a molecular confirmed GJA1 pathogenic variant | | Untested individuals with both ODDD phenotype and known relative with molecular confirmation | | Total individuals with the ODDD phenotype | | |
|---|---|---|---|---|---|---|---|---|---|---|---|
| | | Nucleotide | Protein | Unspecified | Male | Female | Male | Female | Male | Female | Total |
| Gabriel et al. 2011 & Jamsheer et al. 2009 | No | c.31C>T | p.L11F | N/A | 0 | 2 | 0 | 0 | 0% 0 | 100% 2 | 2 |
| Porntaveetus et al. 2017 | No | c.31C>A | p.L11I | N/A | 1 | 0 | 0 | 0 | 100% 1 | 0% 0 | 1 |
| Jamsheer et al. 2014 | No | c.317T>G | p.L106R | N/A | 2 | 0 | 0 | 0 | 100% 2 | 0% 0 | 2 |
| Paznekas et al. 2009 & Nivelon-Chevallier et al. 1981 | No | c.317T>C | p.L106P | N/A | 1 | 0 | 0 | 0 | 100% 1 | 0% 0 | 1 |
| Paznekas et al. 2009 & Paznekas et al. 2003 | No | c.306G>C | p.K102N | N/A | 1 | 2 | 0 | 0 | 33% 1 | 67% 2 | 3 |
| Paznekas et al. 2009; Paznekas et al. 2003; & Wooldridge et al. 1977 | No | c.293A>G | p.Y98C | N/A | 1 | 3 | 1 | 1 | 33% 2 | 67% 4 | 6 |
| Paznekas et al. 2009 | No | c.287T>C | p.V96A | N/A | 0 | 1 | 0 | 0 | 0% 0 | 100% 1 | 1 |
| Wiest et al. 2006 | No | c.287T>A | p.V96E | N/A | 0 | 1 | 0 | 0 | 0% 0 | 100% 1 | 1 |
| Paznekas et al. 2009 & Kjaer et al. 2004 | No | c.286G>A | p.V96M | N/A | 2 | 2 | 0 | 0 | 50% 2 | 50% 2 | 4 |
| Paznekas et al. 2009 & Honkaniemi et al. 2005 | No | c.284A>G | p.H95R | N/A | 0 | 1 | 0 | 1 | 0% 0 | 100% 2 | 2 |
| Paznekas et al. 2009; Paznekas et al. 2003; & Opjordsmoen and Nyberg-Hansen 1980 | No | c.268C>G | p.L90V | N/A | 4 | 0 | 3 | 2 | 78% 7 | 22% 2 | 9 |
| Jamsheer et al. 2014 | No | c.257C>A | p.S86Y | N/A | 0 | 1 | 0 | 0 | 0% 0 | 100% 1 | 1 |
| Pizzuti et al. 2004 | No | c.227G>A | p.R76H | N/A | 1 | 0 | 0 | 0 | 100% 1 | 0% 0 | 1 |
| Izumi et al. 2013 | No | c.226C>T | p.R76C | N/A | 1 | 0 | 0 | 0 | 100% 1 | 0% 0 | 1 |
| Paznekas et al. 2009; Paznekas et al. 2003; & Stanislaw et al. 1998 | No | c.226C>A | p.R76S | N/A | 0 | 2 | 0 | 2 | 0% 0 | 100% 4 | 4 |
| Choi et al. 2018 | No | c.221A>C | p.H74P* | N/A | 1 | 0 | 0 | 0 | 100% 1 | 0% 0 | 1 |
| Paznekas et al. 2009; Richardson et al. 2004; Paznekas et al. 2003; & Gladwin et al. 1997 | No | c.206C>A | p.S69Y | N/A | 0 | 0 | 2 | 5 | 29% 2 | 71% 5 | 7 |
| Paznekas et al. 2009 & Vasconcellos et al. 2005 | No | c.176C>A | p.P59H | N/A | 4 | 4 | 1 | 0 | 56% 5 | 44% 4 | 9 |
| Paznekas et al. 2009 | No | c.145_147dupCAG | p.Q49dup | N/A | 0 | 1 | 0 | 0 | 0% 0 | 100% 1 | 1 |
| Paznekas et al. 2009; Paznekas et al. 2003; Weintraub et al. 1975; & Gellis and Feingold 1974 | No | c.154_156dupTTT | p.F52dup | N/A | 1 | 0 | 1 | 1 | 67% 2 | 33% 1 | 3 |
| Hadjichristou et al. 2017 & Paznekas et al. 2009 | No | c.146A>C | p.Q49P | N/A | 1 | 1 | 0 | 0 | 50% 1 | 50% 1 | 2 |
| Izumi et al. 2013 | No | c.145C>G | p.Q49E | N/A | 0 | 1 | 0 | 0 | 0% 0 | 100% 1 | 1 |
| Paznekas et al. 2009 & Paznekas et al. 2003 | No | c.145C>A | p.Q49K | N/A | 3 | 2 | 0 | 0 | 60% 3 | 40% 2 | 5 |

TABLE 3: Continued.

| Sources | Multiple mutations? | GJA1 mutation — Nucleotide | GJA1 mutation — Protein | Individuals with a molecular confirmed GJA1 pathogenic variant — Unspecified | Male | Female | Untested individuals with both ODDD phenotype and known relative with molecular confirmation — Male | Female | Total individuals with the ODDD phenotype — Male | Female | Total |
|---|---|---|---|---|---|---|---|---|---|---|---|
| Amano et al. 2012; Feller et al. 2008; Paznekas et al. 2009; & Itro et al. 2005 | No | c.142G>A | p.E48K | N/A | 3 | 0 | 0 | 0 | 3 / 100% | 0 / 0% | 3 |
| Jamsheer et al. 2014 | No | c.139G>C | p.D47H | N/A | 0 | 3 | 0 | 0 | 0 / 0% | 3 / 100% | 3 |
| Tumminelli et al. 2016 | No | c.125G>C | p.E42Q | N/A | 1 | 0 | 0 | 0 | 1 / 100% | 0 / 0% | 1 |
| Gabriel et al. 2011 | No | c.120delGGTTGAGTCAGC | p.V41_A44del | N/A | 0 | 1 | 1 | 2 | 1 / 25% | 3 / 75% | 4 |
| Paznekas et al. 2009 & Kellermayer et al. 2005 | Yes (compound heterozygous with GJB2 mutation) | c.121G>C | p.V41L | | | | | | | | |
| | | N/A | p.R127H (GJB2 mutation) | N/A | 0 | 1 | 0 | 0 | 0 / 0% | 1 / 100% | 1 |
| Park et al. 2019; Hayashi et al. 2014; Paznekas et al. 2009; Debeer et al. 2005; & Paznekas et al. 2003 | No | c.119C>T | p.A40V | N/A | 6 | 4 | 4 | 3 | 10 / 59% | 7 / 41% | 17 |
| Wittlieb-Weber et al. 2015 | No | c.175C>T | p.P59S | N/A | 1 | 2 | 0 | 0 | 1 / 33% | 2 / 67% | 3 |
| Attig et al. 2016 | No | c.396_398delAAA | p.I132_K133delinsM | N/A | 3 | 2 | 0 | 0 | 3 / 60% | 2 / 40% | 5 |
| Paznekas et al. 2009 | No | c.19T>G | p.L7V | N/A | 1 | 0 | 0 | 0 | 1 / 100% | 0 / 0% | 1 |
| Himi et al. 2009 | No | c.13A>T | p.S5C | N/A | 0 | 1 | 0 | 0 | 0 / 0% | 1 / 100% | 1 |
| Pace et al. 2019 | No | c.287T>G | p.V96G | N/A | 0 | 1 | 0 | 0 | 0 / 0% | 1 / 100% | 1 |
| | No | c.77T>C | p.L26P | N/A | 0 | 1 | 0 | 0 | 0 / 0% | 1 / 100% | 1 |
| Totals | | | | | 72 | 93 | 52 | 46 | 124 / 47% | 139 / 53% | 263 |

*Unknown which specific individuals tested.

TABLE 4: Eye and ocular adnexa features reported in ODDD.

| Region | Subregion | Features |
|---|---|---|
| Orbit | — | Microphthalmia (110/37%); Hypotelorism (24/8%); Hypertelorism (22/7%); Short axial length (4/1%) |
| Anterior segment | Anterior chamber | Shallow anterior chamber (12/4%); Deep anterior chambers (2/<1%) |
| | Cornea | Microcornea (111/38%); Thick corneas (4/1%); Corneal opacities (3/1%); Corneal farinata (1/<1%); Band keratopathy (1/<1%); Corneal keratosis (1/<1%); Abnormal Descemet's membrane (1/<1%); Anteriorly deviated Schwalbe's line (1/<1%) |
| | Sclera | Blue sclera (1/<1%) |
| | Pupil | Persistent pupillary membranes (13/4%); Eccentric pupils (3/1%) |
| | Lens | Cataracts (17/6%); Lens opacities (2/<1%); White retrolental masses (1/<1%) |
| | Uvea (iris, ciliary body) | Pale/atrophic irides (11/4%); Uveitis (10/3%); General iris abnormalities (7/2%); Synechiae (4/1%); Hypoplastic anterior iris stroma (3/1%); Ciliary body cysts (2/<1%); Flat iris (1/<1%); Iridoschisis (1/<1%); Inferior iris coloboma (1/<1%); Dysplastic iris (1/<1%) |
| Posterior segment | Uvea (choroid) | Thick choroid (2/<1%); Thin choroid (1/<1%) |
| | Vitreous | Vitreous degeneration (1/<1%); Vitreous membrane attachment to optic nerve and lens (1/<1%); Persistent hyperplastic primary vitreous (1/<1%) |
| | Retina/fundus | Dysplastic retina/fundus (3/1%); Pale retina/fundus (2/<1%); Thread-like retinal vasculature (2/<1%); Dystrophic retinal epithelium (1/<1%); Hypoplastic macula (1/<1%); Absent fundal glow with B-scan ultrasound (1/<1%) |
| | Optic disc | Pale/atrophic optic disc (3/1%); Dysplastic optic disc (2/<1%); Ellipsoid optic disc (1/<1%); Optociliary vein presence (1/<1%); Optic disc hypervascularity (1/<1%) |

TABLE 4: Continued.

| | | | | | |
|---|---|---|---|---|---|
| **Ocular adnexa** | Eyelid | Short/narrow palpebral fissures (56/19%) | Epicanthus (36/12%) | Telecanthus (11/4%) | Ptosis (7/2%) | Blepharophimosis (1/<1%) | Entropion (1/<1%) | Ectropion (1/<1%) | Epiblepharon (1/<1%) | Mucosal hypertrophy (1/<1%) |
| | Eyebrow/eyelash | Madarosis (19/6%) | Flared eyebrows (3/1%) (2 medially flared) | Synophyrs (1/<1%) |
| | Nasolacrimal duct | Nasolacrimal duct abnormalities (2/<1%) | Hypolacrimation (1/<1%) |
| **Other** | Refractive errors | Myopia (16/5%) (2 anisometropic) | Hyperopia (8/3%) (2 anisometropic) | Astigmatism (1/<1%) |
| | Eye movement disorders | Strabismus (27/9%) (9 esotropic, 1 exotropic) | Nystagmus (8/3%) | Amblyopia (3/1%) | Duane syndrome (2/<1%) | Brown syndrome (1/<1%) |
| | Additional eye disorders | Glaucoma (51/17%) (4 closed-angle, 1 open-angle) | Paracentral scotoma (1/<1%) |
| | ERG/neurological | Abnormal ERG (2/<1%) | Delayed visual evoked responses (2/<1%) | Occipital subcortical white matter changes (1/<1%) |

TABLE 5: Common *GJA1* mutations with associated eye features.

| Sources | Multiple mutations? | *GJA1* mutation | | Individuals with *GJA1* mutation (confirmed and affected relatives) Total | Associated eye features |
|---|---|---|---|---|---|
| | | Nucleotide | Protein | | |
| Quick and Dobersen 2014; National Center for Biotechnology Information 2020 | Yes | c.605G>A c.717G>A | p.R202H p.R239R | 1 | Microphthalmia (1) |
| Paznekas et al. 2009; Paznekas et al. 2003 | No | c.605G>A | p.R202H | 17 | Microphthalmia (1), microcornea (2) |
| Nishat et al. 2012; Paznekas et al. 2009; Paznekas et al. 2003; and Amador et al. 2008 | No | c.389T>C | p.I130T | 17 | Microphthalmia (4), hypotelorism (6), cataract (1), pale/atrophic optic disc (1), and short palpebral fissures (4) |
| Park et al. 2019; Hayashi et al. 2014; Paznekas et al. 2009; Debeer et al. 2005; and Paznekas et al. 2003 | No | c.119C>T | p.A40V | 17 | Microphthalmia (9), hypertelorism (3), hypotelorism (4), short axial length (4), cataract (1), microcornea (8), thick cornea (4), macular hypoplasia (1), shallow anterior chamber (4), myopia (4), strabismus (6) (1 esotropic), glaucoma (6), and epicanthus (3) |

retina/fundus (*n* = 2), and deep anterior chambers (*n* = 2). Additionally, including this study, the three patients with the p.G22E mutation have the following findings: microphthalmia (*n* = 3), cataracts (*n* = 1), microcornea (*n* = 2), blonde fundus (*n* = 1), persistent pupillary membrane (*n* = 1), deep anterior chamber (*n* = 1), hyperopia (*n* = 1), strabismus (*n* = 2, 1 esotropic), amblyopia (*n* = 1), glaucoma (*n* = 1), short palpebral fissures (*n* = 1), nasolacrimal duct abnormalities (*n* = 1), and epicanthus (*n* = 1) [2, 3, 21, 22].

Some unique genotype-phenotype correlations were noted upon further analysis. Three patients presented with eccentric pupils, but only 2 of these patients were reported with an associated mutation. Both mutations (p.Q49dup and p.Q49P) seem to affect the same amino acid in connexin-43 [3, 61, 72]. Additionally, uveitis was reported in 10 patients, 9 of which were associated with similar mutations. Eight of these patients were within the same study and had the p.H194P mutation, another patient had no molecular confirmation of a *GJA1* mutation, and the other patient was reported with a missense mutation on exon 2 [4, 9, 10, 27, 28]. However, since the majority of these patients were reported within the same study, the apparent genotype-phenotype correlation of p.H194P and uveitis might be due to underreporting of uveitis from other sources with different pathogenic variants or may be due to other factors of the family not identified within the study.

Further analysis of the genotype-phenotype correlation was conducted by pairing the phenotypic manifestations of each mutation with the corresponding defects in the connexin-43 domains. The domains were defined by the amino acid ranges provided on UniProt (P17302–CXA1_HUMAN) [93]. Table 6 [1–3, 5–71, 92, 93] provides a summary of the phenotypes associated with mutations from each domain.

The domains most commonly affected by *GJA1* mutations are the extracellular-1 loop and the cytoplasmic-1 loop of connexin-43, accounting for 19 and 20 mutations, respectively. Disruptions in the extracellular-1 loop presented primarily as microphthalmia (*n* = 32) and microcornea (*n* = 30). A similar pattern can be seen in the cytoplasmic-1 loop, as the most common presentations were microphthalmia (*n* = 20) and microcornea (*n* = 18). Other clinical findings, however, may be able to distinguish mutations resulting from these domains. The next most common findings associated with mutations in the extracellular-1 loop were glaucoma (*n* = 15) and hypertelorism (*n* = 11), as opposed to short palpebral fissures (*n* = 14) and hypotelorism (*n* = 14) for the cytoplasmic-1 loop.

Mutations affecting the cytoplasmic N-terminus and the transmembrane-1 domain shared similar features to the ones in the extracellular-1 and cytoplasmic-1 domains, as microphthalmia and microcornea were the most common clinical findings. However, the mutations in the cytoplasmic N-terminus and transmembrane-1 domain presented with microcornea (*n* = 17 and *n* = 21, respectively) more frequently than microphthalmia (*n* = 5 and *n* = 14, respectively). The opposite pattern is true for the extracellular-1 and cytoplasmic-1 domains.

The mutations in the extracellular-2 loop demonstrate a different phenotypic pattern, as microphthalmia (*n* = 14) occurs the most frequently, while microcornea is less frequent (*n* = 4). Mutations in the transmembrane-2 domain also display a unique pattern, with hypertelorism (*n* = 5) being the most frequent clinical finding. Other domains listed in Table 6 also demonstrate some unique clinical patterns, but this may be due to variability from the small number of samples. The patterns mentioned previously, however, still provide insight into the role of different connexin-43

TABLE 6: Mutant connexin-43 domains and associated phenotype.

| GJA1 mutation | Protein domain (amino acid range) (obtained from UniProt-P17302) | Associated phenotype (no. of individuals) |
|---|---|---|
| p.G2fsX7 (with p.R101X) p.G2V p.L11P p.L11F p.L11I p.L7V p.S5C | Cytoplasmic N-terminus (1-13) | Microcornea (7), microphthalmia (5), epicanthus (4), strabismus (3) (1 esotropic), short palpebral fissures (2), telecanthus (2), amblyopia (1), dysplastic fundus (1), optociliary vein (1), dysplastic optic disc (1), pale/atrophic optic disc (1), persistent pupillary membrane (1), myopia (3), hyperopia (1) (anisometropic), glaucoma (1), ptosis (1), entropion (1), madarosis (1), hypertelorism (1), and cataract (1) |
| p.W25C p. R33X p.I31M p.K23T p.G22E p.G21R p.S18P p.Y17S p.L26P | Transmembrane-1 (14-36) | Microcornea (21), microphthalmia (14), short palpebral fissures (11), persistent pupillary membrane (6), madarosis (6), epicanthus (6), glaucoma (5), anterior iris stroma hypoplasia (3), hypertelorism (2), cataract (2), iris abnormalities (2), blonde fundus (1), iridoschisis (1), deep anterior chamber (1), hyperopia (2), strabismus (7) (3 esotropic), amblyopia (1), nystagmus (1), ptosis (1), epiblepharon (1), nasolacrimal duct obstruction (1), and flared eyebrows (1) (medially flared) |
| p.Q57SfsTer6 p.R76H p.R76C p.R76S p.H74P p.S69Y p.P59H p.Q49dup p.F52dup p.Q49P p.Q49E p.Q49K p.E48K p.D47H p.E42Q p.V41_A44del p.V41L (with p.R127H (GJB2 mutation)) p.A40V p.P59S | Extracellular-1 (37-76) | Microphthalmia (32), microcornea (30), glaucoma (15) (2 closed-angle, 1 open-angle), hypertelorism (11), epicanthus (10), strabismus (9) (3 esotropic), short palpebral fissures (9), iris atrophy (peripupillary) (8), cataract (6), shallow anterior chamber (6), hypotelorism (5), short axial length (4), myopia (4), corneal farinata (4), telecanthus (3), iris abnormalities (2), eccentric pupils (2), persistent pupillary membrane (2), dysplastic fundus (1), dysplastic optic (1), macular hypoplasia (1), synechiae (1), ciliary body cysts (1), deep anterior chamber (1), hyperopia (1), ptosis (1), blepharophimosis (1), madarosis (1), nasolacrimal duct abnormalities (1), and low-voltage ERG (1) |
| p.Y98C p.V96A p.V96E p.V96M p.H95R p.L90V p.S86Y p.V96G | Transmembrane-2 (77-99) | Hypertelorism (5), microcornea (2), microphthalmia (3), glaucoma (3), strabismus (2) (1 esotropic), short palpebral fissures (2), eyelid mucosal hypertrophy (1), telecanthus (1), epicanthus (1), optic disc atrophy (1), hyperopia (1), myopia (1), strabismus (1), paracentral scotoma (1), madarosis (1), and delayed visual evoked potentials (1) |

TABLE 6: Continued.

| GJA1 mutation | Protein domain (amino acid range) (obtained from UniProt-P17302) | Associated phenotype (no. of individuals) |
|---|---|---|
| p.R101X (with p.G2fsX7) p.R101X p.T154N p.T154A p.R148Q p.R148Ter p.M147T p.G143S p.G138D p.G138R p.G138S p.K134N p.K134E p.I130T p.L113P p.E110D p.L106R p.L106P p.K102N p.I132_K133delinsM | Cytoplasmic-1 (100-154) | Microphthalmia (20), microcornea (18), short palpebral fissures (14), hypotelorism (14), glaucoma (9), myopia (7), epicanthus (5), cataract (3), strabismus (3), shallow anterior chamber (3), hypertelorism (2), opaque lens (1), optic disc hypervascularity (1), pale/atrophic optic disc (1), pale irides (1), iris abnormalities (2), astigmatism (1), Duane syndrome (1), ptosis (1), occipital subcortical white matter changes (1), and delayed visual evoked responses (1) |
| p.F169del | Transmembrane-3 (155-177) | Short palpebral fissures (1) |
| p.R202H (with p.R239R) p.R202H p.K206R p.S201F p.H194P | Extracellular-2 (178-208) | Microphthalmia (18), uveitis (8), glaucoma (8), microcornea (4), opaque cornea (2), thick choroid (2), cataract (1), shallow anterior chamber (1), nystagmus (2), and ptosis (1) |
| p.S220Y p.V216L | Transmembrane-4 (209-231) | Microphthalmia (1), glaucoma (1), microcornea (1), and persistent pupillary membrane (1) |
| p.Y230fsX236 | Transmembrane-4 & cytoplasmic C-terminus (209-382) | Hypertelorism (2), hypotelorism (1), and flared eyebrows (2) (1 medially flared) |
| p.R239R (with p.R202H) p.I311P p.C260fsX306 | Cytoplasmic C-terminus (232-382) | Short palpebral fissures (3), epicanthus (2), hypotelorism (2), microcornea (2), pale irides (2), myopia (2), hyperopia (1) (1 anisometropic), corneal opacity (1), microphthalmia (1), retinal dysplasia (1), choroid thinning (1), glaucoma (1), madarosis (1), and loss of flash ERG (1) |
| Missense mutation exon 2 (unspecified) | Unknown | Microphthalmia (1), cataract (1), microcornea (1), uveitis (1), glaucoma (1), epicanthus (1), telecanthus (1), short palpebral fissures (1), and ptosis (1) |

domains in providing phenotypic variability among patients with ODDD.

In conclusion, this report provides a comprehensive review of the eye and ocular adnexa abnormalities that are currently known to be associated with the ODDD phenotype. Limitations of this report include the possibility of an incomplete ophthalmologic evaluation and/or lack of reporting of eye features in all of the evaluated case reports or misdiagnosis in the individuals with the ODDD phenotype without molecular confirmation. As such, it is possible that the reported common eye features within this summary may be over or underrepresented. Ophthalmic manifestations are commonly associated within the phenotype, and a wide spectrum of eye and ocular adnexa structures may be affected. The rarity of this condition provides further incentive to further investigate the phenotype.

## Consent

Consent has been obtained.

# References

[1] A. Dwarakanathan, M. Bhat, S. GN, and S. Shetty, "Missense and deletion mutations in GJA1 causing oculodentodigital dysplasia in two Indian families," *Clinical Dysmorphology*, vol. 24, no. 4, pp. 159–162, 2015.

[2] W. A. Paznekas, S. A. Boyadjiev, R. E. Shapiro et al., "Connexin 43 (GJA1) mutations cause the pleiotropic phenotype of oculodentodigital dysplasia," *American Journal of Human Genetics*, vol. 72, no. 2, pp. 408–418, 2003.

[3] W. A. Paznekas, B. Karczeski, S. Vermeer et al., "GJA1 mutations, variants, and connexin 43 dysfunction as it relates to the oculodentodigital dysplasia phenotype," *Human Mutation*, vol. 30, no. 5, pp. 724–733, 2009.

[4] G. Kayalvizhi, B. Subramaniyan, and G. Suganya, "Clinical manifestations of oculodentodigital dysplasia," *Journal of the Indian Society of Pedodontics and Preventive Dentistry*, vol. 32, no. 4, pp. 350–352, 2014.

[5] D. R. de la Parra and J. C. Zenteno, "A new GJA1 (connexin 43) mutation causing oculodentodigital dysplasia associated to uncommon features," *Ophthalmic Genetics*, vol. 28, no. 4, pp. 198–202, 2007.

[6] R. Richardson, D. Donnai, F. Meire, and M. J. Dixon, "Expression of Gja1 correlates with the phenotype observed in oculodentodigital syndrome/type III syndactyly," *Journal of Medical Genetics*, vol. 41, no. 1, pp. 60–67, 2004.

[7] R. Kellermayer, M. Keller, P. Ratajczak et al., "Bigenic connexin mutations in a patient with hidrotic ectodermal dysplasia," *European Journal of Dermatology*, vol. 15, no. 2, pp. 75–79, 2005.

[8] D. Cavusoglu, N. O. Dundar, P. Arican, B. Ozyilmaz, and P. Gencpinar, "A hypomyelinating leukodystrophy with calcification: oculodentodigital dysplasia," *Acta Neurologica Belgica*, 2019.

[9] N. A. Aminabadi, A. T. Ganji, A. Vafaei, M. Pourkazemi, and S. G. Oskouei, "Oculodentodigital dysplasia: disease spectrum in an eight-year-old boy, his parents and a sibling," *The Journal of Clinical Pediatric Dentistry*, vol. 33, no. 4, pp. 337–341, 2009.

[10] N. A. Aminabadi, M. Pourkazemi, S. G. Oskouei, and Z. Jamali, "Dental management of oculodentodigital dysplasia: a case report," *Journal of Oral Science*, vol. 52, no. 2, pp. 337–342, 2010.

[11] N. Furuta, M. Ikeda, K. Hirayanagi, Y. Fujita, M. Amanuma, and K. Okamoto, "A novel GJA1 mutation in oculodentodigital dysplasia with progressive spastic paraplegia and sensory deficits," *Internal Medicine*, vol. 51, no. 1, pp. 93–98, 2012.

[12] J. S. Quick and M. Dobersen, "Cardiac arrhythmia and death of teenager linked to rare genetic disorder diagnosed at autopsy," *The American Journal of Forensic Medicine and Pathology*, vol. 35, no. 2, pp. 103–105, 2014.

[13] A. Jamsheer, M. Badura-Stronka, A. Sowińska, S. Debicki, K. Kiryluk, and A. Latos-Bieleńska, "A severe progressive oculodentodigital dysplasia due to compound heterozygous GJA1 mutation," *Clinical Genetics*, vol. 78, no. 1, pp. 94–97, 2010.

[14] S. K. Joss, S. Ghazawy, S. Tomkins, M. Ahmed, J. Bradbury, and E. Sheridan, "Variable expression of neurological phenotype in autosomal recessive oculodentodigital dysplasia of two sibs and review of the literature," *European Journal of Pediatrics*, vol. 167, no. 3, pp. 341–345, 2008.

[15] R. J. Richardson, S. Joss, S. Tomkin, M. Ahmed, E. Sheridan, and M. J. Dixon, "A nonsense mutation in the first transmembrane domain of connexin 43 underlies autosomal recessive oculodentodigital syndrome," *Journal of Medical Genetics*, vol. 43, no. 7, article e37, 2006.

[16] A. Gladwin, D. Donnai, K. Metcalfe et al., "Localization of a gene for oculodentodigital syndrome to human chromosome 6q22-q24," *Human Molecular Genetics*, vol. 6, no. 1, pp. 123–127, 1997.

[17] Z. Wang, L. Sun, P. Wang et al., "Novel ocular findings in oculodentodigital dysplasia (ODDD): a case report and literature review," *Ophthalmic Genetics*, vol. 40, no. 1, pp. 54–59, 2019.

[18] M. A. M. van Steensel, L. Spruijt, I. van der Burgt et al., "A 2-bp deletion in theGJA1 gene is associated with oculo-dento-digital dysplasia with palmoplantar keratoderma," *American Journal of Medical Genetics Part A*, vol. 132a, no. 2, pp. 171–174, 2005.

[19] R. J. Gorlin, L. H. Meskin, and J. W. S. Geme, "Oculodentodigital Dysplasia," *The Journal of Pediatrics*, vol. 63, no. 1, pp. 69–75, 1963.

[20] M. Vreeburg, E. A. de Zwart-Storm, M. I. Schouten et al., "Skin changes in oculo-dento-digital dysplasia are correlated with C-terminal truncations of connexin 43," *American Journal of Medical Genetics. Part A*, vol. 143, no. 4, pp. 360–363, 2007.

[21] E. Gumus, "A rare symptom of a very rare disease: a case report of a oculodentodigital dysplasia with lymphedema," *Clinical Dysmorphology*, vol. 27, no. 3, pp. 91–93, 2018.

[22] E. I. Traboulsi and M. M. Parks, "Glaucoma in oculo-dento-osseous dysplasia," *American Journal of Ophthalmology*, vol. 109, no. 3, pp. 310–313, 1990.

[23] T. Wiest, O. Herrmann, F. Stögbauer et al., "Clinical and genetic variability of oculodentodigital dysplasia," *Clinical Genetics*, vol. 70, no. 1, pp. 71-72, 2006.

[24] K. K. Norton, J. C. Carey, and D. H. Gutmann, "Oculodentodigital dysplasia with cerebral white matter abnormalities in a two-generation family," *American Journal of Medical Genetics*, vol. 57, no. 3, pp. 458–461, 1995.

[25] K. W. Park, H. S. Ryu, J. Kim, and S. J. Chung, "Oculodentodigital dysplasia presenting as spastic paraparesis: the first genetically confirmed Korean case and a literature review," *Journal of Movement Disorders*, vol. 10, no. 3, pp. 149–153, 2017.

[26] G. Brice, P. Ostergaard, S. Jeffery, K. Gordon, P. S. Mortimer, and S. Mansour, "A novel mutation in GJA1 causing oculodentodigital syndrome and primary lymphoedema in a three generation family," *Clinical Genetics*, vol. 84, no. 4, pp. 378–381, 2013.

[27] C. Vitiello, P. D'Adamo, F. Gentile, E. M. Vingolo, P. Gasparini, and S. Banfi, "A novel GJA1 mutation causes oculodentodigital dysplasia without syndactyly," *American Journal of Medical Genetics Part A*, vol. 133a, no. 1, pp. 58–60, 2005.

[28] E. M. Vingolo, K. Steindl, R. Forte et al., "Autosomal dominant simple microphthalmos," *Journal of Medical Genetics*, vol. 31, no. 9, pp. 721–725, 1994.

[29] G. F. Judisch, A. Martin-Casals, J. W. Hanson, and W. H. Olin, "Oculodentodigital dysplasia. Four new reports and a literature review," *Archives of Ophthalmology*, vol. 97, no. 5, pp. 878–884, 1979.

[30] P. Debeer, H. van Esch, C. Huysmans et al., "Novel GJA1 mutations in patients with oculo-dento-digital dysplasia (ODDD)," *European Journal of Medical Genetics*, vol. 48, no. 4, pp. 377–387, 2005.

[31] M. Thomsen, U. Schneider, M. Weber, and F. U. Niethard, "The different appearance of the oculodentodigital dysplasia

syndrome," *Journal of Pediatric Orthopaedics. Part B*, vol. 7, no. 1, pp. 23–26, 1998.

[32] R. J. J. van Es, D. Wittebol-Post, and F. A. Beemer, "Oculodentodigital dysplasia with mandibular retrognathism and absence of syndactyly: a case report with a novel mutation in the connexin 43 gene," *International Journal of Oral and Maxillofacial Surgery*, vol. 36, no. 9, pp. 858–860, 2007.

[33] C. T. Schrander-Stumpel, J. B. de Groot-Wijnands, C. de Die-Smulders, and J. P. Fryns, "Type III syndactyly and oculodentodigital dysplasia: a clinical spectrum," *Genetic Counseling*, vol. 4, no. 4, pp. 271–276, 1993.

[34] E. Tasdelen, C. D. Durmaz, and H. G. Karabulut, "Autosomal recessive oculodentodigital dysplasia: a case report and review of the literature," *Cytogenetic and Genome Research*, vol. 154, no. 4, pp. 181–186, 2018.

[35] A. Spaepen, C. Schrander-Stumpel, J. P. Fryns, C. de Die-Smulders, M. Borghgraef, and H. van den Berghe, "Hallermann-Streiff syndrome: clinical and psychological findings in children. Nosologic overlap with oculodentodigital dysplasia?," *American Journal of Medical Genetics*, vol. 41, no. 4, pp. 517–520, 1991.

[36] L. A. Brueton, S. M. Huson, B. Farren, and R. M. Winter, "Oculodentodigital dysplasia and type III syndactyly: separate genetic entities or disease spectrum?," *Journal of Medical Genetics*, vol. 27, no. 3, pp. 169–175, 1990.

[37] O. Orosz, M. Fodor, I. Balogh, and G. Losonczy, "Relative anterior microphthalmos in oculodentodigital dysplasia," *Indian Journal of Ophthalmology*, vol. 66, no. 2, pp. 334–336, 2018.

[38] R. E. Shapiro, J. W. Griffin, and O. C. Stine, "Evidence for genetic anticipation in the oculodentodigital syndrome," *American Journal of Medical Genetics*, vol. 71, no. 1, pp. 36–41, 1997.

[39] T. Kogame, T. Dainichi, Y. Shimomura, M. Tanioka, K. Kabashima, and Y. Miyachi, "Palmoplantar keratosis in oculodentodigital dysplasia with a GJA1 point mutation out of the C-terminal region of connexin 43," *The Journal of Dermatology*, vol. 41, no. 12, pp. 1095–1097, 2014.

[40] S. Nishat, Q. Mansoor, A. Javaid, and M. Ismail, "Oculodentodigital syndrome with syndactyly type III in a Pakistani consanguineous family," *Journal of Dermatological Case Reports*, vol. 6, no. 2, pp. 43–48, 2012.

[41] C. Amador, A. M. Mathews, M. del Carmen Montoya, M. E. Laughridge, D. B. Everman, and K. R. Holden, "Expanding the neurologic phenotype of oculodentodigital dysplasia in a 4-generation Hispanic family," *Journal of Child Neurology*, vol. 23, no. 8, pp. 901–905, 2008.

[42] F. U. Musa, P. Ratajczak, J. Sahu et al., "Ocular manifestations in oculodentodigital dysplasia resulting from a heterozygous missense mutation (L113P) in *GJA1* (connexin 43)," *Eye (London, England)*, vol. 23, no. 3, pp. 549–555, 2009.

[43] T. Loddenkemper, K. Grote, S. Evers, M. Oelerich, and F. Stögbauer, "Neurological manifestations of the oculodentodigital dysplasia syndrome," *Journal of Neurology*, vol. 249, no. 5, pp. 584–595, 2002.

[44] S. C. Kelly, P. Ratajczak, M. Keller, S. M. Purcell, T. Griffin, and G. Richard, "A novel GJA 1 mutation in oculo-dento-digital dysplasia with curly hair and hyperkeratosis," *European Journal of Dermatology*, vol. 16, no. 3, pp. 241–245, 2006.

[45] L. A. Gabriel, R. Sachdeva, A. Marcotty, E. J. Rockwood, and E. I. Traboulsi, "Oculodentodigital dysplasia: new ocular findings and a novel connexin 43 mutation," *Archives of Ophthalmology*, vol. 129, no. 6, pp. 781–784, 2011.

[46] A. Jamsheer, M. Wisniewska, A. Szpak et al., "A novel GJA1 missense mutation in a Polish child with oculodentodigital dysplasia," *Journal of Applied Genetics*, vol. 50, no. 3, pp. 297–299, 2009.

[47] T. Porntaveetus, C. Srichomthong, A. Ohazama, K. Suphapeetiporn, and V. Shotelersuk, "A novel GJA1 mutation in oculodentodigital dysplasia with extensive loss of enamel," *Oral Diseases*, vol. 23, no. 6, pp. 795–800, 2017.

[48] A. Jamsheer, A. Sowińska-Seidler, M. Socha, A. Stembalska, C. Kiraly-Borri, and A. Latos-Bieleńska, "Three novel GJA1 missense substitutions resulting in oculo-dento-digital dysplasia (ODDD) - further extension of the mutational spectrum," *Gene*, vol. 539, no. 1, pp. 157–161, 2014.

[49] A. Nivelon-Chevallier, D. Audry, F. Audry, and R. Dumas, "Oculo-dental-digital dysplasia: report of a case with spastic paraplegia," *Journal de Génétique Humaine*, vol. 29, no. 2, pp. 171–179, 1981.

[50] W. E. Wooldridge, D. D. Anthony, E. R. Olson, G. P. Bates, and T. J. Sammon, "Oculodentodigital dysplasia," *Missouri Medicine*, vol. 74, no. 8, pp. 379–80, 383, 1977, 383.

[51] K. W. Kjaer, L. Hansen, H. Eiberg, P. Leicht, J. M. Opitz, and N. Tommerup, "Novel connexin 43 (GJA1) mutation causes oculo-dento-digital dysplasia with curly hair," *American Journal of Medical Genetics*, vol. 127a, no. 2, pp. 152–157, 2004.

[52] J. Honkaniemi, J. P. Kalkkila, P. Koivisto, V. Kähärä, T. Latvala, and K. Simola, "Letter to the editor: novel GJA1 mutation in oculodentodigital dysplasia," *American Journal of Medical Genetics. Part A*, vol. 139, no. 1, pp. 48-49, 2005.

[53] S. Opjordsmoen and R. Nyberg-Hansen, "Hereditary spastic paraplegia with neurogenic bladder disturbances and syndactylia," *Acta Neurologica Scandinavica*, vol. 61, no. 1, pp. 35–41, 1980.

[54] A. Pizzuti, E. Flex, R. Mingarelli, C. Salpietro, L. Zelante, and B. Dallapiccola, "A homozygous GJA1 gene mutation causes a Hallermann-Streiff/ODDD spectrum phenotype," *Human Mutation*, vol. 23, no. 3, p. 286, 2004.

[55] K. Izumi, A. M. Lippa, A. Wilkens, H. A. Feret, D. McDonald-McGinn, and E. H. Zackai, "Congenital heart defects in oculodentodigital dysplasia: report of two cases," *American Journal of Medical Genetics Part A*, vol. 161a, no. 12, pp. 3150–3154, 2013.

[56] C. L. Stanislaw, C. Narvaez, R. G. Rogers, and C. S. Woodard, "Oculodentodigital dysplasia with cerebral white matter abnormalities: an additional case," *Proceedings of the Greenwood Genetic Cente*, vol. 17, no. 1, pp. 20–24, 1998.

[57] J. Choi, A. Yang, A. Song et al., "Oculodentodigital dysplasia with a novel mutation in GJA1 diagnosed by targeted gene panel sequencing: a case report and literature review," *Annals of Clinical and Laboratory Science*, vol. 48, no. 6, pp. 776–781, 2018.

[58] J. P. Vasconcellos, M. B. Melo, R. B. Schimiti, N. C. Bressanim, F. F. Costa, and V. P. Costa, "A novel mutation in the GJA1 gene in a family with oculodentodigital dysplasia," *Archives of Ophthalmology*, vol. 123, no. 10, pp. 1422–1426, 2005.

[59] D. M. Weintraub, J. L. Baum, and H. M. Pashayan, "A family with oculodentodigital dysplasia," *The Cleft Palate Journal*, vol. 12, pp. 323–329, 1975.

[60] S. S. Gellis and M. Feingold, "Oculodentodigital dysplasia. Picture of the month," *American Journal of Diseases of Children*, vol. 128, no. 1, pp. 81-82, 1974.

[61] C. Hadjichristou, V. Christophidou-Anastasiadou, A. Bakopoulou et al., "Oculo-dento-digital dysplasia (ODDD) due to a GJA1 mutation: report of a case with emphasis on dental manifestations," *The International Journal of Prosthodontics*, vol. 30, no. 3, pp. 280–285, 2017.

[62] K. Amano, M. Ishiguchi, T. Aikawa et al., "Cleft lip in oculodentodigital dysplasia suggests novel roles for connexin43," *Journal of Dental Research*, vol. 91, 7_suppl, pp. S38–S44, 2012.

[63] L. Feller, N. H. Wood, M. D. Sluiter et al., "Report of a black South African child with oculodentodigital dysplasia and a novel GJA1 gene mutation," *American Journal of Medical Genetics Part A*, vol. 146a, no. 10, pp. 1350–1353, 2008.

[64] A. Itro, A. Marra, V. Urciuolo, P. Difalco, and A. Amodio, "Oculodentodigital dysplasia. A case report," *Minerva Stomatologica*, vol. 54, no. 7-8, pp. 453–459, 2005.

[65] G. Tumminelli, I. di Donato, V. Guida, A. Rufa, A. de Luca, and A. Federico, "Oculodentodigital dysplasia with massive brain calcification and a new mutation of GJA1 gene," *Journal of Alzheimer's Disease*, vol. 49, no. 1, pp. 27–30, 2016.

[66] D. Y. Park, S. Y. Cho, D. K. Jin, and C. Kee, "Clinical characteristics of autosomal dominant GJA1 missense mutation linked to oculodentodigital dysplasia in a Korean family," *Journal of Glaucoma*, vol. 28, no. 4, pp. 357–362, 2019.

[67] R. Hayashi, T. Bito, M. Taniguchi-Ikeda, M. Farooq, M. Ito, and Y. Shimomura, "Japanese case of oculodentodigital dysplasia caused by a mutation in the GJA1 gene," *The Journal of Dermatology*, vol. 41, no. 12, pp. 1109-1110, 2014.

[68] C. A. Wittlieb-Weber, K. M. Haude, C. T. Fong, and J. M. Vinocur, "A novel GJA1 mutation causing familial oculodentodigital dysplasia with dilated cardiomyopathy and arrhythmia," *HeartRhythm Case Reports*, vol. 2, no. 1, pp. 32–35, 2016.

[69] A. Attig, M. Trabelsi, S. Hizem et al., "Oculo-dento-digital dysplasia in a Tunisian family with a novel GJA1 mutation," *Genetic Counseling*, vol. 27, no. 3, pp. 433–439, 2016.

[70] M. Himi, T. Fujimaki, T. Yokoyama, K. Fujiki, T. Takizawa, and A. Murakami, "A case of oculodentodigital dysplasia syndrome with novel GJA1 gene mutation," *Japanese Journal of Ophthalmology*, vol. 53, no. 5, pp. 541–545, 2009.

[71] N. P. Pace, V. Benoit, D. Agius et al., "Two novel GJA1 variants in oculodentodigital dysplasia," *Molecular Genetics & Genomic Medicine*, vol. 7, no. 9, article e882, 2019.

[72] U. C. Parashari, S. Khanduri, S. Bhadury, and F. A. Qayyum, "Radiographic diagnosis of a rare case of oculo-dento-digital dysplasia," *South African Journal of Radiology*, vol. 15, no. 4, p. 134, 2011.

[73] P. Beighton, H. Hamersma, and M. Raad, "Oculodento-osseous dysplasia: heterogeneity or variable expression?," *Clinical Genetics*, vol. 16, no. 3, pp. 169–177, 1979.

[74] D. C. Doshi, P. K. Limdi, N. V. Parekh, and N. R. Gohil, "Oculodentodigital dysplasia," *Indian Journal of Ophthalmology*, vol. 64, no. 3, pp. 227–230, 2016.

[75] M. Frasson, N. Calixto, S. Cronemberger, R. A. L. Pessoa de Aguiar, L. L. Leão, and M. J. Burle de Aguiar, "Oculodentodigital dysplasia: study of ophthalmological and clinical manifestations in three boys with probably autosomal recessive inheritance," *Ophthalmic Genetics*, vol. 25, no. 3, pp. 227–236, 2004.

[76] F. D. Gillespie, "A hereditary syndrome: dysplasia oculodentodigitalis," *Archives of Ophthalmology*, vol. 71, no. 2, pp. 187–192, 1964.

[77] D. H. Gutmann, E. H. Zackai, D. McDonald-McGinn, K. H. Fischbeck, and J. Kamholz, "Oculodentodigital dysplasia syndrome associated with abnormal cerebral white matter," *American Journal of Medical Genetics*, vol. 41, no. 1, pp. 18–20, 1991.

[78] G. J. Kurlander, N. W. Lavy, and J. A. Campbell, "Roentgen differentiation of the oculodentodigital syndrome and the Hallermann-Streiff syndrome in infancy," *Radiology*, vol. 86, no. 1, pp. 77–86, 1966.

[79] D. S. Levine, "Delayed gastric emptying and chronic diarrhea in a patient with oculodentodigital dysplasia syndrome," *Journal of Pediatric Gastroenterology and Nutrition*, vol. 5, no. 2, pp. 329–333, 1986.

[80] M. Martínez-García, A. Bustamante-Aragonés, I. Lorda, and M. J. Trujillo-Tiebas, "Displasia oculodentodigital: consejo genético, opciones reproductivas y estudio molecular de un caso clínico referido para diagnóstico preimplantacional," *Medicina Clínica*, vol. 138, no. 13, pp. 592-593, 2012.

[81] J. K. Mills, L. Wheeler, and S. N. Oishi, "A case of familial syndactyly associated with eye and dental abnormalities," *Jaapa*, vol. 28, no. 12, pp. 40–43, 2015.

[82] S. Mosaed, B. H. Jacobsen, and K. Y. Lin, "Case report: imaging and treatment of ophthalmic manifestations in oculodentodigital dysplasia," *BMC Ophthalmology*, vol. 16, no. 1, 2016.

[83] F. Owlia, M. H. Akhavan Karbassi, R. Hakimian, and M. S. Alemrajabi, "A highlighted case for emphasizing on clinical diagnosis for rare syndrome in third world," *Iranian Journal of Child Neurology*, vol. 11, no. 4, pp. 77–80, 2017.

[84] P. Scheutzel, "Oculodentodigital syndrome: report of a case," *Dento Maxillo Facial Radiology*, vol. 20, no. 3, pp. 175–178, 1991.

[85] J. A. Schneider, G. G. Shaw, and D. van Reken, "Congenital heart disease in oculodentodigital dysplasia," *Virginia Medical*, vol. 104, no. 4, pp. 262-263, 1977.

[86] M. G. Schuller, M. L. Barnett, K. Strassburger, D. L. Friedman, and E. M. Sonnenberg, "Oculodentodigital dysplasia," *Oral Surgery, Oral Medicine, and Oral Pathology*, vol. 61, no. 4, pp. 418–421, 1986.

[87] N. L. Sharma, R. C. Sharma, A. Goyal, B. K. Goyal, and K. R. Lakhanpal, "Oculodentolgital dysplasia with cutaneous keratotic papules," *Indian Journal of Dermatology, Venereology and Leprology*, vol. 48, no. 5, pp. 271–273, 1982.

[88] H. S. Sugar, "Oculodentodigital dysplasia syndrome with angle-closure glaucoma," *American Journal of Ophthalmology*, vol. 86, no. 1, pp. 36–38, 1978.

[89] P. Tejada, Y. W. Eduardo, E. Gutiérrez, A. Barceló, and J. Sánchez, "Glaucoma hereditario asociado a displasia oculodentodigital," *Archivos de la Sociedad Española de Oftalmología*, vol. 86, no. 9, pp. 292–294, 2011.

[90] C. J. Thoden, S. Ryoppy, and P. Kuitunen, "Oculodentodigital dysplasia syndrome. Report of four cases," *Acta Paediatrica Scandinavica*, vol. 66, no. 5, pp. 635–638, 1977.

[91] E. I. Traboulsi, B. M. Faris, V. M. D. Kaloustian, J. M. Opitz, and J. F. Reynolds, "Persistent hyperplastic primary vitreous and recessive oculo-dento- osseous dysplasia," *American Journal of Medical Genetics*, vol. 24, no. 1, pp. 95–100, 1986.

[92] National Center for Biotechnology Information, "ClinVar," March 2020, https://www.ncbi.nlm.nih.gov/clinvar/variation/VCV000137482.1.

[93] T. U. Consortium, "UniProt: a worldwide hub of protein knowledge," *Nucleic Acids Research*, vol. 47, no. D1, pp. D506–D515, 2018.

# 29

# Clinical Findings of Melanoma-Associated Retinopathy with anti-TRPM1 Antibody

**Yoichiro Shinohara ⓘ,[1] Ryo Mukai,[1] Shinji Ueno,[2] and Hideo Akiyama[1]**

[1]Department of Ophthalmology, Gunma University School of Medicine, Maebashi, Gunma, Japan
[2]Department of Ophthalmology, Nagoya University School of Medicine, Nagoya, Aichi, Japan

Correspondence should be addressed to Yoichiro Shinohara; shinohara@gunma-u.ac.jp

Academic Editor: Stephen G. Schwartz

*Introduction.* We report the clinical features and clinical course of melanoma-associated retinopathy (MAR), in which autoantibodies against the transient receptor potential cation channel subfamily M member 1 (TRPM1) were detected. *Case Presentation.* A 74-year-old man was referred to our hospital for treatment of bilateral vision loss. The best-corrected visual acuity was 20/100 in the right eye and 20/200 in the left eye. His electroretinogram (ERG) showed a reduced b-wave and a normal dark-adapted a-wave in both eyes. Optical coherence tomography (OCT) revealed loss of the interdigitation zone in both eyes. We strongly suspected MAR based on the markedly reduced b-wave in the ERG and a history of intranasal melanoma. The diagnosis was confirmed after autoantibodies against TRPM1 were detected in his blood serum. Fifteen months later, his ERG remained unchanged, and OCT showed bilateral cystic changes in the internal nuclear layer. The visual acuity in both eyes also remained unchanged. *Conclusions.* Anti-TRPM1 autoantibodies were detected in a patient diagnosed with MAR who had negative flash ERG and retinal microstructural abnormalities, and the impairment did not recover during the follow-up period. Identification of anti-TRPM1 antibodies was helpful in confirming the diagnosis of MAR.

## 1. Introduction

Melanoma-associated retinopathy (MAR) is a disease associated with melanoma that causes dysfunction of retinal ON-bipolar cells [1]. It is a rare disease in Japan, with a lower incidence than in Europe and the United States [2, 3]. Most patients with MAR have night blindness, photopsia, and nephelopsia, but the vision is usually preserved [4]. A negative-type electroretinogram (ERG) in which a normal a-wave and a reduction in the b-wave amplitude are detected is an essential examination for the diagnosis of MAR [5], although misalignment of the outer retinal microstructure in optical coherence tomography (OCT) is a supportive manifestation for the diagnosis. Transient receptor potential cation channel subfamily M member 1 (TRPM1) is an mGluR6-coupled ion channel in the retinal ON-bipolar cell signal transduction pathway [6] and one of the target antigens for patients with MAR [7]. Herein, we report a case of anti-TRPM1 antibody-positive MAR with visual impairment that followed the clinical course, including OCT findings.

## 2. Case Presentation

A 74-year-old Japanese man gradually developed visual disturbances in both eyes. He was referred to our department four months after his symptoms emerged due to an unknown cause. At his first hospital visit, the best-corrected visual acuities of the right and left eyes were 20/100 and 20/200, respectively. Intraocular pressure was normal. Slit-lamp examination and fundus photography yielded normal results in both eyes (Figure 1(a)). Swept-source optical coherence tomography (SS-OCT; DRI OCT-1 Triton, Topcon Corp., Tokyo, Japan) showed loss of interdigitation lines in both eyes (Figure 1(b)). The Goldmann visual field test showed central scotoma in both eyes (Figure 1(c)). MRI showed no specific abnormalities. The

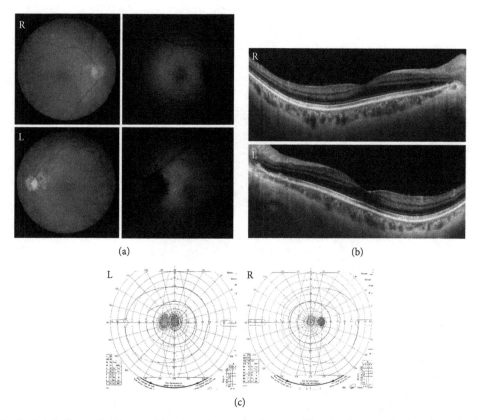

FIGURE 1: Ophthalmological findings of a 74-year-old male patient at the first visit. The visual acuities in the right and left eyes were 20/100 and 20/200, respectively. (a) Fundus photographs and fundus autofluorescence of the patient showing an almost normal fundus. (b) Swept-source optical coherence tomography image showing obscuration of the interdigitation lines in both eyes. (c) The Goldmann visual field test, showing central scotoma in both eyes.

patient had been diagnosed with prostate cancer 9 years ago, and enzalutamide was administered for bone metastases at the initial visit. He had been diagnosed with intranasal melanoma 2 years ago and underwent tumor resection and cervical lymph node dissection. We suspected cancer-associated retinopathy (CAR) based on his medical history, but the anti-recoverin antibody was negative. ERGs were recorded using the RETeval system (LKC Technologies, Gaithersburg, MD, USA) according to the standards of the International Society for Clinical Electrophysiology of Vision. The implicit times and amplitudes of a- and b-waves were automatically analyzed using the software integrated into the RETeval system. The full-field ERGs recorded during the first visit are shown in Figure 2. The rod responses were extinguished, and the rod and cone mixed maximal responses were negative-type ERGs having an a-wave with a normal amplitude and a b-wave with a weaker amplitude than the a-wave in both eyes. The cone responses in the right eye had a square-shaped a-wave and a reduced b-wave amplitude and prolonged implicit time, and those in the left eye were extinguished. The ERGs indicated that the function of retinal ON-bipolar cells was impaired [8]. The amplitudes of the 30-Hz flicker ERGs were almost normal but delayed. Since we suspected MAR from the patient's medical history and ERGs, we used western blot analysis to examine whether anti-TRPM1 antibodies were present in his serum. Serum examinations for the anti-TRPM1 antibody were performed

at Nagoya University, as reported previously [9]. Because the autoantibodies against TRPM1 were positive in this patient's blood sample (Figure 3), he was diagnosed with MAR.

Fifteen months later, the best-corrected visual acuity of both eyes remained unchanged. OCT demonstrated obscuration of the interdigitation lines and cystic changes in the internal nuclear layer (INL) in both eyes (Figures 4(a), 4(b)). The cystic lesions were not detected until the last visit. ERG and Goldmann visual field test results in both eyes essentially remained unchanged for 15 months (Figures 4(c), 4(d)).

## 3. Discussion

We present a case of MAR with negative flash ERG and retinal microstructural abnormalities. Identification of the anti-TRPM1 antibody was helpful in confirming the diagnosis of MAR. The patient was followed up for 15 months, and his visual acuity in one eye was preserved, although it deteriorated slightly in the contralateral eye.

According to previous reports in which changes in visual function were analyzed, visual acuity, color perception, and central visual field were generally preserved in most patients with MAR. However, in this case, the visual acuity of the patient was severely impaired at the initial visit and did not improve during the next 15 months. At the initial visit, SS-OCT was able to detect an irregularity in the

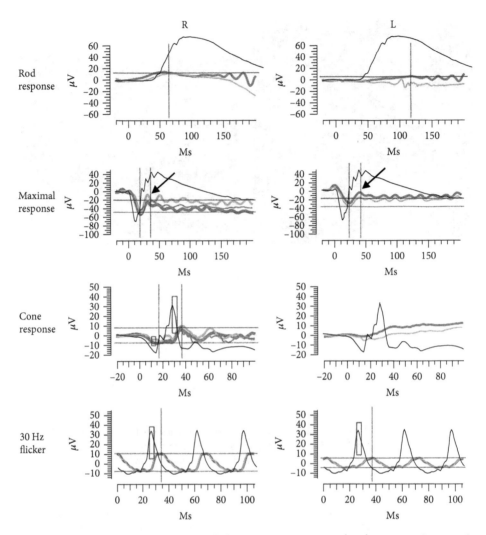

FIGURE 2: Full-field electroretinogram (ERG) of the patient including the rod response, rod and cone mixed maximal response, and 30-Hz flicker response. Yellow, green and blue indicate the first, second, and third responses, respectively. Arrows in the maximal responses show negative-type ERGs in both eyes. Black indicates ERGs from a control eye without any retinal damage.

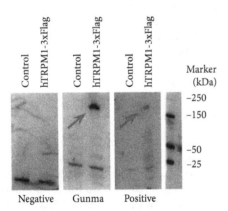

FIGURE 3: Western blot analysis of human TRPM1 antibody using serum from the patient with MAR. Red arrows indicate the hTRPM1-3xFlag protein bands.

interdigitation line, indicating photoreceptor damage, which did not recover during the follow-up period. This damage seemed to correlate with visual disturbances. TRPM1 was

originally identified as a specific protein against melanocytes and has also been reported to be expressed in ON-bipolar cells as a binding protein against mGluR6 [6]. TRPM3 was expressed in high concentrations in the retinal pigment epithelium and inner retina. TRPM1 and TRPM3 have similar sequences [10], and the serum of patients with MAR may cross-react with TRPM1 and TRPM3 [11]. Thus, the patient's serum had a widespread effect on the retina, potentially leading to photoreceptor damage. This response may explain the visual disturbances detected in patients with MAR. At 15 months after the initial visit, OCT revealed a cystic change in the macula (Figure 4(b)). This lesion lies in the INL where bipolar cells are distributed, and it is possible that direct binding of anti-TRPM1 antibody to bipolar cells impairs these cells and leads to cystic changes in the INL. Although fundus fluorescein angiography was not performed in this patient, some CAR patients have been reported to have macular edema due to retinal vasculitis [12]. There was a difference in the ERG amplitude between both eyes of the patient (Figures 2 and 4(d)). All ERGs were performed under similar conditions, and the ERG amplitude

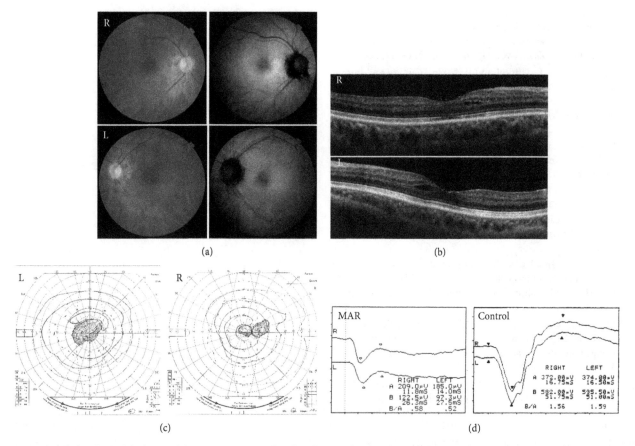

(a)                                                                      (b)

(c)                                                                      (d)

FIGURE 4: Ophthalmological findings of the patient 15 months after the initial visit. The visual acuities in the right and left eyes were 20/120 and 20/200, respectively. (a) Fundus photographs and fundus autofluorescence of the patient showing an almost normal fundus. (b) Optical coherence tomography image showing cyst-like lesions in the internal nuclear layer in both eyes. (c) The Goldmann visual field test, showing a slightly enlarged central scotoma in both eyes. (d) The negative-type waveform with reduced amplitude of the b-wave is unchanged in the maximal response of full-field electroretinogram.

may be correlated with the degree of retinal damage. Retinal damage that could not be assessed by analyzing the retinal structures may be more severe in the left eye than in the right eye of the patient.

Previously, our team reported a correlation between the detection of anti-TRPM1 antibodies and the clinical characteristics of paraneoplastic retinopathy with ON-bipolar cell dysfunction [7]. In this report, autoantibodies against TRPM1 were detected in 5 of the 10 cases. Among these, two had melanoma, and three had lung cancers. Interestingly, in one of the three cases with lung cancer, the negative b-wave and ERG at the initial visit dramatically recovered during the 1-year follow-up. However, in the other two cases, a deteriorated or unchanged b-wave was recorded at the end of the follow-up.

The differences in the clinical courses of each patient can be explained by the variability of recognition sites in anti-TRPM1 antibodies. Some recognition sites can bind to only one specific site, and the binding possibly causes only transient dysfunction of retinal ON-bipolar cells, while other recognition sites can cause severe damage to retinal ON-bipolar cells [7, 13].

In conclusion, this study shows the clinical course of a patient diagnosed with MAR who tested positive for anti-

TRPM1 antibodies. In this case, both visual disturbance and retinal microstructural abnormalities at the initial visit did not recover for 15 months. Anti-TRPM1 antibodies may be useful for confirming the diagnosis of MAR; however, it is important to know the variety of clinical courses in each case with anti-TRPM1 antibodies.

## Acknowledgments

We are grateful to the colleagues of Gunma University, Ota Memorial Hospital, and Nagoya University for their assistance with the acquisition of the data used in this study.

## References

[1] E. L. Berson and S. Lessell, "Paraneoplastic night blindness with malignant melanoma," *American Journal of Ophthalmology*, vol. 106, no. 3, pp. 307–311, 1988.

[2] A. E. Chang, L. H. Karnell, and H. R. Menck, "The National Cancer Data Base report on cutaneous and noncutaneous melanoma: a summary of 84,836 cases from the past decade. The American College of Surgeons Commission on Cancer and the American Cancer Society," *Cancer*, vol. 83, no. 8, pp. 1664–1678, 1998.

[3] K. Murayama, H. Takita, Y. Kiyohara, Y. Shimizu, T. Tsuchida, and S. Yoneya, "Melanoma-associated retinopathy with unknown primary site in a Japanese woman," *Nippon Ganka Gakkai Zasshi*, vol. 110, no. 3, pp. 211–217, 2006.

[4] J. L. Keltner, C. E. Thirkill, and P. T. Yip, "Clinical and immunologic characteristics of melanoma-associated retinopathy syndrome: eleven new cases and a review of 51 previously published cases," *Journal of Neuro-Ophthalmology*, vol. 21, no. 3, pp. 173–187, 2001.

[5] R. Dobson and M. Lawden, "Melanoma associated retinopathy and how to understand the electroretinogram," *Practical Neurology*, vol. 11, no. 4, pp. 234–239, 2011.

[6] C. Koike, T. Obara, Y. Uriu et al., "TRPM1 is a component of the retinal ON bipolar cell transduction channel in the mGluR6 cascade," *Proceedings of the National Academy of Sciences of the United States of America*, vol. 107, no. 1, pp. 332–337, 2010.

[7] S. Ueno, D. Inooka, A. Nakanishi et al., "Clinical course of paraneoplastic retinopathy with anti-TRPM1 autoantibody in JAPANESE cohort," *Retina*, vol. 39, no. 12, pp. 2410–2418, 2019.

[8] M. Kondo and P. A. Sieving, "Primate photopic sine-wave flicker ERG: vector modeling analysis of component origins using glutamate analogs," *Investigative Ophthalmology & Visual Science*, vol. 42, no. 1, pp. 305–312, 2001.

[9] M. Kondo, R. Sanuki, S. Ueno et al., "Identification of autoantibodies against TRPM1 in patients with paraneoplastic retinopathy associated with ON bipolar cell dysfunction," *PLoS One*, vol. 6, no. 5, article e19911, 2011.

[10] R. L. Brown, W. H. Xiong, J. H. Peters et al., "TRPM3 expression in mouse retina," *PLoS One*, vol. 10, no. 2, article e0117615, 2015.

[11] R. M. Duvoisin, T. L. Haley, G. Ren, I. Strycharska-Orczyk, J. P. Bonaparte, and C. W. Morgans, "Autoantibodies in melanoma-associated retinopathy recognize an epitope conserved between TRPM1 and TRPM3," *Investigative Ophthalmology & Visual Science*, vol. 58, no. 5, pp. 2732–2738, 2017.

[12] E. Rahimy and D. Sarraf, "Paraneoplastic and non-paraneoplastic retinopathy and optic neuropathy: evaluation and management," *Survey of Ophthalmology*, vol. 58, no. 5, pp. 430–458, 2013.

[13] W. H. Xiong, R. M. Duvoisin, G. Adamus, B. G. Jeffrey, C. Gellman, and C. W. Morgans, "Serum TRPM1 autoantibodies from melanoma associated retinopathy patients enter retinal on-bipolar cells and attenuate the electroretinogram in mice," *PLoS One*, vol. 8, no. 8, article e69506, 2013.

# 30

# An Adult *Loa loa* Worm in the Upper Eyelid: An Atypical Presentation of Loiasis in the United States

Linnet Rodriguez ⓘD,[1] Julia Michelle White,[1] Nikisha Q. Richards ⓘD,[1] Alan X. You,[2] and Natario L. Couser ⓘD[1,3,4]

[1]Department of Ophthalmology, Virginia Commonwealth University Health System, 401 N 11th St, Richmond, VA 23219, USA
[2]Departments of Internal Medicine and Emergency Medicine, Virginia Commonwealth University Health System, 417 N 11th St, Richmond, VA 23298, USA
[3]Department of Human and Molecular Genetics, Virginia Commonwealth University Health System, 1101 E Marshall St, Richmond, VA 23298, USA
[4]Department of Pediatrics, Virginia Commonwealth University Health System, Children's Hospital of Richmond at VCU, 1000 E Broad St, Richmond, VA 23219, USA

Correspondence should be addressed to Linnet Rodriguez; linnet.rodriguez@vcuhealth.org

Academic Editor: Hiroshi Eguchi

*Purpose*. To report a case of ocular involvement of Loa loa parasite. *Observations*. We present a rare case report of a Loiasis diagnosed in the United States from a patient presenting with subcutaneous migration of an adult worm within an eyelid who was found to have systemic disease with microfilaria in his blood. This is the second report in the United States and the eighth case in published literature worldwide. *Conclusions and Importance*. Due to the relatively mild disease course, Loiasis is relatively ignored in public health in low resource health districts. Understandably, the focus of public health in endemic areas must focus on basic health needs like malnutrition and diseases that entail a greater disease burden. As globalization has increased the amount of trade of physical goods, the effect of immigration also has implications for the spread of infectious disease. Medical practitioners in the United States should be aware of endemic diseases from foreign lands.

## 1. Introduction

*Loa loa* is a common filarial parasite in Western and Central Africa which infects an estimated ten million people or more [1]. Loiasis, the infection caused by this parasite, is asymptomatic in most people infected [2]. Common symptoms of the disease include Calabar swelling, or localized episodes of angioedema, and subconjunctival migration of adult worms [3]. Other ocular structures have also been reported to be affected by Loa loa infection. Therefore, the main objective of this paper is to report a case of Loa loa involvement of an eyelid as it is described below.

## 2. Case Presentation

A 28-year-old healthy male presented to the Emergency Department (ED) with an intermittent "movement sensation" within the left upper eyelid which began 12 hours prior to his presentation.

The patient reported "stinging" pain during the episodic eyelid movements. He denied previous occurrences of this "movement sensation" as well as fever, pruritus, or recent insect bites. Our patient reports possible history of "a tapeworm" in childhood but did not recall any treatment or additional details. Born in Cameroon, the patient immigrated to the United States ten years prior to his presentation. He denied any foreign travel within one year. Two years prior to presentation, he resided in several Caribbean islands including Dominica, Saint Kits, and Barbados.

External examination of the left upper eyelid revealed a subcutaneous thin cylindrical lesion (Figure 1). The patient intermittently noted a painful "movement sensation" of the left upper eyelid. At that time, medical practitioners noted visible episodic movement and slow migration of the subcutaneous lesion. No erythema, edema, or overlying break in the skin was noted. The patient noted that exposure to bright light stopped the "movement sensation" within his eyelid.

General physical exam and complete ophthalmologic exam, including dilated fundoscopy, were unremarkable.

Extraction of the subcutaneous worm was performed in a sterile bedside procedure. Topical anesthesia was applied to the left globe, and local anesthetic was delivered subcutaneously in the eyelid. The location of the worm was marked with ink. A chalazion clamp was placed to aid with excision and confinement of the mobile lesion. A five-millimeter horizontal incision was made just superior to the worm. Blunt dissection was performed to identify the lesion of interest, and the slender 3 cm long white worm was removed (Figure 2, Video 1). The specimen was sent to microbiology and pathology for analysis.

Pathology examination of the gross specimen revealed an adult male *Loa loa* worm. Therefore, this is the first reported case in the United States of a male *Loa loa* worm.

Peripheral blood smear revealed microfilaria. The CBC and BMP were unremarkable except for a mildly elevated ALT of 61. Notably, there was no eosinophilia.

This patient followed with the infectious disease department at our academic medical facility. Microfilarial load of *Loa loa* is being calculated. Onchocerca serologic testing was negative. Patient begun a 21-day-course of oral diethylcarbamazine to decrease the *Loa loa* filarial load. Repeat filarial testing is planned in one year to monitor the disease.

## 3. Discussion

Loiasis is a filarial disease caused by infection with the nematode *Loa loa*. Known colloquially as African eye worm, Loiasis is transmitted to humans by the bites of tabanid flies like *Chrysops silica* and *Chrysops dimidiate*, which introduce larvae into the subcutaneous tissues of human hosts [3]. Over six to twelve months, the larvae develop within human subcutaneous tissues into adult worms, which measure 30-70 millimeters (mm) in length and 0.3-0.5 mm in diameter [3]. Once mature, the adult worms continue traveling through the subcutaneous tissue at rates up to one centimeter per minute [3]. Adult worms have been reported to survive in human tissue for up to 21 years [4]. Immature larvae or microfilariae are released by adult female worms and migrate between the host's bloodstream and lungs in a diurnal pattern [3].

Currently, it is estimated that greater than 10 million people are infected with *Loa loa* [1]. Endemic areas encompass much of Western and Central Africa with the highest prevalence of disease being in Cameroon, Gabon, Equitorial

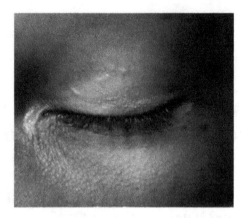

FIGURE 1: External photograph of left periorbital region which demonstrates a thin, serpentine lesion of the left upper eyelid near the eyelid crease.

Guinea, Congo, and the Central African Republic [5]. Though exceedingly common in Western Africa, Loiasis is most often asymptomatic [3]. Symptoms from the disease may emerge years after initial infection [3]. The most common sign of Loiasis is Calabar swellings, which are episodes of localized angioedema most often on the face and extremities [2]. Calabar swellings are caused by a hypersensitivity response to parasitic antigens in subcutaneous tissues [3]. Often painless, Calabar swellings may be painful if involving the joints [3].

A second hallmark of Loiasis is subconjunctival migration of adult worms, which may be associated with conjunctivitis, epiphora, foreign body sensation, and transient eyelid swelling [3]. These symptoms are typically self-limited. While the benign subconjunctival migration of adult *Loa loa* worms is common, other ophthalmic manifestations have been reported, though rarely. Intraocular adult filaria have been noted in the anterior chamber, which may cause corneal edema, uveitis, hypopyon, and secondary cataract formation [6–10]. In patients with disseminated Loiasis and encephalopathy, retinal hemorrhage, retinal artery occlusions, vitreous hemorrhage, and chorioretinitis have been noted [11, 12]. In one case, pathological specimens of the retina showed numerous microfilaria within the retinal vasculature with the concentration of microfilaria corresponding to the degree of retinal edema and hemorrhage [11].

Other more serious but rare systemic complications of Loiasis are reported including meningoencephalitis, hematuria, proteinuria, endomyocardial fibrosis, pleural effusions, arthritis, and lymphangitis [12]. These complications are thought to be due to the inflammatory reaction to microfilarial antigens [11].

To our knowledge, this case represents the second case of periocular subcutaneous *Loa loa* macrofilaria of the eyelid in the United States. Our literature search has only revealed eight similar cases previously recorded in medical literature (the appendix). This is the first male *Loa loa* worm extracted from the periocular subcutaneous tissues. In two of the previously published cases, it was noted that exposure to a bright light source induced movement of the filaria [13, 14]. On

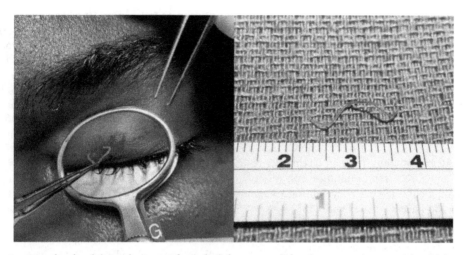

Figure 2: Surgical extraction of male adult Loa loa worm from the left upper eyelid and gross specimen at right which measured 3.2 cm from head to tail.

the contrary, our patient stated that bright light caused cessation of movement of the adult worm.

Diagnosis of *loa loa* may be accomplished by microscopic detection of microfilariae in the peripheral blood. The microfilaria presence in the serum follows a diurnal curve, with a high density between 10:00 and 16:00 [3]. Blood drawn outside this window may yield a false negative result [1]. It is interesting to note that our patient was found to have microfilaria in blood drawn at 20:00. Unfortunately, up to half of *L loa* infected patients do not have detectable microfilariae in their blood, which makes laboratory diagnosis difficult [1]. PCR test is also available in some locations to detect *L loa* specific DNA [3]. Clinical diagnosis may be necessary, and criteria would include exposure to an endemic area, Calabar swelling, and subconjunctival macrofilaria.

Treatment of Loiasis is difficult as its medical treatment poses significant side effects. Coordination of care with an infectious disease or tropical medicine specialist is vital. The first-line treatment, diethylcarbamazine (DEC), utilizes the patient's immune response to kill both microfilaria and adult worms [3]. Complete treatment may require repeated doses. In patients with high loads of microfilaria, DEC treatment entails a significant risk of encephalopathy [1]. Though this side effect is not well understood, it is thought to be due to sudden decomposition of larvae resulting from DEC treatment [1]. Second line treatments include ivermectin and albendazole [1]. Both are limited in efficacy because they only act to kill one life stage of the parasite. Ivermectin treatment is lethal to microfilaria but not adult larvae [3]. In addition, the treatment with ivermectin may also lead to encephalopathy in patients with high microfilarial loads [1]. Albendazole is thought to kill adult parasites by inhibiting microtubule formation and the uptake of glucose, but it does not affect microfilaria [3]. In a few cases in countries with advanced medical systems, apheresis has been used to decrease the burden of microfilaria from the blood which has then allowed for treatment with DEC without adverse effect [15].

There has been no elimination campaign for *Loa loa* due to the relatively low burden of disease caused by the parasite but also due to serious adverse effects from treatment with antihelminthic drugs [16]. Due to the coendemic nature of onchocerciasis and Loiasis, patients treated for either parasitic disease must be tested for the other infection in order to prevent toxic and potentially lethal side effects from medical treatment [3]. Loiasis treatment with DEC is contraindicated in patients coinfected with Onchocerca as the treatment may worsen Onchocercal eye disease [3]. Onchocerciasis treatment with ivermectin may produce severe side effects including encephalopathy, cardiomyopathy, and nephropathy [14, 17]. Patients with a high microfilarial load of *L loa* have been identified as those at highest risk [17].

## 4. Conclusion

Loiasis is an underrecognized and undertreated infectious disease in Central and Western Africa. Though rarely diagnosed in developed nations, practitioners in all medical specialties must be aware of the disease which may present in immigrants and travelers up to 21 years after their initial infection. This case report notes a novel clinical presentation of Loiasis in the United States. A young, healthy male presented with Loiasis ten years after his most recent exposure to an endemic area, Cameroon. He had no hallmark ocular symptoms nor Calabar swelling during the previous ten years, yet he was found to have an adult male *L loa* worm in his eyelid. Microfilaria were noted in his blood sample drawn at night, which is outside the typical midday peak for microfilarial concentration in the blood. Surgical removal of the adult male filaria from the upper eyelid allowed for prompt diagnosis. This is the first case in which a patient noted light to stop filarial movement. Treatment of infection with *Loa loa* requires coordination with infectious disease specialists and can be complicated by incomplete eradication of the filaria and adverse reactions from the treatment.

# Appendix

## Previously Published Cases of Periocular Subcutaneous Adult *Loa loa* in Chronological Order

(1) 32-year-old Zambian woman found to have an asymptomatic female *Loa loa* worm in the left lower eyelid [13]

(2) 23-year-old African student living in Germany presented with "acute, recurrent, multifocal episodes of pain and swelling of his left upper eyelid" for 3 weeks and was found to have a female filaria [18]

(3) 35-year-old Ghanaian male living in the United Kingdom for eight years presented with one day history of left eye redness which had intermittently occurred for the preceding 6 years. A subcutaneous worm was removed from the left upper eyelid [19]

(4) 32-year-old Indian woman presented with a two-month history of "painless vermiform swelling of left upper eyelid" with intermittent "sensation of something crawling". A female *Loa loa* worm was extracted [14]

(5) 60-year-old American man with transient facial swellings had macrofilaria extracted from his left upper eyelid 21 years after travel to Nigeria for a 3-day trip [4]

(6) 32-year-old male patient in Romania presented with left upper eyelid pain, and an adult worm was removed from his left upper eyelid [20]

(7) 31-year-old patient from Cameroon living in France for 8 years who presented for discomfort in eyelid for several weeks found to have microfilaria on blood smear, with removal of parasite from upper pelvis subcutaneous tissue [21]

## Consent

The patient consented to publication of the case in writing.

## References

[1] W. G. Metzger and B. Mordmüller, "Loa loa–does it deserve to be neglected?," *The Lancet Infectious Diseases*, vol. 14, no. 4, pp. 353–357, 2014.

[2] J. J. Padgett and K. H. Jacobsen, "Loiasis: African eye worm," *Transactions of the Royal Society of Tropical Medicine and Hygiene*, vol. 102, no. 10, pp. 983–989, 2008.

[3] J. Kamgno and A. Klion, "Loiasis," in *Hunter's Tropical Medicine and Emerging Infectious Disease*, T. P. Endy, T. Solomon, D. R. Hill, E. T. Ryan, and N. Aronson, Eds., pp. 859–863, Elsevier, Philadelphia, USA, 2019.

[4] E. T. Richardson, R. Luo, D. Fink, T. B. Nutman, J. K. Geisse, and M. Barry, "Transient facial swellings in a patient with a remote African travel history," *Journal of Travel Medicine*, vol. 19, no. 3, pp. 183–185, 2012.

[5] H. G. M. Zouré, S. Wanji, M. Noma et al., "The geographic distribution of Loa loa in Africa: results of large-scale implementation of the Rapid Assessment Procedure for Loiasis (RAPLOA)," *PLoS Neglected Tropical Diseases*, vol. 5, no. 6, 2011.

[6] P. Barua, N. Barua, N. K. Hazarika, and S. Das, "Loa Loa in the anterior chamber of the eye: a case report," *Indian Journal of Medical Microbiology*, vol. 23, no. 1, pp. 59-60, 2005.

[7] A. O. Eballe, E. Epée, G. Koki, D. Owono, C. E. Mvogo, and A. L. Bella, "Intraocular live male filarial Loa loa worm," *Clinical Ophthalmology*, vol. 2, no. 4, pp. 965–967, 2008.

[8] J. Lucot and M. Chovet, "Loase intraoculaire, à propos d'une observation," *La Medicina Tropical*, vol. 32, pp. 523–525, 1972.

[9] O. Osuntokun and O. Olurin, "Filarial worm (Loa loa) in the anterior chamber. Report of two cases," *British Journal of Ophthalmology*, vol. 59, no. 3, pp. 166-167, 1975.

[10] M. Satyavani and K. N. Rao, "Live male adult Loaloa in the anterior chamber of the eye–a case report," *Indian Journal of Pathology & Microbiology*, vol. 36, no. 2, pp. 154–157, 1993.

[11] D. Toussaint and P. Danis, "Retinopathy in generalized Loa-Loa filariasis: a clinicopathological study," *Archives of Ophthalmology*, vol. 74, no. 4, pp. 470–476, 1965.

[12] K. G. Buell, C. Whittaker, C. B. Chesnais et al., "Atypical clinical manifestations of loiasis and their relevance for endemic populations," *Open Forum Infectious Diseases*, vol. 6, no. 11, 2019.

[13] R. C. Chhabra, S. Bhat, and S. M. Shukla, "Occular loiasis in a Zambian woman," *East African Medical Journal*, vol. 66, no. 7, pp. 491–494, 1989.

[14] S. Bhedasgaonkar, R. B. Baile, S. Nadkarni, G. Jakkula, and P. Gogri, "Loa loa macrofilariasis in the eyelid: case report of the first periocular subcutaneous manifestation in India," *Journal of Parasitic Diseases*, vol. 35, no. 2, pp. 230-231, 2011.

[15] L. Muylle, H. Taelman, R. Moldenhauer, R. Van Brabant, and M. E. Peetermans, "Usefulness of apheresis to extract microfilarias in management of loiasis," *British Medical Journal (Clinical Research Ed.)*, vol. 287, no. 6391, pp. 519-520, 1983.

[16] J. Gardon, N. Gardon-Wendel, Demanga-Ngangue, J. Kamgno, J. P. Chippaux, and M. Boussinesq, "Serious reactions after mass treatment of onchocerciasis with ivermectin in an area endemic for _Loa loa_ infection," *Lancet*, vol. 350, no. 9070, pp. 18–22, 1997.

[17] O. Ojurongbe, A. A. Akindele, M. A. Adeleke et al., "Co-endemicity of loiasis and onchocerciasis in rain forest communities in southwestern Nigeria," *PLoS Neglected Tropical Diseases*, vol. 9, no. 3, article e0003633, 2015.

[18] Z. H. Sbeity, A. Jaksche, S. Martin, and K. U. Loeffler, "Loa loa macrofilariasis in the eyelid: case report of the first periocular subcutaneous manifestation in Germany," *Graefe's Archive for Clinical and Experimental Ophthalmology*, vol. 244, no. 7, pp. 883-884, 2006.

[19] G. S. Bowler, A. N. Shah, L. A. Bye, and M. Saldana, "Ocular loiasis in London 2008-2009: a case series," *Eye*, vol. 25, no. 3, pp. 389–391, 2011.

[20] L. Rotaru and C. Serban, "An extremely rare situation–subcutaneously filariasis presented at ED Craiova," *Current Health Sciences Journal*, vol. 40, no. 2, pp. 139-140, 2014.

[21] D. Coeuru, M. Weber, C. Couret, G. Le Meur, and P. Lebranchu, "Subcutaneous upper eyelid Loa Loa macrofilariasis, case report," *Journal Français d'Ophtalmologie*, vol. 41, no. 8, pp. 778–781, 2018.

# 31

# Acute Vitreous and Intraretinal Hemorrhage with Multifocal Subretinal Fluid in Juvenile X-Linked Retinoschisis

**Sidra Ibad,**[1] **Carl S. Wilkins** (iD)**,**[2] **Alexander Pinhas,**[2] **Vincent Sun,**[2] **Matthew S. Wieder** (iD)**,**[2] **and Avnish Deobhakta** (iD)[1,2]

[1]*Icahn School of Medicine at Mount Sinai, One Gustave L. Levy Place, New York, NY, USA*
[2]*New York Eye and Ear Infirmary of Mount Sinai, 310 East 14th Street, Retina Center, New York, NY, USA*

Correspondence should be addressed to Carl S. Wilkins; cswilkins013@gmail.com

Academic Editor: Takaaki Hayashi

*Purpose.* To report a rare case of spontaneous vitreous and intraretinal hemorrhage in a patient with juvenile X-linked retinoschisis which was managed conservatively. *Methods.* Single patient case report. *Introduction.* Juvenile X-linked retinoschisis (JXLR) most often occurs as a result of a genetic defect in the retinoschisin (RS1) gene, causing a separation between the ganglion cell layer and the nerve fiber layer. Spontaneous vitreous hemorrhage has been reported as an uncommon secondary consequence of JXLR. We present a case of spontaneous vitreous and diffuse macular intraretinal hemorrhages in a patient with JXLR which resolved with medical management alone. *Results.* A 23-year-old man with a history of juvenile X-linked retinoschisis presented to the ophthalmic emergency room complaining of acute onset of floaters in his right eye. On examination, the patient was found to have a new vitreous hemorrhage with diffuse intraretinal hemorrhages in his right eye, without new retinal tears or detachment. SD-OCT demonstrated multifocal pockets of subretinal fluid. The genetic testing panel revealed a hemizygous mutation in the RS-1 gene. He was managed conservatively on oral acetazolamide, with the resolution of the subretinal fluid and with both visual and symptomatic improvement. *Conclusions.* Spontaneous vitreous hemorrhage may rarely occur in patients with JXLR, even in the absence of acute retinal tear or detachment. This case demonstrates an atypical presentation of vitreous hemorrhage with diffuse intraretinal hemorrhage and new multifocal areas of subretinal fluid which improved without surgical intervention. Good outcomes may be achieved in these patients with conservative management alone, even in atypical presentations.

## 1. Introduction

With an estimated prevalence ranging from 1 : 15,000 to 30,000, juvenile X-linked retinoschisis (JXLR) is the most common pediatric-onset retinal degeneration. The condition is defined by a characteristic radiating pattern of foveal schisis in nearly all patients, often with a bimodal age distribution in infancy or school-age patients. Other findings include peripheral retinoschisis and pigmentary changes [1]. Complications may arise from vitreoretinal traction, particularly in areas of schisis cavities, including retinal tears and rhegmatogenous retinal detachments (RRD), spontaneous vitreous hemorrhage, and retinal fibrosis. These deleterious secondary findings most commonly present within the first decade of life [2]. There are several prior reports of vitreous hemorrhage in JXLR, either spontaneous or secondary to ret-

inal tear or detachment, treated successfully with surgical intervention [2–4]. We report an atypical case of spontaneous vitreous hemorrhage in JXLR that presented with diffuse intraretinal hemorrhages and formation of multifocal pockets of subretinal fluid, which improved with conservative medical management alone.

## 2. Case Report

A 23-year-old man with a 6-year history of suspected JXLR treated with oral acetazolamide presented to the New York Eye and Ear Infirmary of Mount Sinai with a 3-day history of acute, painless decrease in vision with new floaters in his right eye (OD). Visual acuity on examination was stable from the prior exam at 20/60 bilaterally, with no relative afferent pupillary defect, and normotensive intraocular pressures

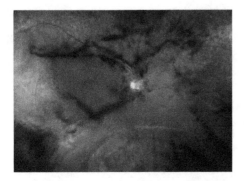

FIGURE 1: Widefield fundus photo of the right eye demonstrating intravitreal hemorrhage, vitreous debris, scattered intraretinal hemorrhage in the macula, and multiple areas of retinoschisis.

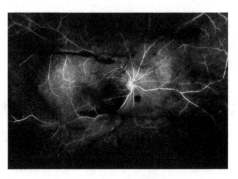

FIGURE 2: Widefield fluorescein angiography of the right eye demonstrating blocked fluorescence from vitreous debris and hemorrhage, with mild decreased perfusion at the areas of retinoschisis, and multiple areas of blocked fluorescence from intraretinal hemorrhage in the macula and near the periphery. There is no visible leakage.

bilaterally. The anterior segment examination was unremarkable. Dilated fundus examination revealed new vitreous debris with hemorrhage, stable areas of retinoschisis temporally and inferiorly with outer retinal holes and areas of vitreoretinal traction, and scattered intraretinal hemorrhages along the arcade within the macula and in the near periphery (Figure 1).

An extrafoveal posterior vitreous detachment (PVD) was noted OD. Widefield fluorescein angiography demonstrated pinpoint areas of late leakage corresponding to new pockets of subretinal fluid, stable mild leakage from vessels at junctional areas of vitreoretinal traction, and nonperfusion at peripheral areas of schisis (Figure 2).

Spectral domain ophthalmic coherence tomography (SD-OCT) demonstrated new, multifocal areas of subretinal cavitation with adjacent hyperreflective foci in the outer plexiform layer corresponding to areas of intraretinal hemorrhage on examination OD (Figures 3(a) and 3(b)).

No retinal tears or detachments were identified in either eye. The decision was made to closely observe the patient with medical management alone.

Serial follow-up examinations revealed the clearing of the vitreous hemorrhage with the resolution of intraretinal hemorrhages (Figure 4).

The peripheral retina remained stable without tears or detachment. Repeat SD-OCT showed the resolution of the subretinal fluid cavities and intraretinal hemorrhages (Figure 5).

The patient was continued on oral acetazolamide 125 mg twice daily, and visual acuity improved to 20/50. An inherited retinal degeneration gene panel (Spark Therapeutics Inc., Philadelphia, PA, USA) was obtained, which identified a hemizygous mutation in the retinoschisin (RS1) gene, confirming the diagnosis of JXLR. The patient remained stable at the 6-month follow-up on medical therapy.

## 3. Discussion

Vitreous hemorrhage is a known complication of JXLR, with or without retinal tear or detachment, and affects a minority of these patients. A wide range of management may be instituted, depending on whether a retinal break is detected or highly likely, and if a sufficient view exists to rule out those

urgent etiologies. Though observational data is relatively sparse, vitreous hemorrhage or retinal detachment has been reported in up to 5% of patients with JXLR, almost always in the first decade of life [1]. These patients often are found to have abnormal vitreous, with 51% of patients reported to have vitreous veils and vitreoretinal traction [2]. Previous reports of vitrectomy in patients with JXLR demonstrated anatomic success in about 80% of surgeries, with coincident vitreous hemorrhage fairly rare at presentation, occurring in only 12% of these patients [3, 4]. We present a case of vitreous hemorrhage accompanied by atypical diffuse intraretinal hemorrhages and multifocal subretinal fluid, all of which were managed with medical management alone with a good outcome.

When vitrectomy is indicated for detachment in JXLR, chronic subretinal fluid or redetachment is common postoperatively, suggesting that despite the initial improvements, final anatomic success may be variable. While most surgeries lead to improved visual acuity, a considerable proportion experience no change or worsening of visual acuity [3, 4]. Vitrectomy remains the gold standard and may require retinectomy and internal limiting membrane (ILM) peeling to achieve reattachment. ILM peeling is controversial due to the formation of retinal breaks via fragile inner laminations but is recommended when surgically feasible. Inner retinal layer retinectomy may provide improved visualization of outer retinal layer breaks, relief of traction, and more complete vitreous removal; however, there is no proven difference in outcomes [5]. Vitreous hemorrhages without retinal breaks may spontaneously resolve; however, acute vitreous hemorrhages with retinal tear or detachment require urgent intervention. Nonsurgical treatments include laser photocoagulation at suspected areas of pathology and carbonic anhydrase inhibitors; however, level one data for these treatments is lacking. Though our patient suffered an acute vitreous hemorrhage at age 28, acute retinal pathology usually manifests in the first decade of life, with rare cases of vitreous hemorrhage reported in infancy [6, 7].

It is important to consider the implications of the genetics of JXLR and the atypical presentation of our patient, particularly in the context of the existing literature. X-linked

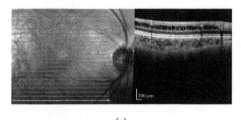 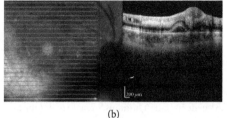

(a)                                                            (b)

FIGURE 3: SD-OCT of the right eye at baseline (a; top) and after acute vitreous hemorrhage (b; bottom). (a) Retinoschisis in the inferior macula. (b) Intraretinal hemorrhage collecting within prior areas of schisis, with a focal serous neurosensory detachment.

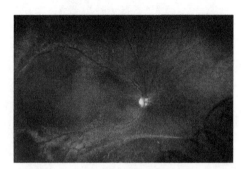

FIGURE 4: Widefield fundus photo of the right eye showing the resolution of vitreous hemorrhage, vitreous debris, and intraretinal macular hemorrhages.

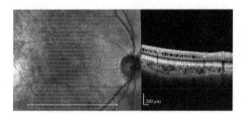

FIGURE 5: SD-OCT of the right eye demonstrating the resolution of subretinal fluid seen in Figure 3.

retinoschisis has a high penetrance with variable phenotypic expression, which complicates the generalizability of interventional studies in guiding treatment paradigms, and may account for the variable outcomes between patients who appear similar anatomically [8]. Our patient developed hemorrhage into preexisting schisis cavities, as well as multifocal subretinal fluid cavities along the presumed areas of prior vitreoretinal traction which likely formed at the moment of release. There is sparse data regarding the rapidity of progression of detachment in these patients secondary to retinal breaks; hence, each patient may be managed differently based on presentation. Significant improvement in subretinal fluid without the presence of a retinal tear may be achieved with carbonic anhydrase inhibitors only, though the current data is limited to observational studies or case reports [9, 10].

Few case series of surgical interventions in these patients exist, though the most commonly reported reason for vitrectomy is RRD [3, 4]. Sen et al. reported the largest case series of 34 eyes with JXLR which underwent surgery for RRD, with only 11% presenting with concomitant vitreous hemorrhage, suggesting that most patients with detachment and JXLR do

not present with this exam finding. Of note, nearly a third of patients in this series underwent a second surgery for redetachment, and 80% achieved final anatomic success, demonstrating overall worse outcomes in these patients compared to vitrectomy for more common causes of RRD [2]. Other interventional series present similar rates of vitreous hemorrhage (12-33%) in these patients, as well as the mean required number of surgeries (1.2-1.8), suggesting similar experience across institutions. The most common reason for anatomic failure in JXLR patients is the development of proliferative vitreoretinopathy [3, 4].

We present a case of JXLR in a 28-year-old male which was complicated by acute hemorrhagic posterior vitreous detachment with intraretinal hemorrhages within schisis cavities and multifocal, pinpoint serous retinal detachments managed with observation. We hypothesize that the prior vitreoretinal traction and abnormally friable tissue in this patient lead to the rupture of the deep capillary plexus during the completion of the PVD. Prior reports of surgical intervention for retinal detachment and vitreous hemorrhage indicate fair anatomic outcomes, though often with multiple procedures needed, and rarely with concomitant presence of vitreous hemorrhage. Without clear identification of a retinal tear in our patient, conservative management was chosen, and a good outcome was achieved without the need for surgery.

## Abbreviations

JXLR:    Juvenile X-linked retinoschisis
RRD:     Rhegmatogenous retinal detachment
OD:      Right eye
OS:      Left eye
PVD:     Posterior vitreous detachment
ILM:     Internal limiting membrane
RS1:     Retinoschisin 1
SD-OCT:  Spectral domain ophthalmic coherence tomography.

## Consent

As all information is anonymous, the patient was not consented.

## Authors' Contributions

All authors (SI, CSW, MSW, AP, VS, AD) contributed to the development, writing, and editing of this manuscript.

# References

[1] S. K. Sikkink, S. Biswas, N. R. A. Parry, P. E. Stanga, and D. Trump, "X-linked retinoschisis: an update," *Journal of Medical Genetics*, vol. 44, no. 4, pp. 225–232, 2007.

[2] F. Simonelli, G. Cennamo, C. Ziviello et al., "Clinical features of X linked juvenile retinoschisis associated with new mutations in the XLRS1 gene in Italian families," *The British Journal of Ophthalmology*, vol. 87, no. 9, pp. 1130–1134, 2003.

[3] P. Sen, A. Agarwal, P. Bhende et al., "Outcome of vitreoretinal surgery for rhegmatogenous retinal detachment in X-linked juvenile retinoschisis," *Indian Journal of Ophthalmology*, vol. 66, no. 12, pp. 1825–1831, 2018.

[4] P. J. Rosenfeld, Flynn HW Jr, H. McDonald et al., "Outcomes of vitreoretinal surgery in patients with X-linked retinoschisis," *Ophthalmic Surgery and Lasers*, vol. 29, no. 3, pp. 190–197, 1998.

[5] C. D. Regillo, W. S. Tasman, and G. C. Brown, "Surgical management of complications associated with X-linked retinoschisis," *Archives of Ophthalmology*, vol. 111, no. 8, pp. 1080–1086, 1993.

[6] Y. Iordanous and T. G. Sheidow, "Vitrectomy for X-linked retinoschisis: a case report and literature review," *Canadian Journal of Ophthalmology*, vol. 48, no. 4, pp. e71–e74, 2013.

[7] J. J. Lee, J. H. Kim, S. Y. Kim, S. S. Park, and Y. S. Yu, "Infantile vitreous hemorrhage as the initial presentation of X-linked juvenile retinoschisis," *Korean Journal of Ophthalmology*, vol. 23, no. 2, pp. 118–120, 2009.

[8] B. T. Savoie and P. J. Ferrone, "Complicated congenital retinoschisis," *Retinal Cases & Brief Reports*, vol. 11, Supplement 1, pp. S202–S210, 2017.

[9] R. S. Molday, U. Kellner, and B. H. F. Weber, "X-linked juvenile retinoschisis: clinical diagnosis, genetic analysis, and molecular mechanisms," *Progress in Retinal and Eye Research*, vol. 31, no. 3, pp. 195–212, 2012.

[10] A. Sadaka and R. A. Sisk, "Dramatic regression of macular and peripheral retinoschisis with dorzolamide 2 % in X-linked retinoschisis: a case report," *Journal of Medical Case Reports*, vol. 10, no. 1, p. 142, 2016.

# 32

# Intraoperative Cycling Pressure Variation in the Treatment of Central Retinal Artery Occlusion

## A. Altun ⓘ

*Department of Ophthalmology, Bahcesehir University, Istanbul, Turkey*

Correspondence should be addressed to A. Altun; aaltun06@gmail.com

Academic Editor: Cristiano Giusti

A 45-year-old male presented to the clinic of ophthalmology with central retinal artery occlusion (CRAO). There was no response to medical treatment, ocular massage, and anterior chamber paracentesis. CRAO was resolved by pars plana vitrectomy and intraoperative cycling pressure variation. The best-corrected visual acuity improved to 20/100 on the first day and to 20/20 on the first month, postoperatively.

## 1. Introduction

Central retinal artery occlusion (CRAO) is an ophthalmological emergency because the sudden and catastrophic vision loss might be permanent. Perfusion of the retinal ganglion cell layer is provided by end-artery circulation of the retinal artery [1]. In CRAO, infarction develops in the inner retina and retinal ganglion cells [2]. Providing rapid and early reperfusion is vital in CRAO.

Many medical and surgical treatment methods have been defined for the management of CRAO. Digital ocular massage [3], acetazolamide [4], intravenous mannitol [5], oral pentoxifylline [6], inhalation of 10% carbogen [7], sublingual isosorbide dinitrate [8], intravenous methylprednisolone [9], intravenous or intra-arterial recombinant tissue plasminogen activator [2], hyperbaric oxygen [10], anterior chamber paracentesis [11], and Nd:YAG (neodymium-doped yttrium aluminum garnet) laser embolectomy/embolysis [12] are the most known alternatives.

Technological advances in microsurgery have recently led to the more frequent application of vitreoretinal surgical interventions in the management of CRAO [13]. In this paper, we aimed to present a case with CRAO resolved by pars plana vitrectomy (PPV) and intraoperative cycling pressure variation, which did not respond to medical treatment, ocular massage, and anterior chamber paracentesis.

## 2. Patient and Methods

A 45-year-old male patient was presented to the clinic of ophthalmology with an advanced level of visual acuity loss that started suddenly in his right eye 1 hour ago. Informed consent was obtained from the patient for all treatment and surgical procedures. Complete ophthalmologic examination and fundus fluorescein angiography (FFA) were performed preoperatively and postoperatively.

Sublingual 10 mg isosorbide dinitrate (Isordil, Actavis, Turkey) and oral 100 mg acetylsalicylic acid (Coraspin, Bayer AG, Germany) were given to the patient, and ocular massage was performed to the eye immediately. Anterior chamber paracentesis was performed 2 hours later. Transconjunctival sutureless 25-gauge PPV (AA) was performed to the right eye. After core vitrectomy, the posterior hyaloid was detached with the help of triamcinolone acetonide (Kenacort, Deva, Turkey).

Intraoperative cycling pressure variation was induced in a five-second period with 650 mmHg venturi pump power in the closest position to the optic nerve head (Constellation, Alcon, USA). The same application was done at 15-second intervals. Intraocular pressure adjustment of the device was determined to be 35 mmHg during active suction and 15 mmHg between the intervals with continuing infusion. Intraoperative cycling pressure variation on the optic nerve head was repeated until blood flow in the central retinal artery was observed.

FFA imaging was performed again on the first day, postoperatively. Blood analysis, transesophageal echocardiography, and carotid artery Doppler ultrasonography were also performed for etiological evaluation. The patient was recommended to continue taking 100 mg of acetylsalicylic acid postoperatively. The patient was followed up for 1 month in the postoperative period.

## 3. Results

The best-corrected visual acuity (BCVA) was no light perception in the right eye and 20/20 in the left eye. There was relative afferent pupillary defect in the right eye. In biomicroscopic examination, anterior segment findings were within normal limits in both eyes. Funduscopic examination showed retinal edema with arteriolar attenuation and cherry spot appearance in the right eye (Figure 1). In FFA, retinal blood flow in the right eye was found to be very low (Figure 2). Funduscopic findings of the left eye were within normal limits. Intraocular pressures (IOP) were 15 mmHg and 16 mmHg in the right and left eyes, respectively.

After ocular massage and anterior chamber paracentesis, there was no improvement in visual acuity and funduscopic findings. At the end of vitrectomy, there was no blood flow in the central retinal artery. In the eleventh active suction period, it was observed that the blood flow in the retinal artery started again, intraoperatively. On the first postoperative day, control FFA imaging revealed that edema and arterial attenuation in the retina disappeared (Figure 3) and retinal blood flow in the right eye was equally similar to the left eye (Figure 4). BCVA improved to 20/100 on the first day. During follow-up, BCVA in the right eye improved to 20/40 on the first week and to 20/20 on the first month, postoperatively.

All of the blood test results (partial thromboplastin time, activated partial thromboplastin time, international normalized ratio, and complete blood count) were within normal limits. Echocardiography showed no focus of thromboembolism in the heart. Only two atherosclerotic plaques were detected on the right side in Doppler ultrasonography of the internal carotid artery.

## 4. Discussion

Central retinal artery occlusion (CRAO) is an ophthalmic emergency that can cause significant and irreversible visual impairment. Although FFA is the gold standard in diagnosis, funduscopic examination findings (retinal edema, cherry red spot) and the presence of relative afferent pupillary defects are also helpful. Although it is more common in men, the incidence of CRAO is approximately 1 per 100,000 people [14]. The most common cause of occlusion is embolism, and the content of emboli could be cholesterol, calcium, and platelet-fibrin. The source of cholesterol and platelet-fibrin containing emboli is usually the heart or internal carotid artery [15]. In our case, there were two atherosclerotic in the right internal carotid artery.

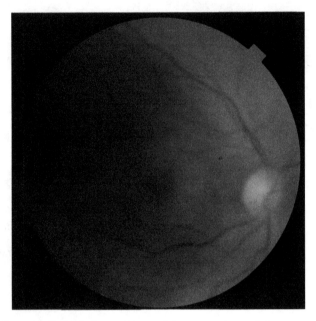

FIGURE 1: Retinal edema with arteriolar attenuation and cherry spot appearance in the right eye.

Although experimental studies show that permanent damage in the retina develops to complete occlusion in 90 minutes, in the presence of incomplete occlusion, vision regain could be achieved after delays of 8 to 24 hours, and this period may be extended in cases where macular perfusion is maintained by the cilioretinal artery [14]. In our case, although the occlusion level was high, retinal perfusion was sustained, albeit very little. Although 3 hours have passed, the apparent vision regain may be related to ongoing perfusion, albeit weak.

Cycling pressure variation of the IOP may be successful in some cases in order to move or dislodge the thromboembolism. For this purpose, different methods have been defined in the literature. Ocular massage [3], anterior chamber paracentesis [11], intravenous mannitol or acetazolamide, and topical antiglaucoma drugs [4, 5] are the main alternatives. We initially applied ocular massage to the eye, since it was a noninvasive option. When there was no success with ocular massage, we performed anterior chamber paracentesis in the operating room.

Inhalation of 10% carbogen or sublingual isosorbide dinitrate could be applied to induce vasodilatation in the retinal artery. Isosorbide dinitrate is a preferred molecule in the treatment of angina pectoris and heart failure today. Nitrate-derived drugs cause relaxation in venous vessels rather than arteries. This may be the reason for their low effectiveness in CRAO. Pentoxifylline is a methylxanthine derivative that is called "a rheologic modifier" for its effects on increasing the deformability of red blood cells and used for the treatment of intermittent claudication. Pentoxifylline has been used in a limited number of cases in the treatment of CRAO but is not preferred today due to its low efficacy [16].

Another noninvasive method is Nd:YAG laser embolectomy/embolysis. In a meta-analysis that Man et al. conducted to investigate 13 cases in the literature where the Nd:YAG

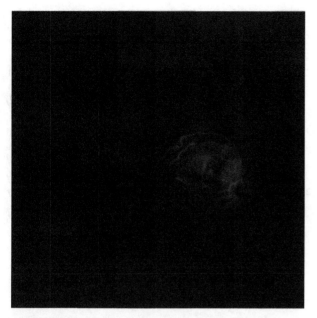

FIGURE 2: Preoperative low retinal perfusion in the right eye.

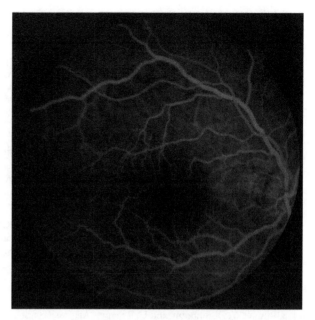

FIGURE 4: Postoperative retinal reperfusion of the right eye.

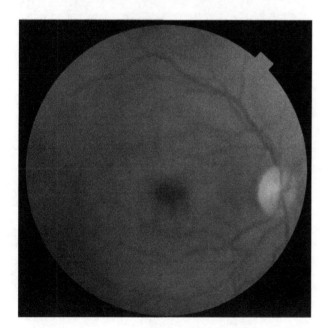

FIGURE 3: Postoperative fundus photograph of the right eye.

artery massage in a patient that was unresponsive to medical treatment and had branch retinal artery occlusion for 5 days [20]. Lu et al. reported that they achieved success by retrieving embolus with microsurgical forceps in a case with branch retinal artery occlusion [21]. In a study of 10 patients with CRAO, Almeida et al. reported that they massaged the retinal artery in the optic nerve head with a "special probe" after PPV and achieved three or more lines of improvement in BCVA in six cases [22]. The reason that Lu et al. achieved limited visual success in their study may be due to traumatic neuropathy developing in the optic nerve head during massage. Nadal et al. reported that vitrectomy with intrasurgical control of ocular hypotony may be effective in the treatment of CRAO [23].

In our case, CRAO was resolved with PPV and intraoperative cycling pressure variation. To induce cycling pressure variation, we performed active suction from a point very close to the optic nerve head. This application may be unreasonable due to the hydrostatic pressure effect mechanism. To avoid optic nerve trauma, active suction could also be performed in the vitreous cavity away from the optic nerve head.

## 5. Conclusion

In cases with central retinal artery occlusion that does not respond to digital ocular massage and medical treatment, PPV and intraoperative cycling pressure variation on the optic nerve head could be a successful and nontraumatic method in providing reperfusion of the retina.

## References

[1] A. Michalinos, S. Zogana, E. Kotsiomitis, A. Mazarakis, and T. Troupis, "Anatomy of the Ophthalmic Artery: A Review concerning Its Modern Surgical and Clinical Applications," *Anatomy Research International*, vol. 2015, Article ID 591961, 8 pages, 2015.

laser was applied for CRAO, they reported that there was visual improvement in most of the cases, the common complication was vitreous hemorrhage, and high pulse energy may be detrimental [12]. In our case, we did not prefer the Nd:YAG laser since the exact location of the embolus was not clear in funduscopic imaging or examination.

In cases when medical and noninvasive methods fail, operational interventions may be required [17, 18]. In a study of 13 cases with CRAO, Kadonosono et al. reported that they applied a tissue plasminogen activator into the retinal artery to achieve arterial cannulation after PPV and provided significant visual success [19]. Takata et al. also reported similar success in their two-case presentation [13]. Lin et al. reported that BCVA improved to 20/25 with vitrectomy and retinal

[2] B. Mac Grory, P. Lavin, H. Kirshner, and M. Schrag, "Thrombolytic therapy for acute central retinal artery occlusion," *Stroke*, vol. 51, no. 2, pp. 687–695, 2020.

[3] D. Schmidt, "Ocular massage in a case of central retinal artery occlusion the successful treatment of a hitherto undescribed type of embolism," *European Journal of Medical Research*, vol. 5, no. 4, pp. 157–164, 2000.

[4] O. Duxbury, P. Bhogal, G. Cloud, and J. Madigan, "Successful treatment of central retinal artery thromboembolism with ocular massage and intravenous acetazolamide," *Case Reports*, vol. 2014, article bcr-2014-207943, 2014.

[5] A. Chronopoulos and J. S. Schutz, "Central retinal artery occlusion-a new, provisional treatment approach," *Survey of Ophthalmology*, vol. 64, no. 4, pp. 443–451, 2019.

[6] L. Incandela, M. R. Cesarone, G. Belcaro, and R. Steigerwalt, "Treatment of vascular retinal disease with pentoxifylline: a controlled, randomized trial," *Angiology*, vol. 53, Supplement 1, pp. S31–S34, 2002.

[7] S. B. Fowler, "Carbogen in the management of a central retinal artery occlusion," *Insight*, vol. 37, no. 4, pp. 10-11, 2012.

[8] S. Rumelt, Y. Dorenboim, and U. Rehany, "Aggressive systematic treatment for central retinal artery occlusion," *American Journal of Ophthalmology*, vol. 128, no. 6, pp. 733–738, 1999.

[9] V. Biousse, F. Nahab, and N. J. Newman, "Management of acute retinal ischemia: follow the guidelines!," *Ophthalmology*, vol. 125, no. 10, pp. 1597–1607, 2018.

[10] B. S. Bagli, S. G. Çevik, and M. T. Çevik, "Effect of hyperbaric oxygen treatment in central retinal artery occlusion," *Undersea & Hyperbaric Medicine*, vol. 45, no. 4, pp. 421–425, 2018.

[11] T. S. Youn, P. Lavin, M. Patrylo et al., "Current treatment of central retinal artery occlusion: a national survey," *Journal of Neurology*, vol. 265, no. 2, pp. 330–335, 2018.

[12] V. Man, I. Hecht, M. Talitman et al., "Treatment of retinal artery occlusion using transluminal Nd:YAG laser: a systematic review and meta-analysis," *Graefe's Archive for Clinical and Experimental Ophthalmology*, vol. 255, no. 10, pp. 1869–1877, 2017.

[13] Y. Takata, Y. Nitta, A. Miyakoshi, and A. Hayashi, "Retinal endovascular surgery with tissue plasminogen activator injection for central retinal artery occlusion," *Case Rep Ophthalmol.*, vol. 9, no. 2, pp. 327–332, 2018.

[14] W. Farris and J. R. Waymack, "Central retinal artery occlusion," in *StatPearls*, StatPearls Publishing, Treasure Island (FL), 2020.

[15] S. S. Hayreh, "Central retinal artery occlusion," *Indian Journal of Ophthalmology*, vol. 66, no. 12, pp. 1684–1694, 2018.

[16] L. L. Brunton, H. D. Randa, and B. C. Knollmann, *Goodman and Gilman's The Pharmacological Basis of Therapeutics*, McGraw-Hill Education, New York, USA, 13th edition, 2018.

[17] F. Matonti, L. Hoffart, S. Nadeau, J. Hamdan, and D. Denis, "Surgical embolectomy for central retinal artery occlusion," *Canadian Journal of Ophthalmology*, vol. 48, no. 2, pp. e25–e27, 2013.

[18] J. García-Arumí, V. Martinez-Castillo, A. Boixadera, A. Fonollosa, and B. Corcostegui, "Surgical embolus removal in retinal artery occlusion," *The British Journal of Ophthalmology*, vol. 90, no. 10, pp. 1252–1255, 2006.

[19] K. Kadonosono, S. Yamane, M. Inoue, T. Yamakawa, and E. Uchio, "Intra-retinal arterial cannulation using a microneedle for central retinal artery occlusion," *Scientific Reports*, vol. 8, no. 1, p. 1360, 2018.

[20] C. J. Lin, C. W. Su, H. S. Chen, W. L. Chen, J. M. Lin, and Y. Y. Tsai, "Rescue vitrectomy with blocked artery massage and bloodletting for branch retinal artery occlusion," *Indian Journal of Ophthalmology*, vol. 65, no. 4, pp. 323–325, 2017.

[21] N. Lu, N. L. Wang, G. L. Wang, X. W. Li, and Y. Wang, "Vitreous surgery with direct central retinal artery massage for central retinal artery occlusion," *Eye (London, England)*, vol. 23, no. 4, pp. 867–872, 2009.

[22] D. R. P. Almeida, Z. Mammo, E. K. Chin, and V. B. Mahajan, "SURGICAL EMBOLECTOMY FOR FOVEA-THREATENING ACUTE RETINAL ARTERY OCCLUSION," *Retinal Cases & Brief Reports*, vol. 10, no. 4, pp. 331–333, 2016.

[23] J. Nadal, A. Ding Wu, and M. Canut, "Vitrectomy with intrasurgical control of ocular hypotony as a treatment for central retina artery occlusion," *Retina*, vol. 35, no. 8, pp. 1704-1705, 2015.

# 33

# Management of Acute Posterior Multifocal Placoid Pigment Epitheliopathy (APMPPE): Insights from Multimodal Imaging with OCTA

**Mariana A. Oliveira🆔,[1] Jorge Simão,[1] Amélia Martins,[1] and Cláudia Farinha[1,2,3]**

[1]*Department of Ophthalmology, Centro Hospitalar e Universitário de Coimbra (CHUC), Coimbra, Portugal*
[2]*Coimbra Institute for Clinical and Biomedical Research, Faculty of Medicine, University of Coimbra (iCBR-FMUC), Coimbra, Portugal*
[3]*Association for Innovation and Biomedical Research on Light and Imaging (AIBILI), Coimbra, Portugal*

Correspondence should be addressed to Mariana A. Oliveira; mariana.alg.oliveira@gmail.com

Academic Editor: J. Fernando Arevalo

A 28-year-old man presented to the emergency room with blurred vision in the right eye for two days. He reported a preceding flu-like illness one week earlier. His best-corrected visual acuity (BCVA) was 20/40 in the right eye and 20/25 in the left eye. There was no anterior chamber inflammation or vitritis in either eye. He presented multiple yellowish-white placoid lesions in the posterior pole, some involving the foveal area, bilaterally. General examination and systemic investigation were unremarkable. Multimodal evaluation with fluorescein angiography, indocyanine green angiography, and spectral domain and optical coherence tomography angiography (OCTA) were consistent with the diagnosis of acute posterior multifocal placoid pigment epitheliopathy. Due to centromacular involvement with decreased BCVA, treatment with oral methylprednisolone was started after infectious causes were ruled out. After two weeks, the patient presented functional and anatomical improvement. OCTA showed partial reperfusion of the choriocapillaris in the affected areas, in both eyes.

## 1. Introduction

Chorioretinal diseases may be a diagnostic challenge, and multimodal imaging is a strong resource in the management of these entities. This report describes the clinical course of a man with acute posterior multifocal placoid pigment epitheliopathy (APMPPE), documented by a multimodal approach, and especially with the recent introduction of OCTA in the clinical practice.

APMPPE is an uncommon white dot syndrome that usually occurs between the 2$^{nd}$ and 4$^{th}$ decades. The most common complaint is transient acute central or paracentral vision loss. First described by Gass in 1968 [1], it affects man and woman equally and is characterized by multiple whitish-yellow inflammatory lesions at the outer retina, retinal pigment epithelium, and choroid [2]. The etiopathogenetic mechanism of this entity is still not entirely clarified;

however, it seems that the primary insult occurs at the level of inner choroid/choriocapillaris with retinal changes occurring secondarily [3, 4]. Some authors even discuss the current name of this entity, advocating for a change to choroidopathy rather than epitheliopathy [5].

We report a case of APMPPE with centromacular involvement, treated with systemic corticotherapy, with ocular fundus lesions and choriocapillaris reperfusion in optical coherence tomography angiography (OCTA), thus corroborating the predominant role of hypoperfusion of choriocapillaris in the etiopathogenesis of this disease.

## 2. Case Presentation

A fit-and-well 28-year-old man presented to our emergency room with a 2-day history of blurred vision in his right eye. He mentioned he always had lower VA in his left eye, and

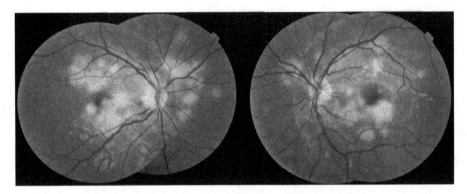

FIGURE 1: Bilateral presentation of fundus examination. Color fundus photography images show multiple bilateral yellow-white placoid lesions, at the level of external retina, posterior to the equator, and a slight fade of the edges of the optic nerve.

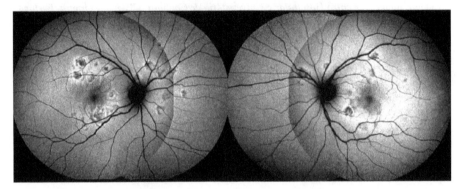

FIGURE 2: Bilateral fundus autofluorescence. Images show hypoautoflourescence corresponding to the placoid lesions, with a hyperautofluorescent edge.

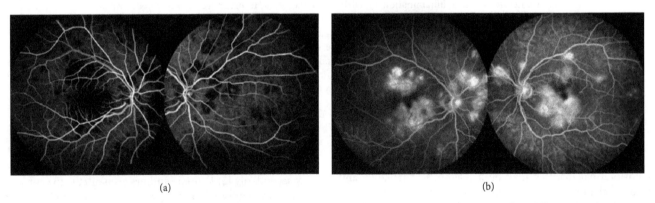

(a)                                        (b)

FIGURE 3: Representative fluorescein angiography (FA) images. FA typically showing early hypofluorescent placoid lesions (a) that become hyperfluorescent in the mid and late phases of the angiogram (b).

no prior history of ocular disease was reported. He had presented with myalgia and headache one week earlier, which resolved spontaneously. His BCVA was 20/40 in the right eye and 20/25 in the left eye. Slit-lamp biomicroscopy was unremarkable. Dilated fundus examination exhibited a hyperemic optic disc, peripapillary edema, and multiple yellowish-white placoid lesions in the posterior pole, some involving the foveal area, bilaterally (Figure 1). General examination was unremarkable.

Fundus autofluorescence (FAF) showed hypoautofluorescent lesions with an area of relative hyperautofluorescence along their edge (Figure 2). Hypofluorescence at the placoid lesions in the early phase that changed to hyperfluorescence at the late phases was evident on fluorescein angiography (FA) (Figures 3(a) and 3(b)). Indocyanine green angiography (ICGA) evidenced hypofluorescence of placoid lesions from early to late phases (Figures 4 and 5(a)). OCT (Avanti RTVue-XR 100, Optovue Inc., Fremont, CA) demonstrated bilateral focal areas of disruption of the ellipsoid layer and hyperreflectivity in the outer retina, primarily localizing to the outer nuclear layer (ONL) but also being seen at the level of the outer plexiform layer (Figure 5(c)). These features were

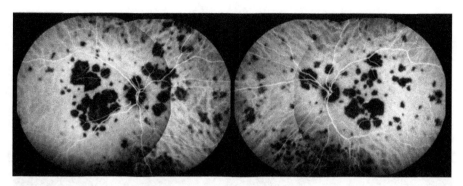

FIGURE 4: Representative indocyanine green angiography (ICGA) images. ICGA evidences hypofluorescence through the entire angiogram, corresponding to the placoid lesions.

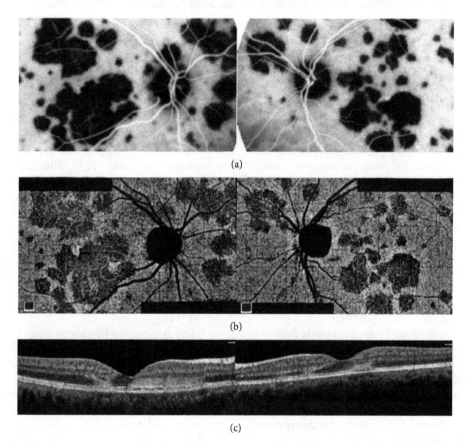

(a)

(b)

(c)

FIGURE 5: Multimodal evaluation of placoid lesions. (a) Indocyanine green angiography (ICGA) shows hypofluorescence corresponding to the placoid lesions; (b) optical coherence tomography (OCT) angiography demonstrates choriocapillaris ischemia in the corresponding lesions seen on ICGA; (c) OCT exhibiting hyperreflectivity from the outer plexiform layer to the RPE with normal retinal thickness.

more evident in the right eye. OCTA revealed significant hypoperfusion at the level of the choriocapillaris in the active lesions bilaterally (Figure 5(b)).

Due to the potential association with central nervous system (CNS) abnormalities, the patient was observed by the Department of Neurology. Neurologic examination, cranioencephalic-computerized tomography, and cervical and transcranial Doppler ultrasonography were unremarkable.

Extensive work-up to rule out other pathologies that could mimic APMPPE, including infectious diseases, was performed. This included serology for syphilis, herpes simplex

1 and 2, cytomegalovirus, Epstein-Barr, varicella zoster, Borrelia, HIV 1 and 2, and QuantiFERON-TB Gold test, which were all negative for active infection. Complete blood count, angiotensin conversion enzyme, hepatic enzymes, renal function, and thorax X-ray were unremarkable. C-reactive protein and sedimentation velocity were increased (3.86 mg/dL and 31 mm/h, respectively).

Regarding the differential diagnosis, we excluded syphilis, tuberculosis, other infectious causes, Vogt–Koyanagi–Harada disease, and sarcoidosis, based on the history, the results of laboratory tests, and the lack of systemic findings.

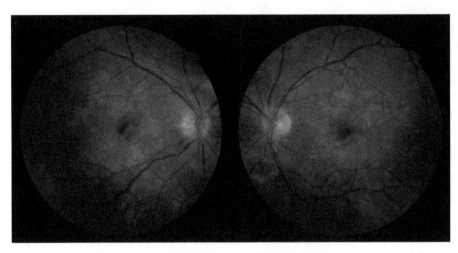

FIGURE 6: Bilateral presentation of fundus examination, after two weeks of follow-up. Color fundus photography images show the placoid lesions in resolution.

The presence of a previous viral prodrome, the young age, and the multiple yellowish-white placoid lesions in the posterior pole pointed to an inflammatory choriocapillaropathy. The morphology of the lesions helped in the discrimination of the white dot syndrome, as the placoid conformation with lesions bigger than 125 $\mu$m with a low degree of inflammation was in favor of APMPPE or serpiginous choroiditis. However, the choroiditis' geographical pattern with centrifugal extension from the peripapillary region typical of serpiginous choroiditis was not observed [6]. Instead, the deep multiple yellowish-white placoid lesions in the posterior pole associated with a minimal vitreous inflammation in a young healthy male with a negative QuantiFERON-TB Gold test are favorable of the diagnosis of APMPPE. The fact that the lesions resolved over time without recurrences was also in favor of this diagnosis. There are relentless serpiginous and ampiginous forms that can mimic APMPPE.

The placoid lesions in APMPPE spontaneously resolve in most cases, and VA usually recovers within a few months [7]. However, there are reports of permanent changes and therapy with corticosteroids may have a role when there is foveal involvement, advanced age, unilateral disease, and recurrences or risk of central nervous system vasculitis [8]. Due to centromacular involvement, the patient started treatment with 1 mg/kg/day of methylprednisolone.

After two weeks, the patient presented functional and anatomical improvement. BCVA was 20/30 in his right eye and 20/22 in the left eye. Slit-lamp examination remained unremarkable, and at dilated fundus examination, it was possible to note placoid macular lesions in resolution (Figure 6). No de novo lesions were observed. SD-OCT demonstrated resolution of macular edema and focal atrophy of outer retinal layers corresponding to the previous hyperreflective areas (Figure 7). OCTA showed reperfusion of the choriocapillaris in the affected placoid areas, in both eyes (Figure 8).

At this time, methylprednisolone was tapered off to 48 mg/day and a reevaluation was scheduled to two weeks later. Unfortunately, the patient missed these and the subsequent appointments. A head magnetic resonance imaging requested by the neurology department was also missed.

## 3. Discussion

Acute posterior multifocal placoid pigment epitheliopathy is a nongranulomatous chorioretinitis of uncertain origin that occurs in healthy young adults. Frequently, as we observed in our patient, a viral prodrome precedes the onset of ophthalmologic symptoms [1, 7]. This fact raises the question of an infectious agent as the trigger for the illness [9–11].

Although the ophthalmic findings may reflect RPE involvement, accumulating evidence indicates that the primary lesion is posterior to this and choroidal perfusion is abnormal. Secondary ischemic changes would produce disruption of the pigment epithelium, resulting in typical placoid lesions [12, 13]. Nowadays, OCTA allows visualization of the rarefaction of the choriocapillary at corresponding placoid lesions seen in the fundus at the acute stage of the disease [14].

There is a picture developed that APMPPE is an acute, autolimited monophasic inflammatory illness with a typical clinical pattern, sometimes with profound loss of vision, but usually with remarkable visual recovery despite substantial residual scarring of the RPE [1, 15]. Though subtotal recovery of VA is usual, many patients have long-term visual symptoms and some have significant residual field defects [7]. Eyes without initial foveal involvement evidence final better functional prognosis (87.5% have a BCVA higher than 20/25 versus 39.2% when there is foveal involvement) [16, 17]. In fact, a report of 33 eyes with APMPPE observed that in the 7 eyes in which VA failed to recover to better than 20/80, all had foveal involvement. They also presented one of the following atypical features: age older than 60 years, unilaterality, an interval before involvement of the second eye of at least 6 months, and recurrence of the disease [18]. In rare cases, typical signs are also associated with progressive deterioration, with widespread severe choroidal atrophy after apparent clinical healing of the placoid lesions [19].

In this case, we did not observe uncharacteristic features, although foveal involvement was initially present. For this reason, we initiated therapy with oral corticosteroid. Data

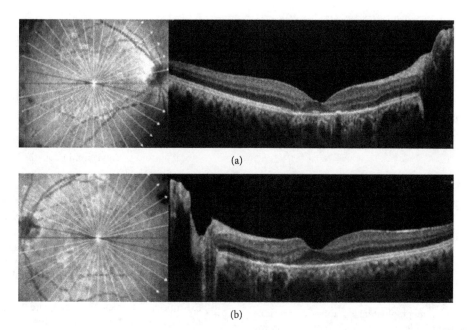

(a)

(b)

FIGURE 7: Optical coherence tomography of the right (a) and left (b) eyes after two weeks of follow-up. OCT demonstrated resolution of macular edema and focal atrophy of outer retinal layers, from the outer plexiform layer to the retinal pigmented epithelium, corresponding to the previous hyperreflective areas.

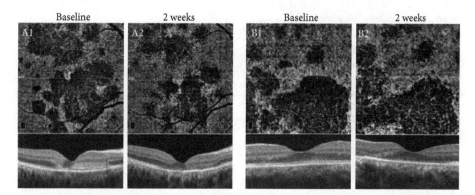

FIGURE 8: Optical coherence tomography angiography (OCTA) images at the level of choriocapillaris revealing focal areas of hypoperfusion in the right (A1 and A2) and left (B1 and B2) eyes. After two weeks, the area of hypoperfusion at the level of the choriocapillaris improved and the thinning of the outer retina in spectral domain optical coherence tomography persisted.

from literature does not provide clear information regarding the use of oral corticosteroids. Cases describing the use of steroids advocate it is possible that it modifies the natural course of lesions, although the role of this treatment in the eventual resolution of this clinical condition remains speculative, that is, the choroidal reperfusion may also occur spontaneously in the course of the disease, without steroids [12, 16, 20]. When there is central nervous system involvement, it is stated that intravenous corticosteroids associated with immunosuppressive therapy should be considered. In a case series of patients with APMPPE and SNC lesions, all patients were submitted to treatment with corticosteroids and in some of them, VA decreased when they were tapered off [8].

A recent publication distinguished 4 phases of APMPPE based on multimodal imaging: choroidal, chorioretinal, transitional, and resolution [4]. Lesions in phase 1 (choroidal) can resolve without any morphological sequelae. Our patient

presented in phase 2, as there was evidence of classic active lesion on FA with early hypofluorescence and late hyperfluorescence, persistent hypocyanescence of lesions across ICGA frames, and choroidal hypoperfusion on OCTA. There was also loss of structural integrity and hyperreflectivity of the outer retinal layers including RPE, ellipsoid layer, and ELM on SD-OCT and predominant hypoautofluorescent of APMPPE lesions noted on FAF.

As we observed with OCTA, the reperfusion of choriocapillaris was only partial and can occur in a centripetally pattern from the outer edge of the APMPPE lesion. This was also previously described [4]. In the follow-up visit, persistent thinning of the outer retina was visible on SD-OCT with hyporeflectivity at the level of RPE, which was consistent with phase 4 in these areas.

Multimodal imaging provides valuable information about the clinical course of APMPPE. Despite the utility of

FA and ICGA images for monitoring disease activity and the very typical pattern, these are invasive techniques, and due to the blocking effects, they do not allow to locate the depth of the primary lesion or to characterize it. On the other hand, OCTA enhances understanding of the hypoperfusion choriocapillaris involvement of lesions, noninvasively. In our case, we could identify previously described progression patterns of this entity and document good response to treatment by a noninvasive method.

# References

[1] J. D. M. Gass, "Acute posterior multifocal placoid pigment epitheliopathy," *Archives of Ophthalmology*, vol. 80, no. 2, pp. 177–185, 1968.

[2] D. A. Quillen, J. B. Davis, J. L. Gottlieb et al., "The white dot syndromes," *American Journal of Ophthalmology*, vol. 137, no. 3, pp. 538–550, 2004.

[3] R. Dolz-Marco, D. Sarraf, V. Giovinazzo, and K. B. Freund, "Optical coherence tomography angiography shows inner choroidal ischemia in acute posterior multifocal placoid pigment epitheliopathy," *Retinal Cases & Brief Reports*, vol. 11, pp. S136–S143, 2017.

[4] T. R. Burke, C. J. Chu, S. Salvatore et al., "Application of OCT-angiography to characterise the evolution of chorioretinal lesions in acute posterior multifocal placoid pigment epitheliopathy," *Eye*, vol. 31, no. 10, pp. 1399–1408, 2017.

[5] A. Y. Zhang, I. C. Han, and M. F. Goldberg, "Renaming of acute posterior multifocal placoid pigment epitheliopathy (APMPPE) to acute multifocal placoid choroidopathy (AMP-C)," *JAMA Ophthalmology*, vol. 135, no. 3, p. 185, 2017.

[6] H. Nazari Khanamiri and N. A. Rao, "Serpiginous choroiditis and infectious multifocal serpiginoid choroiditis," *Survey of Ophthalmology*, vol. 58, no. 3, pp. 203–232, 2013.

[7] M. D. Wolf, W. L. Alward, and J. C. Folk, "Long-term visual function in acute posterior multifocal placoid pigment epitheliopathy," *Archives of Ophthalmology*, vol. 109, no. 6, pp. 800–803, 1991.

[8] H. S. O'Halloran, J. R. Berger, W. B. Lee et al., "Acute multifocal placoid pigment epitheliopathy and central nervous system involvement: nine new cases and a review of the literature," *Ophthalmology*, vol. 108, no. 5, pp. 861–868, 2001.

[9] S. J. Ryan and A. E. Maumenee, "Acute posterior multifocal placoid pigment epitheliopathy," *American Journal of Ophthalmology*, vol. 74, no. 6, pp. 1066–1074, 1972.

[10] P. J. Fitzpatrick and D. M. Robertson, "Acute posterior multifocal placoid pigment epitheliopathy," *Archives of Ophthalmology*, vol. 89, no. 5, pp. 373–376, 1973.

[11] P. Azar Jr., R. S. Gohd, D. Waltman, and K. A. Gitter, "Acute posterior multifocal placoid pigment epitheliopathy associated with an adenovirus type 5 infection," *American Journal of Ophthalmology*, vol. 80, no. 6, pp. 1003–1005, 1975.

[12] A. F. Deutman, J. A. Oosterhuis, T. N. Boen-Tan, and A. L. Aan de Kerk, "Acute posterior multifocal placoid pigment epitheliopathy. Pigment epitheliopathy of choriocapillaritis?," *The British Journal of Ophthalmology*, vol. 56, no. 12, pp. 863–874, 1972.

[13] W. S. Holt, C. D. J. Regan, and C. Trempe, "Acute posterior multifocal placoid pigment epitheliopathy," *American Journal of Ophthalmology*, vol. 81, no. 4, pp. 403–412, 1976.

[14] R. Kinouchi, N. Nishikawa, A. Ishibazawa, and A. Yoshida, "Vascular rarefaction at the choriocapillaris in acute posterior multifocal placoid pigment epitheliopathy viewed on OCT angiography," *International Ophthalmology*, vol. 37, no. 3, pp. 733–736, 2017.

[15] N. P. Jones, "Acute posterior multifocal placoid pigment epitheliopathy," *The British Journal of Ophthalmology*, vol. 79, no. 4, pp. 384–389, 1995.

[16] T. Fiore, B. Iaccheri, S. Androudi et al., "Acute posterior multifocal placoid pigment Epitheliopathy," *Retina*, vol. 29, no. 7, pp. 994–1001, 2009.

[17] T. V. Roberts and P. Mitchell, "Acute posterior multifocal placoid pigment epitheliopathy: a long-term study," *Australian and New Zealand Journal of Ophthalmology*, vol. 25, no. 3, pp. 277–281, 1997.

[18] S. Pagliarini, B. Piguet, T. J. Ffytche, and A. C. Bird, "Foveal involvement and lack of visual recovery in APMPPE associated with uncommon features," *Eye*, vol. 9, no. 1, pp. 42–47, 1995.

[19] S. Daniele, C. Daniele, F. Orcidi, and A. Tavano, "Progression of choroidal atrophy in acute posterior multifocal placoid pigment epitheliopathy," *Ophthalmologica*, vol. 212, no. 1, pp. 66–72, 1998.

[20] T. H. Kirkham, T. J. Ffytche, and M. D. Sanders, "Placoid pigment epitheliopathy with retinal vasculitis and papillitis," *The British Journal of Ophthalmology*, vol. 56, no. 12, pp. 875–880, 1972.

# 34

# Case Series of Perforated Keratomycosis after Laser-Assisted In Situ Keratomileusis

Taher Eleiwa ⓘ,[1,2] Eyup Ozcan ⓘ,[1,3] Samar Abdelrahman,[4] Omar Solyman,[5] Abdelrahman M. Elhusseiny ⓘ,[6] Gehad Youssef,[2] and Ahmed Bayoumy[2]

[1]Bascom Palmer Eye Institute, Miller School of Medicine, University of Miami, Miami, FL, USA
[2]Department of Ophthalmology, Faculty of Medicine, Benha University, Egypt
[3]Net Eye Medical Center, Gaziantep, Turkey
[4]Department of Clinical Pathology, Faculty of Medicine, Benha University, Egypt
[5]Department of Ophthalmology, Texas Childrens Hospital, Baylor College of Medicine, Houston, TX, USA
[6]Department of Ophthalmology, Kasr Al-Ainy Hospitals, Cairo University, Cairo, Egypt

Correspondence should be addressed to Taher Eleiwa; tahereleiwa87@gmail.com

Academic Editor: Claudio Campa

*Background.* Fungal keratitis is an extremely rare complication of laser vision correction resulting in poor visual outcomes. Amniotic membrane transplantation should be kept in mind in eyes with corneal perforation prior to penetrating keratoplasty. *Aim.* To assess the outcomes of multilayered fresh amniotic membrane transplantation (MLF-AMT) in patients with severe keratomycosis after laser-assisted in situ keratomileusis (LASIK). *Study design.* Hospital-based prospective interventional case series. *Methods.* Five eyes of 5 patients were included in the study. All cases underwent microbiological scrapings from residual bed and intrastromal injections of amphotericin (50 mcg/mL), with flap amputation if needed, followed by topical 5% natamycin and 0.15% amphotericin. MLF-AMT was performed after corneal perforation. Later, penetrating keratoplasty (PK) was performed when corneal opacity compromised visual acuity. The outcome measures were complete resolution of infection, corneal graft survival, and best-corrected visual acuity (BCVA). *Results.* The mean age of patients was $22 \pm 1.2$ years with 4/5 (80%) were females. The mean interval between LASIK and symptom onset was $8.8 \pm 1$ day, and the mean interval between symptom onset and referral was $14 \pm 1.4$ days. Potassium hydroxide (KOH) smears showed filamentous fungi, and Sabouraud's medium grew Aspergillus in all cases. Melted flaps were amputated in 4 (80%) cases. MLF-AMT was performed in all cases due to corneal perforation after a mean time of $12.4 \pm 1.2$ days of antifungals. In all cases, complete resolution of infection was seen $26 \pm 1.8$ days after MLF-AMT, and optical PK was done at a mean of 2.4 months later. No postoperative complications after MLF-AMT or PK were observed, with a 0% incidence of corneal graft rejection, and a final BCVA ranged from 20/20 to 20/80 after a mean follow-up of $14 \pm 1.1$ months. *Conclusion.* MLF-AMT is a safe and valid option to manage corneal perforation during keratmycosis treatment to avoid emergency therapeutic keratoplasty.

## 1. Introduction

Laser-assisted in situ keratomileusis (LASIK) has become the leading laser vision correction method in the last two decades. Besides its high accuracy and predictability, infectious keratitis after LASIK has been reported as a rare and devastating complication [1–3]. In the survey of American Cataract and Refractive Surgery (ASCRS), the prevalence of microbial keratitis was reported as a rate of 0.034% in more than 300,000 procedures, and 10% of those cultured microorganisms were fungal agents [4]. Fungal keratitis is a vision-threatening condition that may cause corneal melting and perforation [5, 6]. Although variable applications of antifungals, such as fluconazole, natamycin, amphotericin B, and voriconazole have been implemented, their efficacy is limited because of the fungistatic nature of most of topical antifungals with poor penetration to the deeper corneal layers, and the development of drug resistance [6]. Therefore, therapeutic keratoplasty (TPK) is usually required to protect the integrity of the globe and improve visual acuity [7]. However, recurrence of fungal infections and low graft survival rates after TPK are still challenging [8–10].

In this prospective interventional case series, we evaluated the procedure of multilayered fresh amniotic membrane transplantation (MLF-AMT) prior to penetrating keratoplasty (PK) in patients with severe fungal keratitis after LASIK. The outcome measures were complete resolution of infection, corneal graft survival, and best-corrected visual acuity.

## 2. Case Report

*2.1. Methods.* Our study included all patients with refractory microbiologically diagnosed keratomycosis after LASIK who presented to our outpatient clinic at Benha University hospital, from January 2017 to July 2018. Cases were referred to our hospital after doing LASIK surgery elsewhere. This study was approved by the Institutional Review Board of Benha University hospital, and informed consents were taken from all patients in accordance with the Declaration of Helsinki. Patients having coincident viral or bacterial keratitis, recent eye trauma, recent contact lens use, and previous ocular pathology with any systemic illness were excluded from the study.

At admission, a full history was taken, including age, gender, and time intervals after LASIK surgery till the start of complaint, referral to our department. Clinical data recorded included best-corrected visual acuity (BCVA), clinical features of corneal infiltrate, ocular tension, anterior chamber (AC) inflammatory activity, and corneal perforation characteristics.

At the first visit, under topical anesthesia, a flap lift was done; then, collection of specimens from underneath the flap, the residual stromal bed, AC hypopyon, and amputated parts of macerated flaps was done and sent for microbiological analysis. Processing of all samples was performed according to a standardized protocol in an operating room under complete aseptic measures [11]. 10% potassium hydroxide (KOH) wet mount was reported immediately, and once fungal etiology was verified, amphotericin (50 mcg/mL) interface wash, with intrastromal injection, was performed in the same sitting. Then, according to the antifungal sensitivity tests, topical 5% natamycin and amphotericin 0.15% with oral itraconazole were given in all patients. MLF-AMT was indicated for corneal perforation and AC collapse.

Fresh human amniotic membrane (AM) was acquired from women who were seronegative for viral hepatitis, human immunodeficiency virus, and syphilis before undergoing elective caesarean section. Membranes were manually peeled from the underlying placental tissue and washed in 0.9% normal saline 4 times, then rinsed once in 0.025% sodium hypochlorite. After trimming the amnion along with the underlying chorion into pieces (5 × 5 cm$^2$ in size), it was stored in normal saline containing penicillin (50,000 U) and streptomycin (1 gm/400 cc of saline) at 4°C not surpassing a period of 48 h. During the surgery, the amnion was bluntly separated from the chorion and rinsed in gentamicin containing normal saline before usage.

Under peribulbar anesthesia, debridement of the necrotic tissue at the ulcer base was done, and samples were sent for microbial analysis. The AM was adjusted to fit the ulcer dimensions and put one layer superimposed on another layer afterwards, all with stromal face down. Using interrupted 10/0 nylon sutures, all layers were secured in place. The AC was reformed, and the hypopyon was aspirated and sent for cultures. At the end of the surgery, amphotericin 50 mcg/mL was injected subconjunctivally, and gentamycin eye ointment was applied. After that, the antifungal frequency was either maintained or tapered according to the clinical scenario. In follow-up visits, the dimensions of stromal infiltrates and the height of AC hypopyon were documented. Patients were assessed daily until reepithelialization and absence of AC leak were observed. Sutures were removed after 2 weeks.

Elective PK was performed subsequently after complete resolution of infection if the AM filled stroma is obscuring the visual axis. All PKs were done by one surgeon under peribulbar anesthesia with supplementary intravenous (IV) sedation. The donor grafts were 0.5 mm larger than the recipient's corneal flap. Corneal flaps were not removed prior to trephination. Hessburg-Barron trephines were used, and corneal grafts were secured in place with 16 interrupted 10–0 nylon sutures. Postoperatively, patients were prescribed topical ofloxacin 0.3%, prednisolone acetate 1% eye drops, preservative-free lubricant eye drops, and antiglaucoma medications if needed. Topical steroids were tapered gradually over one year. Topography-guided selective suture removal was commenced 3-6 months postoperatively.

Complete resolution of infection and restoration of functioning vision were the study outcome measures.

## 3. Results

Our study included 5 eyes of 5 patients presented with post-LASIK keratomycosis. Table 1 summarized the demographics and the clinical characteristics of study participants. The mean age of the patients was $22 \pm 1.2$ (median, 22; range, 19-26) years. The mean duration between LASIK and symptoms onset was $8.8 \pm 1$ (median, 8; range, 7-12) days, the mean duration from start of symptoms and presentation to us was $14 \pm 1.4$ (median, 15; range, 10-18) days, and the mean duration between $1^{st}$ visit and AMT was $12.4 \pm 1.2$ (median, 12; range, 10-16) days. Steroids were halted by the primary surgeons when infectious keratitis was questioned, and they were prescribed topical antibiotics and antifungal drops. However, case #5 was initially misdiagnosed as diffuse lamellar keratitis (DLK) and treated with steroid wash and increasing the frequency of topical prednisolone acetate 1%.

The presenting BCVA, clinical features, and antifungal treatment approaches are demonstrated in Table 2. KOH wet mount showed septate fungal hyphae in specimens collected from all patients. Aspergillus fumigatus was detected in all eyes after 72 hours of culture. The LASIK flap was melted and had to be amputated in all eyes except case #3 (Figure 1). Fungal hyphae were seen via microscopic examination of the amputated flap in those cases. Intracameral injection of amphotericin was not done in cases (1, 3, 4) due to high ocular tension. Oral acetazolamide was given to

TABLE 1: Clinical characteristics of patients.

| Cases | Age (Y) | Gender | Period between LASIK and C/O (D) | Period between onset of C/O and referral (D) | Time to fresh multilayered AMT: indication (D) | Period between AMT and complete resolution of infection (D) | Period between AMT and PK (M), indication of PK | Total follow-up time (M) |
|---|---|---|---|---|---|---|---|---|
| 1 | 19 | Female | 7 | 10 | 2.5 mm perforation (14) | 22 | 2, amniotic membrane filled stroma interfering with vision | 12 |
| 2 | 22 | Male | 12 | 16 | 3.5 mm perforation (10) | 27 | 2, amniotic membrane filled stroma interfering with vision | 14 |
| 3 | 20 | Female | 10 | 15 | 3.5 mm perforation (16) | 24 | 3, amniotic membrane filled stroma interfering with vision | 15 |
| 4 | 26 | Female | 7 | 12 | 4 mm perforation (12) | 29 | 2, amniotic membrane filled stroma interfering with vision | 12 |
| 5 | 24 | Female | 8 | 18 | 4.5 mm perforation (10) | 32 | 3, amniotic membrane filled stroma interfering with vision | 18 |

cases (1, 3, 4, and) due to high ocular tension. Case #5 was injected twice intrastromally (5 days apart) due to diffuse dense infiltrates with peripheral satellites (Figure 2). MLF-AMT was performed in all cases after corneal perforation. After AMT, topical amphotericin B 0.15% (every 2 hours) and atropine sulfate 1% (twice daily) were resumed. Specimens collected at time of AMT came back positive for Aspergillus fumigatus. Complete resolution of infection, reepithelialization of corneal surface, and restoration of corneal thickness were seen within $26 \pm 1.8$ (median, 27; range, 22-32) days after AMT in all cases. Topical treatment was continued for 1 week and tapered over 2 weeks after full resolution of infection. Elective PK was performed uneventfully in all eyes, 2.4 (median, 2; range, 2-3) months after AMT. The final BCVA ranged from 20/20 to 20/80 at an average follow-up of $14 \pm 1.1$ (median, 14; range, 12-18) months.

## 4. Discussion

LASIK is the most commonly performed refractive surgery for the correction of ametropia. It merges the precision of excimer laser photoablation and the benefits of maintaining the integrity of Bowman's layer and the covering corneal epithelium, decreasing the risk of postprocedure corneal inflammation [12].

Although infection after LASIK, especially fungal infection, is a rare complication, it has serious consequences as visual impairments are not uncommon after infection [13]. Published reports on infections following LASIK found that severe visual acuity reductions were significantly more associated with keratomycosis rather than bacterial and mycobacterial infections [14]. Biomechanically weakening, lack of commercially available antifungal eye drops, usage of steroids [15], and delayed diagnosis might be held responsible for the aggressive course of fungal keratitis after LASIK. It is noteworthy to mention that the high rate of treatment failure in eyes with Aspergillus species may be attributed to the perpendicular growth pattern of fungal filaments that made the infection penetrate quickly deep into the corneal layers [12]. Also, the discrepancy between infection and postoperative sterile keratitis must be made cautiously for vital therapeutic decisions. Misdiagnosis of the infection as inflammation can aggravate the current clinical illness and deteriorate the prognosis (case #5, Figure 2) [3]. Several treatment options have been disclosed in literature such as flap amputation, AMT, and PK along with antifungals. Here, we reported five cases of keratomycosis after LASIK and a stepwise therapeutic plan to reach the optimal outcomes.

Antimicrobial penetration, particularly antifungal drops, may be insufficient to reach infections that lie at the interface or deeper in the stroma owing to the sequestered nature of infections following LASIK [13, 16, 17]. Therefore, it is commended to lift and reposition flap earlier during the course of infection for culture, scraping, and irrigating the stromal bed especially when the infiltrate involves the interface to help better antimicrobial penetration and removes the sequestered nidus for the infection [13, 17]. For case #5, we did intrastromal injections of amphotericin-B ($50 \mu g/ml$) twice to increase the ocular concentration of the antifungal therapy enough to be effective in the abolition of the deep corneal infection, and according to Garcia et al., this concentration does not appear to be detrimental to corneal keratocytes or endothelial cells [17]. In addition, we used intracameral injections of amphotericin B at a concentration of $5 \mu g$ in 0.1. Yoon et al. postulated that there is no difference in treatment success rates between intracameral amphotericin-B and conventional treatment; however, intracameral injections can decrease time to resolution of hypopyon and time to improvement in the treatment of keratomycosis [18].

Flap amputation was performed in our series except in one case at the initial presentation. Flap amputation may limit the extent of corneal injury caused by the infection and increases drug penetration. Mittal et al. reported a complete resolution of keratomycosis with interface wash

TABLE 2: Clinical and microbiological features of patients.

| Cases | Medical and surgical interventions | Indication for fresh multilayered AMT | Culture | Initial clinical signs | Presenting BCVA | Prior medical history and surgical interventions | Final BCVA |
|---|---|---|---|---|---|---|---|
| 1 | Flap amputation, amphotericin B 50 mcg/ml (interface wash, intrastromal injection), topical (amphotericin B 0.15%, natamycin 5%), oral (itraconazole, doxycycline, acetazolamide) | 2.5 mm perforation | Aspergillus fumigatus | Lid edema, chemosis, ciliary injection, cornea (hypothesia, central interface infiltrates 3x3 mm, endothelial plaque, heaped up 3 mm hypopyon, dehiscent LASIK flap), T++ | 20/200 | Topical (moxifloxacin, natamycin, vancomycin, ceftazidime), oral (doxycycline, acetazolamide), LASIK, subconjunctival injection of vancomycin, ceftazidime | 20/20 |
| 2 | Flap amputation, amphotericin B 50 mcg/ml (interface wash, intrastromal and intracameral injection), topical (amphotericin B 0.15%, natamycin 5%), oral (itraconazole, doxycycline) | 3.5 mm perforation | Aspergillus fumigatus | Lid edema, chemosis, ciliary injection, cornea (hypothesia, central interface infiltrates 4 × 4 mm, endothelial plaque, heaped up hypopyon, macerated LASIK flap), Tn | CF close to the face | Topical (moxifloxacin, natamycin, vancomycin, ceftazidime), LASIK, subconjunctival injection of vancomycin, ceftazidime | 20/40 |
| 3 | Amphotericin B 50 mcg/ml (interface wash, intrastromal injection), topical (amphotericin B 0.15%, natamycin 5%), oral (itraconazole, doxycycline, acetazolamide) | 3.5 mm perforation | Aspergillus fumigatus | Lid edema, chemosis, ciliary injection, cornea (hypothesia, inferior interface infiltrates 4 × 2 mm, endothelial plaque, heaped up 1 mm hypopyon, healthy LASIK flap), T++ | HM | Topical (moxifloxacin, natamycin, vancomycin, amikacin), oral (doxycycline), LASIK, subconjunctival injection of vancomycin, amikacin | 20/40 |
| 4 | Flap amputation, amphotericin B 50 mcg/ml (interface wash, intrastromal injection), topical (amphotericin B 0.15%, natamycin 5%), oral (itraconazole, doxycycline) | 4 mm perforation | Aspergillus fumigatus | Lid edema, chemosis, ciliary injection, cornea (hypothesia, central interface infiltrates 5 × 4 mm, endothelial plaque, heaped up 1.5 mm hypopyon, macerated LASIK flap), T+ | CF close to the face | Topical (moxifloxacin, vancomycin, ceftazidime, natamycin), oral (acetazolamide), LASIK, subconjunctival injection of vancomycin, ceftazidime | 20/20 |
| 5 | Flap amputation, amphotericin B 50 mcg/ml (interface wash, intrastromal and intracameral injection twice), topical (amphotericin B 0.15%, natamycin 5%), oral (itraconazole, doxycycline) | 4.5 mm perforation | Aspergillus fumigatus | Lid edema, ciliary injection, cornea (hypothesia, central interface infiltrates 6 × 5.5 mm, endothelial plaque, peripheral satellites, heaped up 3 mm hypopyon, melted LASIK flap), Tn | HM | Topical (moxifloxacin, natamycin, vancomycin, ceftazidime), oral (fluconazole, vitamin C, doxycycline), LASIK, Interface wash with (steroid, moxifloxacin, BSS), subconjunctival injection of vancomycin, ceftazidime | 20/80 |

using voriconazole with selective flap amputation followed by topical and systemic antifungal treatment [19]. It is noteworthy to mention that failure of the abovementioned treatment has been reported which was attributed to delayed diagnosis [19]. This could be in agreement with our series who failed medical therapy and flap amputation due to relatively late presentation.

AM promotes epithelialization and exhibits antifibrotic, anti-inflammatory, antiangiogenic, and antimicrobial features [20]. There are few reports in the literature that used AM to reestablish globe integrity in cases of perforated keratitis following refractive surgery. AMT stops aqueous humor seepage, seals the corneal defect, and restores AC depth in cases of perforations acting as efficient tectonic support [21,

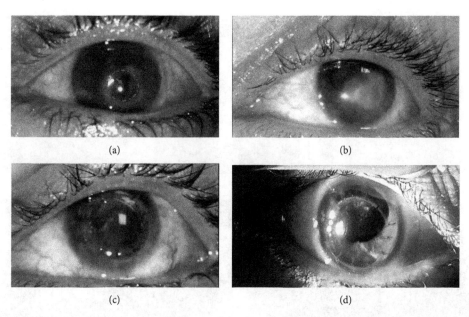

(a)
(b)
(c)
(d)

FIGURE 1: Slit-lamp photos of case #3 showing. (a) Descemetocele and perforation with iris prolapse and inferior AC loss 11 days after intrastromal amphotericin injection. (b) Corneal opacity and epithelialized corneal surface 5 weeks after multilayered fresh amniotic membrane transplantation. (c) Clear full-thickness corneal graft secured with interrupted 10/0 nylon sutures (1$^{st}$ postoperative day). (d) Healthy corneal graft 9 months after PK.

22]. Also, a ML-AMT using an AM placed in the stromal ulcer provides an alternative to collagen and supplies stromal layers while the overhanging AM graft provides a basement membrane for proper epithelialization [23]. We preferred ML-AM grafts than single layer grafts in managing perforations as a single layer of AM degrades in few weeks which is not a sufficient time for stromal layers to regenerate and fill the defect [24]. In many studies cryopreserved AM was used but in our series we preferred using fresh AMs. Although fresh and preserved AMs have been found to be equally effective when transplanted onto the ocular surface according to Adds et al. [24], Hori et al. demonstrated that viable human amniotic epithelial cells in fresh grafts elicit beneficial effects on the secretion of anti-inflammatory factors, which are otherwise decreased in eyes with infectious keratitis [25, 26]. AMT timing in fungal keratitis is critical, and its application in acute phases of fungal keratitis is controversial. Besides its promoting effect on epithelial healing and mechanical barrier effects, AM may alter the host response against fungi by scavenging the anti-inflammatory cells, including their reactive oxygen species [27]. Therefore, AMT should be considered when the infection is controlled or imminent corneal perforation is suspected [28, 29]. In our series, we used the fresh ML-AMT prior to PK in perforated corneas with active keratomycosis to promote healing and to increase the survival rates of elective corneal transplant. We report 100% resolution of infection and 0% incidence of graft rejection over a mean follow-up of 14 ± 1.4 months.

Compared with visual rehabilitation, the prognosis of PK differs markedly when performed for therapeutic or tectonic reasons. Robaei et al. demonstrated that planned PKs have significantly higher clear graft survival compared with emergency PKs in inflamed tissue [26]. 5-year graft survival rate was 90% for scheduled PKs versus 51% for surgery on kerati-

tis [26]. Maier et al. indicated that TPK that was performed for infectious keratitis exhibited more graft failures than elective keratoplasties [29]. Xie et al. reported a graft rejection rate of 38.5% after TPK in eyes with corneal perforation due to fungal keratitis [30]. Hoffman et al. reported that AMT has decreased the inflammation in severe infectious keratitis and helped to avoid an emergency keratoplasty [31]. They achieved a graft survival rate of 90% over the median 20 months follow-up duration with elective keratoplasty [31], compared to a 2-year graft survival rate of 10.6% after therapeutic keratoplasty performed in fungal keratitis in another study [9]. In our series, after termination of the inflammatory condition of the eye and assessments verified progressive integration of the AM tissues within the cornea, an elective PK was performed to offset residual corneal scarring and improve the visual outcomes. Thus, replacing emergent high-risk keratoplasties by normal risk keratoplasties increase success rate with better visual outcome and no recurrence of infection. Shi et al. reported a rate of 6.34% recurrence in patients with fungal keratitis who underwent keratoplasties [7]. They reported that steroid use before transplantation, corneal perforation, and the presence of hypopyon increases the risk of recurrence significantly. We reported no recurrence in our series, which could be attributed to anterior chamber wash, and intrastromal/subconjunctival injection using amphotericin B that were done during AMT surgery.

Our study has some limitations. First, the lack of serological donor tests 3 months after preparation of fresh AM. Second, all cases in the present study had isolated fungal keratitis, so the effect of fresh AMs was not studied in bacterial or viral keratitis. Third, despite encouraging, our results stem from 5 cases only; however, we hope that other teams replicate our results in their own populations.

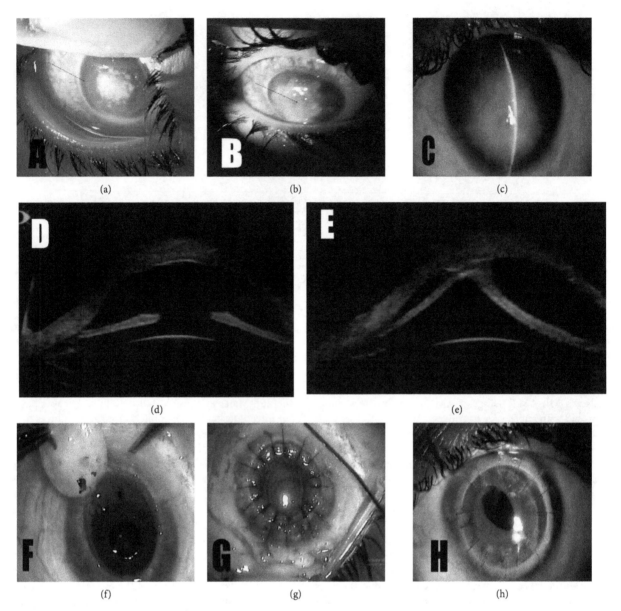

FIGURE 2: (a) Slit-lamp photo of case #5 at 1st visit showing ciliary injection, central dense interface infiltrates with peripheral satellites within the edge of the flap (arrow) and hypopyon. (b) Slit-lamp photo 48 hours after flap amputation and 2nd intrastromal amphotericin injection showing diffuse dense infiltrate with evolving descemetocele (arrow). (c) Slit-lamp photo, 3 weeks after sutures removal, showing: quiet eye, epithelialized cornea, stroma filled with amniotic membrane, and formed anterior chamber (AC). (d) Ultrabiomicrosopic (UBM) image of anterior segment showing: restored corneal thickness and formed AC. (e) UBM image of anterior segment showing inferior peripheral anterior synechia (PAS). (f, g) Intraoperative pictures captured during penetrating keratoplasty (PK) showing removal of the trephined cornea and release of the PAS at 6 o'clock position (f), corneal graft secured with interrupted 10/0 nylon sutures (g). (h) Slit-lamp photos 5 months after PK showing clear and healthy corneal graft.

In conclusion, fungal keratitis is a vision-threatening complication of LASIK that could be presented with early onset of symptoms in the early postoperative days. Fresh ML-AMT represents a viable method of treatment to promote healing and prevent further melting of corneal tissue induced by fungal keratitis which helps avoid an emergency PK and improves the final visual consequences of a sequential PK in the secondarily quiet eye. Further studies using larger sample sizes and longer follow-up are required to indicate the safety and efficacy.

## Authors' Contributions

All authors attest that they meet the current ICMJE criteria for authorship.

## References

[1] M. A. Chang, S. Jain, and D. T. Azar, "Infections following laser in situ keratomileusis: an integration of the published literature," *Survey of Ophthalmology*, vol. 49, no. 3, pp. 269–280, 2004.

[2] W. L. Chen, Y. Y. Tsai, J. M. Lin, and C. C. Chiang, "Unilateral Candida parapsilosis interface keratitis after laser in situ keratomileusis: case report and review of the literature," *Cornea*, vol. 28, no. 1, pp. 105–107, 2009.

[3] H. Taylan Sekeroglu, E. Erdem, K. Yar, M. Yagmur, T. R. Ersoz, and A. Uguz, "A rare devastating complication of LASIK: bilateral fungal keratitis," *Journal of Ophthalmology*, vol. 2010, Article ID 450230, 4 pages, 2010.

[4] R. Solomon, E. D. Donnenfeld, D. T. Azar et al., "Infectious keratitis after laser in situ keratomileusis: results of an ASCRS survey," *Journal of Cataract and Refractive Surgery*, vol. 29, no. 10, pp. 2001–2006, 2003.

[5] A. Chowdhary and K. Singh, "Spectrum of fungal keratitis in North India," *Cornea*, vol. 24, no. 1, pp. 8–15, 2005.

[6] I. P. Kaur, C. Rana, and H. Singh, "Development of effective ocular preparations of antifungal agents," *Journal of Ocular Pharmacology and Therapeutics*, vol. 24, no. 5, pp. 481–494, 2008.

[7] N. V. Florcruz and J. R. Evans, "Medical interventions for fungal keratitis," *Cochrane Database of Systematic Reviews*, vol. 4, no. article CD004241, 2015.

[8] W. Shi, T. Wang, L. Xie et al., "Risk factors, clinical features, and outcomes of recurrent fungal keratitis after corneal transplantation," *Ophthalmology*, vol. 117, no. 5, pp. 890–896, 2010.

[9] J. Mundra, R. Dhakal, A. Mohamed et al., "Outcomes of therapeutic penetrating keratoplasty in 198 eyes with fungal keratitis," *Indian Journal of Ophthalmology*, vol. 67, no. 10, pp. 1599–1605, 2019.

[10] S.-E. Ti, J. A. Scott, P. Janardhanan, and D. T. H. Tan, "Therapeutic keratoplasty for advanced suppurative keratitis," *American Journal of Ophthalmology*, vol. 143, no. 5, pp. 755–762.e2, 2007.

[11] B. Rautaraya, S. Sharma, S. Kar, S. Das, and S. K. Sahu, "Diagnosis and treatment outcome of mycotic keratitis at a tertiary eye care center in eastern India," *BMC Ophthalmology*, vol. 11, no. 1, p. 39, 2011.

[12] X. Dong, W. Shi, Q. Zeng, and L. Xie, "Retracted: Roles of adherence and matrix metalloproteinases in growth patterns of fungal pathogens in cornea," *Current Eye Research*, vol. 30, no. 8, pp. 613–620, 2009.

[13] F. Llovet, V. de Rojas, E. Interlandi et al., "Infectious keratitis in 204 586 LASIK procedures," *Ophthalmology*, vol. 117, no. 2, pp. 232–238, 2010.

[14] M. Moshirfar, J. D. Welling, V. Feiz, H. Holz, and T. E. Clinch, "Infectious and noninfectious keratitis after laser in situ keratomileusis: occurrence, management, and visual outcomes," *Journal of Cataract and Refractive Surgery*, vol. 33, no. 3, pp. 474–483, 2007.

[15] E. C. Jamerson, A. M. Elhusseiny, R. H. ElSheikh, T. K. Eleiwa, and Y. M. El Sayed, "Role of matrix metalloproteinase 9 in ocular surface disorders," *Eye & Contact Lens*, vol. 46, pp. S57–S63, 2020.

[16] Q. Peng, M. P. Holzer, P. H. Kaufer, D. J. Apple, and K. D. Solomon, "Interface fungal infection after laser in situ keratomileusis presenting as diffuse lamellar keratitis: a clinico-pathological report," *Journal of Cataract and Refractive Surgery*, vol. 28, no. 8, pp. 1400–1408, 2002.

[17] E. Garcia-Valenzuela and C. D. Song, "Intracorneal injection of amphotericin B for recurrent fungal keratitis and endophthalmitis," *Archives of Ophthalmology*, vol. 123, no. 12, pp. 1721–1723, 2005.

[18] K.-C. Yoon, I.-Y. Jeong, S.-K. Im, H.-J. Chae, and S.-Y. Yang, "Therapeutic effect of intracameral amphotericin B injection in the treatment of fungal keratitis," *Cornea*, vol. 26, no. 7, pp. 814–818, 2007.

[19] V. Mittal, R. Jain, R. Mittal, and V. S. Sangwan, "Post-laser in situ keratomileusis interface fungal keratitis," *Cornea*, vol. 33, no. 10, pp. 1022–1030, 2014.

[20] M. Nubile, P. Carpineto, M. Lanzini, M. Ciancaglini, E. Zuppardi, and L. Mastropasqua, "Multilayer amniotic membrane transplantation for bacterial keratitis with corneal perforation after hyperopic photorefractive keratectomy: case report and literature review," *Journal of Cataract and Refractive Surgery*, vol. 33, no. 9, pp. 1636–1640, 2007.

[21] K. Hanada, J. Shimazaki, S. Shimmura, and K. Tsubota, "Multilayered amniotic membrane transplantation for severe ulceration of the cornea and sclera," *American Journal of Ophthalmology*, vol. 131, no. 3, pp. 324–331, 2001.

[22] J. Liu, L. Li, and X. Li, "Effectiveness of cryopreserved amniotic membrane transplantation in corneal ulceration: a meta-analysis," *Cornea*, vol. 38, no. 4, pp. 454–462, 2019.

[23] P. Prabhasawat, N. Tesavibul, and W. Komolsuradej, "Single and multilayer amniotic membrane transplantation for persistent corneal epithelial defect with and without stromal thinning and perforation," *The British Journal of Ophthalmology*, vol. 85, no. 12, pp. 1455–1463, 2001.

[24] P. J. Adds, C. J. Hunt, and J. K. Dart, "Amniotic membrane grafts, "fresh" or frozen? A clinical and in vitro comparison," *The British Journal of Ophthalmology*, vol. 85, no. 8, pp. 905–907, 2001.

[25] J. Hori, M. Wang, K. Kamiya, H. Takahashi, and N. Sakuragawa, "Immunological characteristics of amniotic epithelium," *Cornea*, vol. 25, 10, Supplement 1, pp. S53–S58, 2006.

[26] D. Robaei, N. A. Carnt, and J. K. Dart, "Acanthamoeba keratitis in the UK–a case series of 196 patients," *Clinical and Experimental Ophthalmology*, vol. 41, pp. 28–29, 2013.

[27] D. Lockington, P. Agarwal, D. Young, M. Caslake, and K. Ramaesh, "Antioxidant properties of amniotic membrane: novel observations from a pilot study," *Canadian Journal of Ophthalmology*, vol. 49, no. 5, pp. 426–430, 2014.

[28] W. C. Park and S. C. Tseng, "Modulation of acute inflammation and keratocyte death by suturing, blood, and amniotic membrane in PRK," *Investigative Ophthalmology & Visual Science*, vol. 41, no. 10, pp. 2906–2914, 2000.

[29] P. Maier, D. Bohringer, and T. Reinhard, "Clear graft survival and immune reactions following emergency keratoplasty," *Graefe's Archive for Clinical and Experimental Ophthalmology*, vol. 245, no. 3, pp. 351–359, 2007.

[30] L. Xie, H. Zhai, and W. Shi, "Penetrating keratoplasty for corneal perforations in fungal keratitis," *Cornea*, vol. 26, no. 2, pp. 158–162, 2007.

[31] S. Hoffmann, N. Szentmary, and B. Seitz, "Amniotic membrane transplantation for the treatment of infectious ulcerative keratitis before elective penetrating keratoplasty," *Cornea*, vol. 32, no. 10, pp. 1321–1325, 2013.

# 35

# Idiopathic Acute Exudative Polymorphous Vitelliform Maculopathy: Insight into Imaging Features and Outcomes

Sónia Torres-Costa ⓘ,[1] Susana Penas,[1,2] Ângela Carneiro,[1,2] Renato Santos-Silva,[1,2] Rodolfo Moura,[1] Elisete Brandão,[1] Fernando Falcão-Reis,[1,2] and Luís Figueira[1,3,4]

[1]Department of Ophthalmology, Centro Hospitalar Universitário de São João, Porto, Portugal
[2]Department of Surgery and Physiology, Faculty of Medicine, University of Porto, Porto, Portugal
[3]Department of Pharmacology and Therapeutics, Faculty of Medicine of the University of Porto, Porto, Portugal
[4]Center for Drug Discovery and Innovative Medicines (MedInUP), University of Porto, Porto, Portugal

Correspondence should be addressed to Sónia Torres-Costa; sonia.torres.costa@gmail.com

Academic Editor: J. Fernando Arevalo

The authors describe imagiological findings in idiopathic exudative polymorphous vitelliform maculopathy. A 41-year-old woman complained of bilateral blurry vision. Best-corrected visual acuity was 20/20 bilaterally. Bilateral small serous neurosensory detachments in the fovea were seen at fundoscopy and confirmed by spectral-domain optical coherence tomography. Fluorescein angiography was unremarkable. Indocyanine green angiography presented discrete hyperfluorescent spots on the posterior pole. Later, more bleb-like lesions with a vitelliform appearance and hyperautofluorescent on blue fundus autofluorescence were detected. One year later, a complete resolution of the fluid was observed. To conclude, multimodal evaluation of patients with idiopathic exudative polymorphous vitelliform maculopathy is essential for the correct diagnosis of this disease.

## 1. Introduction

Idiopathic exudative polymorphous vitelliform maculopathy (IEPVM) is a rare disease, described by Gass in 1988 [1]. Only 20 additional idiopathic cases have been reported, but several paraneoplastic or infection-related cases have been described [1–4]. Age at presentation varies, ranging from 13 to 69 years, and both genders are affected [2]. This pathology is characterized by blurred vision, a mild decrease in visual acuity, and sometimes headaches [2]. Patients present with multiple yellow-white, morphologically variable lesions at the level of the retinal pigment epithelium (RPE) and serous neurosensory detachments (SND) with polymorphous subretinal yellowish deposits [1].

Although a decrease in photoreceptor function usually persists over time, this disorder has a good visual prognosis, with visual acuity improvement as resolution of macular edema progresses [2, 5].

Here, we describe the clinical findings and multimodal features of IEPVM during one year of follow-up.

## 2. Case Report

We report the case of a 41-year-old white female patient who presented to our Emergency Department complaining of bilateral blurry vision for five days. Best-corrected visual acuity (BCVA) was 20/20 in both eyes. Anterior chamber examination and intraocular pressure were unremarkable. Fundoscopy showed small SND in the fovea bilaterally, with no signs of inflammation or optic nerve changes (Figures 1(a) and 1(a1)). Spectral-domain optical coherence tomography (SD-OCT) confirmed the foveal SND (Figures 2(a) and 2(a1)), with no internal reflectivity. Blue fundus autofluorescence (FAF) (Figures 3(a) and 3(a1)) and fluorescein angiography (Figures 4(a) and 4(a1)) were unremarkable and indocyanine green angiography presented very discrete

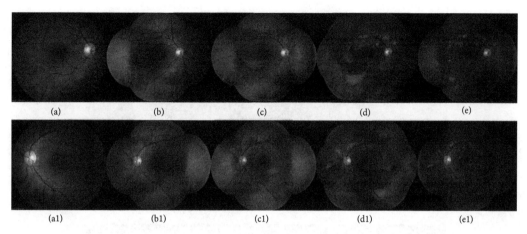

FIGURE 1: Right and left eye sequential color fundus photographs. At presentation, bilateral subfoveal serous retinal detachments were identified at the posterior pole (a and a1). One month after the onset of the visual symptoms, multifocal yellowish subretinal material was observed along the vascular temporal arcades (b and b1). Two months later, there is coalescence of the multiple lesions with progressive precipitation of vitelliform material (c and c1). Progressively, at the macular region, a large vitelliform detachment with a "pseudohypopyon" appearance and multiple vitelliform lesions with a honeycomb-like pattern appeared at the posterior pole. In this phase, the vitelliform material acquired a more yellowish coloration due to progressive accumulation (d and d1). One year after diagnosis, complete resolution of fluid with progressive reduction of curvilinear yellowish deposits could be seen.

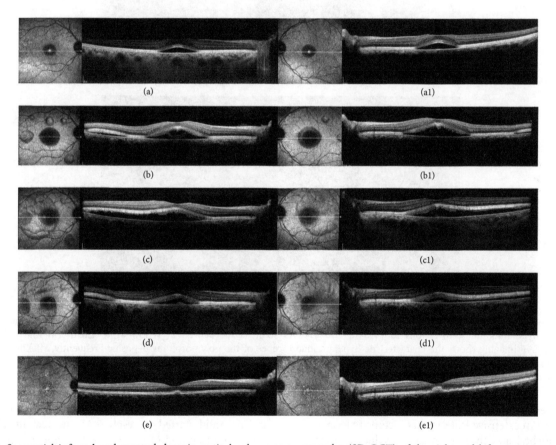

FIGURE 2: Sequential infrared and spectral domain optical coherence tomography (SD-OCT) of the right and left eyes. At presentation, bilateral subfoveal serous retinal detachment was present (a and a1). One month later, there was progression of bilateral macular subretinal fluid with the appearance of new small bleb-like serous retinal detachments along vascular arcades; SD-OCT showed a large serous neurosensory retinal detachment with remarkable thickening of the photoreceptor layer associated with the accumulation of amorphous material in the subretinal space (b and b1). Two months later, it is possible to observe the coalescence of the lesions. External limiting membrane and ellipsoid integrity was preserved (c and c1). At six months, SD-OCT revealed a marked reduction of the serous component in the detachments, and progressive shedding of the photoreceptor layer with more amorphous material accumulated in the subretinal space (d and d1). One year after diagnosis, a complete resolution of subretinal fluid with persistence of small vitelliform material deposits could be seen. It is possible to notice that the ellipsoid and external limiting membrane were slight disrupted.

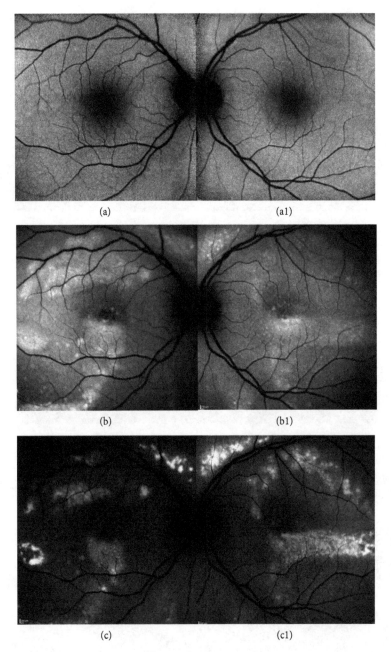

FIGURE 3: Right and left eye blue fundus autofluorescence (FAF) at presentation and eight months later. Initially, there was no significant evidence of hyperautofluorescent lesions in FAF (a and a1). As soon as the subretinal yellow-white vitelliform material starts to accumulate, FAF imaging shows the characteristic hyperautofluorescence of the polymorphous deposits. Frequently, vitelliform material precipitates along the inferior margins of the serous detachments, forming curvilinear deposits (b and b1). One year after diagnosis, FAF demonstrated a progressive reduction in hyperautofluorescence (c).

hyperfluorescent spots in the posterior pole (Figures 4(b) and 4(b1)). An extensive workup that included blood analysis and cerebral and thoracic imaging excluded infectious, inflammatory, or neoplastic causes.

One month later, more bleb-like lesions were detected, acquiring a yellowish coloration, with a vitelliform appearance, that were hyperautofluorescent on FAF. SD-OCT showed multiple SND with internal hyperreflective deposits. Full-field electroretinography was normal, but electrooculography revealed an Arden ratio reduction to 1.38 in the right eye and 1.44 in the left eye. Six months later, the vitelliform

detachments progressed to a "pseudohypopyon" appearance, and the fluid started to resolve. At one year of follow-up, complete resolution of the fluid with regression of deposits can be seen (Figures 1(e) and 1(e1)).

## 3. Discussion

Multimodal evaluation, a long follow-up time and high clinical suspicion are essential for the establishment of the correct diagnosis of patients with IEPVM. As we described in this clinical case, it was only possible to observe the

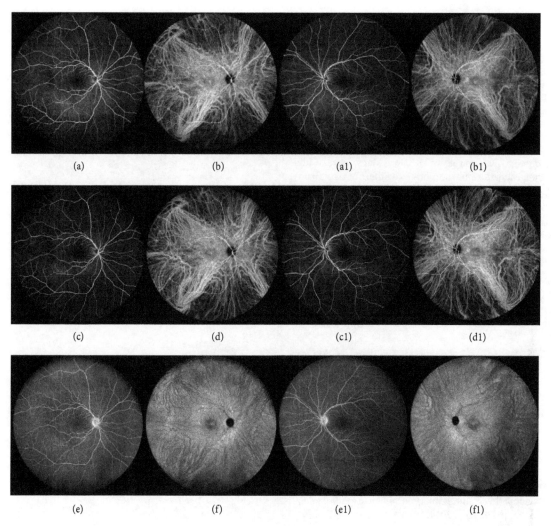

FIGURE 4: Right and left eye wide field fluorescein angiography (FA) and indocyanine green angiography (ICGA). At presentation, FA (a and a1) had an innocent aspect without any leakage or pooling evidence. ICGA (b and b1) presented very discrete hyperfluorescent spots in the posterior pole. Similarly, one month later, in early (c and c1) and late (e and e1) phases, FA remained relatively silent. Of note, ICGA revealed small hyperfluorescent points around vascular arcades in early (d and d1) and, more evidently, in late phases (f and f1).

appearance of vitelliform lesions, characteristically hyperautofluorescent on FAF, after one month of follow-up. Although the clinical features of IEPVM are being increasingly described in current literature, there is little information regarding its pathogenesis. More recently, it has been suggested that the autofluorescent material in IEPVM is derived not only from lipofuscin but also from indigestible components of phagocytized photoreceptor outer segments, which accumulate as a result of the lack of apposition of the retina to the RPE [1]. Some authors hypothesized that a possible variation in the chemical composition in the subretinal space is present in the course of the disease. According to this hypothesis, there is initially a transudate, resulting from the impaired RPE, that subsequently becomes enriched with lipofuscin and from photoreceptor outer segment shedding [1]. This theory is supported by FAF, in which a progressive increase in autofluorescence is noted as higher deposition of lipofuscin and indigestible components of phagocytized photoreceptor outer segments occurs.

Currently, there is no consensus as to whether prompt systemic or intraocular therapy with steroids or intraocular antivascular endothelial growth factor drugs could improve the clinical course. In fact, most results originated from isolated case reports and case series [1, 6].

Regardless of the chosen treatment, gradual visual recovery occurs over time, but electrophysiologic abnormalities may persist [1].

The presence of clinical and imagiological findings suggestive of exudative polymorphous vitelliform maculopathy warrants additional investigations to carefully exclude other underlying masquerading diseases and specifically paraneoplastic syndromes, as they are sometimes associated with this disorder [1].

Although IEPVM presents similarities with vitelliform macular dystrophy, no mutations in BEST1 or peripherin/RDS have been described [1]. Rarely, recurrence or secondary choroidal neovascularization can occur, reinforcing the importance of following these patients [1].

## Disclosure

This case report was presented at the 19th EURETINA Congress, 5-8 September 2019, Paris, France, and at the 61th Portuguese Ophthalmology Congress, 5-8 December 2018, Vilamoura, Portugal.

## References

[1] I. Barbazetto, K. K. Dansingani, R. Dolz-Marco et al., "Idiopathic acute exudative polymorphous vitelliform maculopathy: clinical spectrum and multimodal imaging characteristics," *Ophthalmology*, vol. 125, no. 1, pp. 75–88, 2018.

[2] D. Massaro, A. Pece, F. Pichi et al., "A case of acute exudative polymorphous vitelliform maculopathy: follow-up and widefield spectral-domain optical coherence tomography," *European Journal of Ophthalmology*, vol. 25, no. 5, pp. e91–e94, 2015.

[3] S. A. Al-Dahmash, C. L. Shields, C. G. Bianciotto, A. J. Witkin, S. R. Witkin, and J. A. Shields, "Acute exudative paraneoplastic polymorphous vitelliform maculopathy in five cases," *Ophthalmic Surgery, Lasers, and Imaging*, vol. 43, no. 5, pp. 366–373, 2012.

[4] B. Wolff, S. Mrejen, K. B. Freund, C. Titah, and M. Mauget-Faysse, "A case of neurosyphilis revealed by acute exudative polymorphous vitelliform maculopathy," *Ophthalmic Surgery, Lasers & Imaging Retina*, vol. 45, pp. e29–e31, 2014.

[5] P. Kozma, K. G. Locke, Y. Z. Wang, D. G. Birch, and A. O. Edwards, "Persistent cone dysfunction in acute exudative polymorphous vitelliform maculopathy," *Retina*, vol. 27, no. 1, pp. 109–113, 2007.

[6] A. Scupola, E. Abed, M. G. Sammarco et al., "Intravitreal dexamethasone implant for acute exudative polymorphous vitelliform maculopathy," *European Journal of Ophthalmology*, vol. 24, no. 5, pp. 803–807, 2014.

# 36

# Faster Recovery of Internal Ophthalmoplegia than External Ophthalmoplegia in a Miller Fisher Variant of Guillain-Barre Syndrome

**Golla Abhinav,**[1] **Jorge Gamez Jr.,**[1] **Michael C. Yang,**[1] **Tetyana Vaysman** ⓘ,[2] **Michelle von Gunten,**[1] **and Antonio Liu** ⓘ[1]

[1]*Department of Neurology, Adventist Health White Memorial, Los Angeles, California, USA*
[2]*Department of Internal Medicine, University of Maryland, Cheverly, Maryland, USA*

Correspondence should be addressed to Antonio Liu; liuak@ah.org

Academic Editor: Huban Atilla

We present a case of classic Miller Fisher Syndrome (MFS) variant of Guillain-Barre Syndrome (GBS) with detailed description in the difference between the internal and external ophthalmoplegia. They are different in their onset, duration, and recovery.

## 1. Introduction

MFS variant of GBS is associated with both the internal and external ophthalmoplegia [1]. Prior studies have noted that the defect in pupillary reactivity can vary with time [2]. With the pupillometer (NeurOptics NPi®-200), it is now possible to accurately and consistently measure pupillary size and reactivity. Ultimately, this device allows clinicians to objectively quantify pupillary function with the standardized Neurological Pupil Index (NPi) Pupil Reactivity Assessment Scale.

The pupillometer is an easy-to-use, handheld device that can be used at bedside. It is loaded with a SmartGuard cartridge and held up to the patient's eye. The device accurately and consistently measures pupillary size and reactivity speed. The Neurological Pupil Index (NPi) Pupil Reactivity Assessment Scale scores range from 0 to 4.9. A score of 0 represents a nonreactive, immeasurable, or atypical response. A score of less than 3.0 indicates abnormal ("sluggish") reactivity. A score of 3.0-4.9 indicates normal ("brisk") reactivity. Additionally, a NPi score difference that is greater than or equal to 0.7 between the right- and left-eye measurements suggests a pupillary abnormality.

Currently, the literature describing the rate of recovery of the internal and external ophthalmoplegia in MFS is scarce.

We present a case of antibody-proven MFS with the classic pattern of descending weakness. Notably, our patient's internal ophthalmoplegia developed prior to external ophthalmoplegia and also resolved much earlier.

## 2. Case Presentation

A 44-year-old right-hand-dominant male with no significant past medical history presented to the emergency department with two days of difficulty speaking and loss of balance, stating "my voice is just different." The patient endorsed having severe diarrhea two weeks prior and had also received the influenza vaccine six months prior to admission. Upon presentation, the patient's vital signs were within normal limits. Upon interview, examiners did not appreciate any aphasia, but the patient's speech possessed a notable nasal quality. Upon physical examination, the patient required major assistance to ambulate. All physical symptoms were acute in nature; he was previously working, ambulating, and completing activities of daily living without any issues.

Initial exam of extraocular movements revealed minimal deficits in left-eye abduction and horizontal nystagmus that changed direction with lateral gaze in either direction. Over the next three days, the patient's minor ocular movement deficits progressed into severe external ophthalmoplegia in

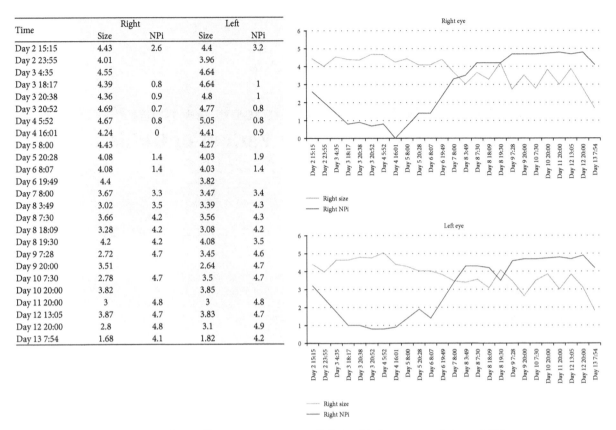

| Time | Right | | Left | |
|------|-------|-----|------|-----|
|      | Size  | NPi | Size | NPi |
| Day 2 15:15 | 4.43 | 2.6 | 4.4 | 3.2 |
| Day 2 23:55 | 4.01 |     | 3.96 |     |
| Day 3 4:35  | 4.55 |     | 4.64 |     |
| Day 3 18:17 | 4.39 | 0.8 | 4.64 | 1 |
| Day 3 20:38 | 4.36 | 0.9 | 4.8 | 1 |
| Day 3 20:52 | 4.69 | 0.7 | 4.77 | 0.8 |
| Day 4 5:52  | 4.67 | 0.8 | 5.05 | 0.8 |
| Day 4 16:01 | 4.24 | 0   | 4.41 | 0.9 |
| Day 5 8:00  | 4.43 |     | 4.27 |     |
| Day 5 20:28 | 4.08 | 1.4 | 4.03 | 1.9 |
| Day 6 8:07  | 4.08 | 1.4 | 4.03 | 1.4 |
| Day 6 19:49 | 4.4  |     | 3.82 |     |
| Day 7 8:00  | 3.67 | 3.3 | 3.47 | 3.4 |
| Day 8 3:49  | 3.02 | 3.5 | 3.39 | 4.3 |
| Day 8 7:30  | 3.66 | 4.2 | 3.56 | 4.3 |
| Day 8 18:09 | 3.28 | 4.2 | 3.08 | 4.2 |
| Day 8 19:30 | 4.2  | 4.2 | 4.08 | 3.5 |
| Day 9 7:28  | 2.72 | 4.7 | 3.45 | 4.6 |
| Day 9 20:00 | 3.51 |     | 2.64 | 4.7 |
| Day 10 7:30 | 2.78 | 4.7 | 3.5 | 4.7 |
| Day 10 20:00| 3.82 |     | 3.85 |     |
| Day 11 20:00| 3    | 4.8 | 3 | 4.8 |
| Day 12 13:05| 3.87 | 4.7 | 3.83 | 4.7 |
| Day 12 20:00| 2.8  | 4.8 | 3.1 | 4.9 |
| Day 13 7:54 | 1.68 | 4.1 | 1.82 | 4.2 |

FIGURE 1: Daily pupillometry measurements. Relationship between pupil size and NPi.

all directions. During this time, he also developed bilateral ptosis. Pupillary size and reactivity were measured daily using the pupillometer. During hospital day one and two, pupillary function remained relatively normal (right NPi 2.6 "borderline sluggish," left NPi 3.2 "brisk"). However, on hospital day three, pupillometer readings suggested that the patient's pupils were "sluggish" bilaterally (right NPi 0.7, left NPi 0.8) (Figure 1).

The table shows the recorded pupil size and corresponding NPi score over the course of the patient's admission. The adjacent graphs represent the recorded measurements through time (the gray lines indicate pupil size (in mm), blue line indicates right NPi, and red line indicates left NPi).

Throughout the hospital course, the patient's nasal tone remained unchanged, but he developed moderate to severe dysarthria and minimal to moderate dysphagia. The patient's extremity and truncal ataxia continued to worsen, and he subsequently required moderate assistance with a walker to ambulate. Sensation to light touch, temperature (ice examination), and proprioception remained intact. However, he reported tingling and "skin tightness" that persisted for over one week. The patient never developed urinary or bowel incontinence. He denied shortness of breath, maintained a normal vital capacity, and exhibited normal arterial blood gas studies.

Ganglioside antibody panel was sent out on hospital day one and resulted on hospital day ten, which was remarkable for elevated antibody levels (Asialo-GM1 Ab 279, GD1a Ab 52, and GQ1b Ab 273). Due to a high suspicion for

an autoimmune neuromuscular disease, plasma exchange was initiated on hospital day three. A total of five plasmapheresis treatments were administered. The patient developed orthostatic hypotension on several occasions that led to two syncopal episodes, both within an hour of plasma exchange treatment. Pupillary reactivity recovered within four days of symptom onset (by hospital day seven); however, it took several weeks for external ophthalmoplegia to resolve (Figure 1). The patient was discharged home on hospital day twenty. At the time of discharge, his external ophthalmoplegia persisted with only partial recovery. Six weeks after discharge, the patient's symptoms had completely resolved and antibody levels had normalized (Asialo-GM1 Ab 50, GD1a Ab 18, and GQ1b Ab 48).

## 3. Discussion

Miller Fisher Syndrome (MFS) is a rare variant of Guillain-Barre Syndrome (GBS), occurring in 1-7% of GBS cases worldwide [3] and 5% of GBS cases in Western countries [4]. Early ocular findings of MFS and GBS include ophthalmoplegia, diplopia, and pupillary abnormalities (internal ophthalmoplegia)—all of which have been well described in the literature. However, at the time of authorship, the natural history of pupillary deficits and external ophthalmoplegia in MFS has not yet been objectively described in the literature.

The literature contains many references of MFS presentation, with both a typical triad of ophthalmoplegia, areflexia, and ataxia and atypical variants of MFS different in combination of symptoms. Kaymakamzade et al. have reported an interesting case of atypical MFS in a 17-year-old male patient, confirmed by raised titers of anti-GQ1b antibodies with an early onset of external ophthalmoplegia following by internal ophthalmoplegia and characterized by mydriasis and decreased reactivity to light [5]. Lopez et al. [6] have described a case of a 74-year-old woman with a sole presentation of internal ophthalmoplegia evidenced by nonreactive midsized pupils with preserved visual acuity as initial manifestation of MFS. The patient developed external ophthalmoplegia, mild ataxia, and hyporeflexia by the second day of the initial presentation and full resolution in two months [6]. These cases are interesting in demonstrating sequence of presentation, whereas out investigation is unique in focusing on difference in onset, duration, and recovery rate between the internal and external ophthalmoplegia.

This case report demonstrates that the internal and external ophthalmoplegia can occur together in MFS but are independent of each other in terms of onset, severity, and duration. Man [1] describes the case of a 46-year-old patient with total internal and external ophthalmoplegia as the initial presenting symptoms of MFS, confirmed with serum-positive anti-GQ1b antibodies. Serum anti-GQ1b antibodies are associated with GBS and MFS. GQ1b is a ganglioside that is commonly found in cell membranes of cranial nerves that innervate extraocular muscles (oculomotor, trochlear, and abducens nerve), confirmed by immunohistochemical studies [7]. Evidence strongly suggests that the ophthalmoparesis in MFS results from a direct action of anti-GQ1b antibodies on the presynaptic neuromuscular junction (NMJ) between cranial nerves and extraocular muscles [8]. Anti-GQ1b antibodies bind to presynaptic receptors which trigger a large release of acetylcholine and ultimately impair NMJ function [8]. Additionally, GQ1b gangliosides are also found in the ciliary ganglion, which is a presynaptic ganglion responsible for pupillary sphincter and ciliary muscle control [8]. These mechanisms may explain the prevalence of the internal and external ophthalmoplegia in MFS and GBS.

The use of a pupillometer in our presented case allowed for objective measurements of pupillary size and reactivity over the disease course of MFS. The patient's pupillary reactivity worsened acutely on hospital day three and resolved after four days (hospital day seven) (Figure 1). External ophthalmoplegia reached its nadir on hospital day seven, continued to persist on hospital day twenty with only minor improvement, and eventually resolved after several weeks. The patient's symptoms were completely resolved by the six-week follow-up appointment after discharge. This case report of Miller Fisher Syndrome (MFS), with positive anti-GQ1b antibodies, objectively documents the natural history of the internal and external ophthalmoplegia and demonstrates that these two entities can be independent of each other with regard to disease onset, severity, and duration.

## Consent

Informed written consent was obtained from the patient for publication of this case report.

## References

[1] B. L. Man, "Total internal and external ophthalmoplegia as presenting symptoms of Miller Fisher syndrome," *Case Reports*, vol. 2014, 2014.

[2] G. Gupta and A. Liu, "Atypical Miller Fisher syndrome with anisocoria and rapidly fluctuating pupillary diameter," *Case Reports in Neurological Medicine*, vol. 2015, Article ID 472843, 2 pages, 2015.

[3] J. W. Teener, "Miller Fisher's syndrome," *Seminars in Neurology*, vol. 32, no. 5, pp. 512–516, 2012.

[4] M. M. Dimachkie and R. J. Barohn, "Guillain-Barré syndrome and variants," *Neurologic Clinics*, vol. 31, no. 2, pp. 491–510, 2013.

[5] B. Kaymakamzade, F. Selcuk, A. Koysuren, A. I. Colpak, S. E. Mut, and T. Kansu, "Pupillary involvement in Miller Fisher syndrome," *Neuro-Ophthalmology*, vol. 37, no. 3, pp. 111–115, 2013.

[6] T. Lopez, S. Mur, A. M. Gutierrez Alvarez, and C. Jimemez, "Oftalmoplejía interna como comienzo de un síndrome de Miller-Fisher," *Neurología*, vol. 29, no. 8, pp. 504-505, 2014.

[7] A. Chiba, S. Kusunoki, H. Obata, R. Machinami, and I. Kanazawa, "Serum anti-GQ1b IgG antibody is associated with ophthalmoplegia in Miller Fisher syndrome and Guillain-Barré syndrome: clinical and immunohistochemical studies," *Neurology*, vol. 43, no. 10, pp. 1911–1917, 1993.

[8] J. B. Winer, "Guillan Barre syndrome," *Molecular pathology*, vol. 54, pp. 381–385, 2001.

# Permissions

The contributors of this book come from diverse backgrounds, making this book a truly international effort. This book will bring forth new frontiers with its revolutionizing research information and detailed analysis of the nascent developments around the world.

We would like to thank all the contributing authors for lending their expertise to make the book truly unique. They have played a crucial role in the development of this book. Without their invaluable contributions this book wouldn't have been possible. They have made vital efforts to compile up to date information on the varied aspects of this subject to make this book a valuable addition to the collection of many professionals and students.

This book was conceptualized with the vision of imparting up-to-date information and advanced data in this field. To ensure the same, a matchless editorial board was set up. Every individual on the board went through rigorous rounds of assessment to prove their worth. After which they invested a large part of their time researching and compiling the most relevant data for our readers.

The editorial board has been involved in producing this book since its inception. They have spent rigorous hours researching and exploring the diverse topics which have resulted in the successful publishing of this book. They have passed on their knowledge of decades through this book. To expedite this challenging task, the publisher supported the team at every step. A small team of assistant editors was also appointed to further simplify the editing procedure and attain best results for the readers.

Apart from the editorial board, the designing team has also invested a significant amount of their time in understanding the subject and creating the most relevant covers. They scrutinized every image to scout for the most suitable representation of the subject and create an appropriate cover for the book.

The publishing team has been an ardent support to the editorial, designing and production team. Their endless efforts to recruit the best for this project, has resulted in the accomplishment of this book. They are a veteran in the field of academics and their pool of knowledge is as vast as their experience in printing. Their expertise and guidance has proved useful at every step. Their uncompromising quality standards have made this book an exceptional effort. Their encouragement from time to time has been an inspiration for everyone.

The publisher and the editorial board hope that this book will prove to be a valuable piece of knowledge for researchers, students, practitioners and scholars across the globe.

# List of Contributors

**Padmanaban Meleth and Sameer Iqbal**
Vitreoretinal Services, Chaithanya Eye Hospital and Research Institute, Trivandrum, India

**Manoj Soman, Jay U. Sheth and Unnikrishnan Nair**
Vitreoretinal Services, Chaithanya Eye Hospital and Research Institute, Trivandrum, India
Chaithanya Innovation in Technology and Eyecare (Research), Trivandrum, India

**Vamsee Neerukonda, Swetha Dhanireddy and Samuel Alpert**
SUNY Upstate Medical University, Department of Ophthalmology, Syracuse, NY, USA

**Anny M. S. Cheng**
Florida International University, Herbert Wertheim College of Medicine, Miami, FL, USA

**Han Y. Yin**
SUNY Upstate Medical University, Department of Ophthalmology, Syracuse, NY, USA
Florida International University, Herbert Wertheim College of Medicine, Miami, FL, USA

**Matthew K. Adams and Christina Y. Weng**
Department of Ophthalmology, Baylor College of Medicine, 6565 Fannin Street, NC-205, Houston, TX 77030, USA

**Yanru Chen and Minghan Li**
Xiamen University Affiliated Xiamen Eye Center, Xiamen, Fujian 36100, China
Fujian Key Laboratory of Ocular Surface and Corneal Diseases, Xiamen, Fujian 36100, China

**Mingyan Wei and Qian Chen**
Department of Ophthalmology, Xiang'an Hospital of Xiamen University, Xiamen, Fujian 36102, China
Fujian Provincial Key Laboratory of Ophthalmology and Visual Science, Xiamen, Fujian 36102, China
Eye Institute of Xiamen University, Xiamen, Fujian 36102, China
School of Medicine, Xiamen University, Xiamen, Fujian 36102, China

**M. M. Shamim, M. Whaley and A. B. Sallam**
Department of Ophthalmology, Harvey and Bernice Jones Eye Institute, University of Arkansas for Medical Sciences (UAMS) Medical Center, Little Rock, Arkansas, USA

**H. Rana**
Hospitalist, UAMS Medical Center, Little Rock, Arkansas, USA

**S. K. Jeffus**
Department of Pathology, UAMS Medical Center, Little Rock, Arkansas, USA

**S. Bhatti**
Department of Oncology, Winthrop P. Rockefeller Cancer Institute, UAMS Medical Center, Little Rock, Arkansas, USA

**Bishow Raj Timalsina, Gulshan Bahadur Shrestha and Madhu Thapa**
Department of Ophthalmology, B.P. Koirala Lions Centre for Ophthalmic Studies, Kathmandu, Nepal

**Somnath Chakraborty**
Retina Institute of Bengal, Siliguri, India

**Jay Umed Sheth**
Surya Eye Institute and Research Center, Mumbai, India

**Aashish Raj Pant**
Department of Oculofacial Plastic Surgery, Mechi Eye Hospital, Jhapa, Nepal

**Rinkal Suwal**
Department of Optometry, B.P. Eye Foundation, Hospital for Children, Eye, ENT and Rehabilitation Services (CHEERS), Bhaktapur, Nepal

**Purushottam Joshi**
Department of Vitreo-Retina, Mechi Eye Hospital, Jhapa, Nepal

**Santosh Chaudhary**
Department of Ophthalmology, B.P. Koirala Institute of Health Sciences, Dharan, Nepal

**Yousuf Siddiqui**
University of Minnesota Medical School, University of Minnesota, 420 Delaware St SE, Minneapolis, MN 55455, USA

**Olufemi E. Adams, Michael A. Simmons, Justin Yamanuha and Dara D. Koozekanani**
Department of Ophthalmology and Visual Neurosciences, University of Minnesota, 516 Delaware Street SE, Minneapolis, MN 55455, USA

**Christian Nieves-Ríos**
Ponce Health Sciences University, Department of Surgery, Ponce, PR, USA

**Guillermo A. Requejo Figueroa, Sofía C. Ayala Rodríguez, Alejandra Santiago-Díaz, Eduardo J. Rodriguez-Garcia, Alejandro L. Perez, Erick Rivera-Grana and Armando L. Olive**
University of Puerto Rico School of Medicine, Department of Ophthalmology, Medical Sciences Campus, San Juan, PR, USA

**Adriana C. Figueroa-Díaz and Rafael Martín-García**
University of Puerto Rico School of Medicine, Department of Dermatology, Medical Sciences Campus, San Juan, PR, USA

**Grazia Maria Cozzupoli, Daniele Gui, Valerio Cozza, Claudio Lodoli, Mariano Alberto Pennisi, Aldo Caporossi and Benedetto Falsini**
Fondazione Policlinico Universitario A. Gemelli, Universit`a Cattolica del S. Cuore, Rome, Italy

**Shoko Ubukata, Tatsuya Mimura, Emiko Watanabe, Koichi Matsumoto, Makoto Kawashima, Kazuma Kitsu, Mai Nishio and Atsushi Mizota**
Department of Ophthalmology, Teikyo University School of Medicine, Tokyo 173-8605, Japan

**Mojtaba Abrishami, Ramin Daneshvar, Nasser Shoeibi, Hamid Reza Heidarzadeh and Seyedeh Maryam Hosseini**
Eye Research Center, Mashhad University of Medical Sciences, Mashhad, Iran

**Neda Saeedian**
Department of Internal Medicine, Faculty of Medicine, Mashhad University of Medical Sciences, Mashhad, Iran

**Augusto Magalhães, Jorge Meira, Ana Maria Cunha, Raul Jorge Moreira and Jorge Breda**
Departament of Ophthalmology, Centro Hospitalar Universitário de São João, Porto, Portugal

**Elisa Leão-Teles**
Reference Centre of Inherited Metabolic Diseases, Centro Hospitalar Universitário de São João, Porto, Portugal

**Manuel Falcão and Fernando Falcão-Reis**
Departament of Ophthalmology, Centro Hospitalar Universitário de São João, Porto, Portugal
Department of Surgery and Physiology, Faculty of Medicine of University of Porto, Porto, Portugal

**Alessandro Abbouda, Simone Bruschi and Maria Pia Paroli**
Department of Ophthalmology, Sapienza University, Umberto I Hospital, Rome, Italy

**Irene Abicca**
IRCCS-Fondazione Bietti, Rome, Italy

**Federico Ricci and Gianluca Aloe**
UOSD Retinal Pathology PTV Foundation Policlinico Tor Vergata University, Rome, Italy

**Shaikha Aldossari and Amani Al Bakri**
King Khaled Eye Specialist Hospital, Riyadh, Saudi Arabia

**Yumna Kamal**
King Abdulaziz University, Jeddah, Saudi Arabia

**Hassaan Asif, Zhuangjun Si, Steven Quan, Pathik Amin, David Dao, Lincoln Shaw, Dimitra Skondra and Mary Qiu**
Department of Ophthalmology and Visual Science, University of Chicago, Chicago, Illinois, USA

**Rika Tsukii, Yuka Kasuya and Shinji Makino**
Department of Ophthalmology, Jichi Medical University, Shimotsuke, Tochigi, Japan

**Annahita Amireskandari and Andrew Bean**
Department of Ophthalmology and Visual Sciences, West Virginia University, Morgantown, WV, USA

**Ivan J. Lee and Thomas Mauger**
Department of Ophthalmology, West Virginia University School of Medicine, WVU Eye Institute, 1 Medical Center Dr., Morgantown, WV 26506, USA

**Logan Vander Woude, Ramak Roohipour and Gibran Syed Khurshid**
Department of Ophthalmology, University of Florida, USA

**Maria A. Mavrommatis**
Department of Ophthalmology, Icahn School of Medicine at Mount Sinai, 1 Gustave L. Levy Pl, New York, NY 10029, USA

**Sarah A. Avila and Richard France**
Department of Ophthalmology, Icahn School of Medicine at Mount Sinai, 1 Gustave L. Levy Pl, New York, NY 10029, USA
James J Peters VA Medical Center, Department of Ophthalmology, 130 W Kingsbridge Rd, Bronx, NY 10468, USA

**Anadi Khatri, Satish Timalsena and Sudhir Gautam**
Birat Eye Hospital, Biratnagar, Nepal

**Muna Kharel**
Nepalese Army Institute of Health Sciences, Kathmandu, Nepal

**Kursiah Mohd Razali**
Department of Ophthalmology, Hospital Raja Permaisuri Bainun, Jalan Raja Ashman Shah, 30450 Ipoh, Perak, Malaysia

**Mushawiahti Mustapha**
Department of Ophthalmology, Hospital Canselor Tuanku Muhriz, Jalan Yaacob Latif, Bandar Tun Razak, 56000 Cheras, Kuala Lumpur, Malaysia

**Prem Ananth Palaniappan and Fairuz Amran**
Institute for Medical Research, Jalan Pahang, 50588 Kuala Lumpur, Wilayah Persekutuan Kuala Lumpur, Malaysia

**Satheitra Rajandran**
Department of Ophthalmology, Hospital Raja Permaisuri Bainun, Jalan Raja Ashman Shah, 30450 Ipoh, Perak, Malaysia
Department of Ophthalmology, Hospital Canselor Tuanku Muhriz, Jalan Yaacob Latif, Bandar Tun Razak, 56000 Cheras, Kuala Lumpur, Malaysia

**Chandni Pradhan**
Mechi Eye Hospital, Birtamod-9, Jhapa, Nepal

**Simanta Khadka**
Bharatpur Eye Hospital, Bharatpur-10, Chitwan, Nepal

**Mohsen Farvardin, Mohammad Hassan Jalalpour and Mohammad Reza Khalili**
Poostchi Ophthalmology Research Center, Department of Ophthalmology, School of Medicine, Shiraz University of Medical Sciences, Shiraz, Iran

**Golnoush Mahmoudinezhad**
Hamilton Glaucoma Center, Shiley Eye Institute, Viterbi Family Department of Ophthalmology, University of California San Diego, La Jolla, CA, USA

**Fereshteh Mosavat and Soheila Aleyasin**
Division of Allergy and Immunology, Department of Pediatrics, School of Medicine, Shiraz University of Medical Sciences, Shiraz, Iran

**Hamidreza Jahanbani-Ardakani**
Department of Ophthalmology, School of Medicine, Shiraz University of Medical Sciences, Shiraz, Iran
Student Research Committee, Shiraz University of Medical Sciences, Shiraz, Iran

**Nathan Pirakitikulr, Ann Q. Tran and Wendy W. Lee**
Division of Oculofacial Plastic and Reconstructive Surgery, Bascom Palmer Eye Institute, University of Miami-Miller School of Medicine, Miami, FL, USA

**Armando L. Garcia and Sander R. Dubovy**
Florida Lions Ocular Pathology Laboratory, Bascom Palmer Eye Institute, University of Miami Miller School of Medicine, Miami, FL, USA

**Virang Kumar**
Virginia Commonwealth University School of Medicine, Richmond, VA, USA

**Natario L. Couser**
Department of Ophthalmology, Virginia Commonwealth University Health System, 401 N 11th St, Richmond, VA 23219, USA
Department of Human and Molecular Genetics, Virginia Commonwealth University Health System, 1101 E Marshall St, Richmond, VA 23298, USA
Department of Pediatrics, Virginia Commonwealth University Health System, Children's Hospital of Richmond at VCU, 1000 E Broad St, Richmond, VA 23219, USA

**Arti Pandya**
Department of Pediatrics, Division of Genetics and Metabolism, School of Medicine, University of North Carolina at Chapel Hill, Chapel Hill, NC, USA

**Yoichiro Shinohara, Ryo Mukai and Hideo Akiyama**
Department of Ophthalmology, Gunma University School of Medicine, Maebashi, Gunma, Japan

**Shinji Ueno**
Department of Ophthalmology, Nagoya University School of Medicine, Nagoya, Aichi, Japan

**Linnet Rodriguez, Julia Michelle White and Nikisha Q. Richards**
Department of Ophthalmology, Virginia Commonwealth University Health System, 401 N 11th St, Richmond, VA 23219, USA

**Alan X. You**
Departments of Internal Medicine and Emergency Medicine, Virginia Commonwealth University Health System, 417 N 11th St, Richmond, VA 23298, USA

**Sidra Ibad**
Icahn School of Medicine at Mount Sinai, One Gustave L. Levy Place, New York, NY, USA

**Carl S. Wilkins, Alexander Pinhas, Vincent Sun and Matthew S. Wieder**
New York Eye and Ear Infirmary of Mount Sinai, 310 East 14th Street, Retina Center, New York, NY, USA

**Avnish Deobhakta**
Icahn School of Medicine at Mount Sinai, One Gustave
L. Levy Place, New York, NY, USA
New York Eye and Ear Infirmary of Mount Sinai, 310
East 14th Street, Retina Center, New York, NY, USA

**A. Altun**
Department of Ophthalmology, Bahcesehir University,
Istanbul, Turkey

**Mariana A. Oliveira, Jorge Simão and Amélia Martins**
Department of Ophthalmology, Centro Hospitalar e
Universitário de Coimbra (CHUC), Coimbra, Portugal

**Cláudia Farinha**
Department of Ophthalmology, Centro Hospitalar e
Universitário de Coimbra (CHUC), Coimbra, Portugal
Coimbra Institute for Clinical and Biomedical Research,
Faculty of Medicine, University of Coimbra (iCBR-
FMUC), Coimbra, Portugal
Association for Innovation and Biomedical Research
on Light and Imaging (AIBILI), Coimbra, Portugal

**Taher Eleiwa**
Bascom Palmer Eye Institute, Miller School of Medicine,
University of Miami, Miami, FL, USA
Department of Ophthalmology, Faculty of Medicine,
Benha University, Egypt

**Gehad Youssef and Ahmed Bayoumy**
Department of Ophthalmology, Faculty of Medicine,
Benha University, Egypt

**Eyup Ozcan**
Bascom Palmer Eye Institute, Miller School of Medicine,
University of Miami, Miami, FL, USA
Net Eye Medical Center, Gaziantep, Turkey

**Samar Abdelrahman**
Department of Clinical Pathology, Faculty of Medicine,
Benha University, Egypt

**Omar Solyman**
Department of Ophthalmology, Texas Childrens
Hospital, Baylor College of Medicine, Houston, TX,
USA

**Abdelrahman M. Elhusseiny**
Department of Ophthalmology, Kasr Al-Ainy
Hospitals, Cairo University, Cairo, Egypt

**Sónia Torres-Costa, Rodolfo Moura and Elisete
Brandão**
Department of Ophthalmology, Centro Hospitalar
Universitário de São João, Porto, Portugal

**Susana Penas, Ângela Carneiro and Renato Santos-
Silva**
Department of Ophthalmology, Centro Hospitalar
Universitário de São João, Porto, Portugal
Department of Surgery and Physiology, Faculty of
Medicine, University of Porto, Porto, Portugal

**Luís Figueira**
Department of Ophthalmology, Centro Hospitalar
Universitário de São João, Porto, Portugal
Department of Pharmacology and Therapeutics,
Faculty of Medicine of the University of Porto, Porto,
Portugal
Center for Drug Discovery and Innovative Medicines
(MedInUP), University of Porto, Porto, Portugal

**Golla Abhinav, Jorge Gamez Jr., Michael C. Yang,
Michelle von Gunten and Antonio Liu**
Department of Neurology, Adventist Health White
Memorial, Los Angeles, California, USA

**Tetyana Vaysman**
Department of Internal Medicine, University of
Maryland, Cheverly, Maryland, USA

# Index

Printed in the USA
CPSIA information can be obtained
at www.ICGtesting.com
JSHW051510111223
53612JS00005B/79